and Health Care in Britain

Health and Health Care in Britain

Third Edition

Rob Baggott

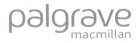

Learning Resources Centre

13247514

First edition 1994
Reprinted three times
Second edition 1998
Reprinted five times
Third edition 2004

First published 2004 by
PALGRAVE MACMILLAN
Houndmills, Basingstoke, Hampshire RG21 6XS and
175 Fifth Avenue, New York, N.Y. 10010
Companies and representatives throughout the world

PALGRAVE MACMILLAN is the global academic imprint of the Palgrave Macmillan division of St. Martin's Press, LLC and of Palgrave Macmillan Ltd. Macmillan® is a registered trademark in the United States, United Kingdom and other countries. Palgrave is a registered trademark in the European Union and other countries.

ISBN-13: 978–0–333–96158–2 hardback
ISBN-10: 0–333–96158–7 hardback
ISBN-13: 978–0–333–96159–9 paperback
ISBN-10: 0–333–96159–5 paperback

This book is printed on paper suitable for recycling and made from fully managed and sustained forest sources.
Logging, pulping and manufacturing processes are expected to conform to the environmental regulations of the country of origin.

A catalogue record for this book is available from the British Library.

10   9   8   7   6   5
13 12 11 10 09 08 07

Printed in China

To Debbie, Mark, Danny and Melissa

Contents

List of Figures, Tables and Exhibits

Figures

Tables

Exhibits

Preface and Acknowledgements

Spare a thought for those sad individuals who write about contemporary policy developments, especially those – such as myself – misguided enough to take an interest in health policy. In recent years the torrent of government initiatives in this field has swollen to biblical proportions, making it almost impossible to put pen to paper, let alone assess the consequences. Most previous books on the NHS and health policy are now of historical interest – they tell the reader little about today's terrain. This includes my own previous edition of *Health and Health Care in Britain*, which was published as recently as February 1998. To persist with the metaphor, it is as if the plains have been flooded and the coastline changed, and a new map is therefore urgently needed.

But, paradoxically, the same old dilemmas and issues, familiar to readers of previous editions of this book, remain. How can health care resources be more efficiently allocated? What is the most appropriate balance of power between centre and locality in the NHS? Should the NHS work more closely with the private sector? What is the most appropriate balance between community and institutional care? Should public health be given higher priority? How can accountability be improved? Moreover, health issues and the NHS remain high on the political agenda, and the consequences of this remain much the same. Indeed, one reason why the NHS has faced so many changes in recent years is because of its political profile. Media interest in the state of the NHS and in health issues remains insatiable, and those responsible for health policy and service provision are acutely aware of this.

And yet I am grateful for the opportunity to work on a third edition. The previous editions have been well received, and have become standard reading on many health policy and management courses. Thank you to all those readers – tutors and students – who have made positive comments about the book. I hope the new edition satisfies your need for an updated version.

As usual, I should like to acknowledge a large number of people for their help, though the ultimate responsibility for the book remains mine alone. First of all, I should like to thank my wife, Debbie, and our children, Mark, Danny and Melissa, who have endured the usual consequences of an academic project on family life. I am also grateful to many colleagues, in particular Katherine Hooper, the Administrator of the Health Policy Research Unit, for her assistance in tracking down sources and her help in preparing this manuscript for publication. Similarly, thanks to HPRU co-director, Professor Judith Allsop, for her support and advice, and to our close colleague, Dr Kathryn Jones, HPRU Research Fellow. Other De Montfort staff who have helped out with various advice or bits of information include Helen Bentley, Professor David Buchanan, Dr Merrill Clarke, Dr Lorraine Culley, Professor Martyn Denscombe, Dr Simon Dyson, Nicky Drucquer, Professor Louise Fitzgerald, Professor Steven Leach, Jackie Leatham, Dr Sally Ruane, Paul Pleasance, and Martin Williams. I should also like to thank former colleagues Di Tofts, Ellen Carter, and Julie Prowse. Thanks also to Professor David Wilson, Dean of the Business and Law Faculty at De Montfort, for his advice and support over the years.

The book has also drawn on advice and information supplied by others. These include Professor Mike Saks, pro vice-chancellor at the University of Lincoln, and a former colleague at De Montfort; Dr Shirley McIver, Judith Smith and Dr John Glasby of the Health Services Management Centre at Birmingham University; Professor Keiron Walshe of the Health Services Management Unit at the University of Manchester; Colin Palfrey of the University of Wales at Swansea; Colin Morgan, from the University of Glamorgan, Professor Michael Moran of Manchester University; Bruce Wood, formerly of the same institution; and Ann Wall and Barry Owen, formerly of Sheffield Hallam University. I have also appreciated the help and support of colleagues in the Political Studies Association Health Group, including Dr Alison Hann, Dr Ian Greener, Professor Stephen Harrison, Dr Chris Nottingham, Dr Fiona O'Neill, Professor Calum Paton, Dr Stephen Peckham and Dr Martin Powell. I should also like to thank my contacts in the NHS for their observations and anecdotes, which generated valuable insights and helped me to see beyond 'the ivory tower'.

There are a number of acknowledgements related to the reproduction of material with permission. Thanks to Dr James Le Fanu and Time Warner for the reproduction of information from *The Rise and Fall of* Modern *Medicine* which appears in Figure 2.1. To Professor John Appleby for permission to use the data from *Five Year Health Check: A Review of Government Policy 1997–2002* (Table 6.1). To HM Treasury for the reproduction of a table from the Wanless Report (Table 6.2). To Laing and Buisson for allowing me to reproduce a table from their *Healthcare Market Review 2001/2* (Table 6.3). To Rebecca Rosen for the use of material (in Chapter 8) drawn from a report on *Access to Health Care: Taking Forward the Findings of a Scoping Exercise*. To the OECD for the use of data in Figures 6.1 and 6.2. Finally, to WHO European Region for permission to use text adapted from *Health 21: The Health Policy Framework for the WHO European Region*.

Finally, thanks to my editor at Palgrave, Jon Reed, for his advice, support and encouragement, to my copy editor, Kate Possnett, for guiding me through the final stages, and to Steven Kennedy, who persuaded me to write the first edition of *Health and Health Care in Britain* back in the early 1990s.

Rob Baggott
Leicester, June 2004

List of Abbreviations

ACHCEW	Association of Community Health Councils for England and Wales
AHA	Area Health Authority
AIDS	Acquired immune deficiency syndrome
AMI	Acute myocardial infarction
BMA	British Medical Association
BMI	Body mass index
BPA	Basic practice allowance
BSE	Bovine spongiform encephalopathy
CAM	Complementary and alternative medicine
CAT	Computerised axial tomography
CCST	Certificate of Completion of Specialist Training
CFISSA	Centrally Funded Initiatives and Services and Special Allocations
CFS	Chronic fatigue syndrome
CHAI	Commission for Healthcare Audit and Inspection (now known as the Healthcare Commission)
CHC	Community Health Council
CHD	Coronary heart disease
CHI	Commission for Health Improvement
CIP	Cost improvement programme
CJD	Creutzfeldt-Jakob disease
CMO	Chief Medical Officer
CMT	Clinical management team
CNO	Chief Nursing Officer
COMA	Committee on the Medical Aspects of Food and Nutrition Policy
CPD	Continuing professional development
CPPIH	Commission for Patient and Public Involvement in Health
CPRS	Central Policy Review Staff
CRAG	Clinical Resource and Audit Group
CSBS	Clinical Standards Board for Scotland
CSCI	Commission for Social Care Inspection
DALY	Disability adjusted life year
DEFRA	Department for Environment, Food and Rural Affairs
DfES	Department for Education and Skills

DGH	District general hospital
DGM	District general manager
DHA	District health authority
DHSS	Department of Health and Social Security
DMT	District management team
DMU	Directly managed units
DoH	Department of Health
DsPH	Directors of Public Health
DTC	Diagnostic and treatment centre
DWP	Department for Work and Pensions
EBM	Evidence-based medicine
EBP	Evidence-based practice
ECR	Extra-contractual referral
EHS	Emergency hospital service
ENT	Ear, nose and throat
ERG	External reference group
EU	European Union
FACS	Fair Access to Care Services
FCE	Finished consultant episode
FHSA	Family Health Services Authority
FPC	Family Practitioner Committee
FPS	Family Practitioner Services
FSA	Food Standards Agency
GDP	Gross domestic product
GHS	General Household Survey
GMC	General Medical Council
GM	Genetically modified
GMS	General medical services
GOC	General Optical Council
GP	General practitioner
GPA	Good practice allowance
GPF	General practice fundholder
GSCC	General Social Care Council
HAI	Hospital-acquired infection
HAZ	Health Action Zone
HCHS	Hospital and Community Health Services
HEA	Health Education Authority
HEI	Higher education institution
HFA	Health for All
HImP	Health improvement programme
HISS	Hospital information support systems
HIV	Human immunodeficiency virus
HMC	Hospital Management Committee

HMO	Health Maintenance Organisation
HRG	Healthcare resource group
HRT	Hormone replacement therapy
HSCWB	Health, social care and well-being
HSSB	Health Services Supervisory Board
HTA	Health technology assessment
HTBS	Health Technology Board for Scotland
ICAS	Independent Complaints Advocacy Service
ICT	Information and communication technology
IHSM	Institute for Health Services Management
IPPR	Institute for Public Policy Research
ISTC	Independent sector treatment centre
IT	Information technology
JCB	Joint Commissioning Board
JIP	Joint investment plan
LDP	Local delivery plan
LHB	Local health board
LHCC	Local Health Care Co-operative
LHG	Local health group
LIFT	Local improvement finance trust
LPG	Local planning group
LSP	Local strategic partnership
MAFF	Ministry of Agriculture, Fisheries and Food
MAT	Modernisation action team
ME	Myalgic encephalomyelitis
MHCO	Managed health care organisation
MIT	Minimally invasive therapy
MOH	Medical Officer of Health
MoH	Ministry of Health
MRI	Magnetic resonance imaging
MRSA	Methicillin-resistant staphylococcus aureus
NAHAT	National Association of Health Authorities and Trusts
NAO	National Audit Office
NCAA	National Clinical Assessment Authority
NCEPOD	National Confidential Enquiry into Perioperative Deaths
NCSC	National Care Standards Commission
NCT	National Childbirth Trust
NCVO	National Council for Voluntary Organisations
NEAT	New and Emerging Applications of Technology
NELH	National Electronic Library for Health
NHI	National Health Insurance
NHS	National Health Service
NHSE	National Health Service Executive

NHSME	National Health Service Management Executive
NICE	National Institute for Clinical Excellence
NNS	Neighbourhood nursing service
NSF	National Service Framework
NVQ	National Vocational Qualification
ODPM	Office of the Deputy Prime Minister
OECD	Organisation for Economic Co-operation and Development
ONS	Office for National Statistics
OPCS	Office for Population Censuses and Surveys
OSC	Overview and Scrutiny Committee
PAC	Public Accounts Committee
PAF	Performance Assessment Framework
PALS	Patient Advice and Liaison Service
PCG	Primary care group
PCT	Primary care trust
PDS	Personal dental service
PET	Positron emission tomography
PFI	Private finance initiative
PHCT	Primary health care team
PMS	Personal medical services
PPIF	Patient and Public Involvement Forum
PVS	Persistent vegetative state
QALY	Quality adjusted life year
R&D	Research and development
RAWP	Resource Allocation Working Party
RCN	Royal College of Nursing
RCT	Randomised controlled trial
RGM	Regional general manager
RHA	Regional Health Authority
RHB	Regional Hospital Board
RMI	Resource management initiative
SARS	Severe acute respiratory syndrome
SEHD	Scottish Executive Health Department
SGT	Self-governing trust
SHA	Special health authority
SIGN	Scottish Intercollegiate Guidelines Network
SMR	Standardised mortality ratio
SSI	Social Services Inspectorate
STD	Sexually transmitted disease
STG	Special transitional grant
StHA	Strategic health authority
TB	Tuberculosis
TOPSS	Training Organisation for the Personal Social Services

TPP	Total purchasing pilot
TQM	Total quality management
UKCC	UK Central Council (for Nursing, Midwifery and Health Visiting)
UNICEF	United Nations International Children's Emergency Fund
VFMU	Value For Money Unit
WDC	Workforce Development Confederation
WHO	World Health Organisation
WRVS	Women's Royal Voluntary Service

Health and Illness

Present standards of health in Britain are relatively high, not only in comparison with past generations, but also internationally. Britain in the new millennium is a comparatively healthy place in which to be born and to live. However, the focus upon overall standards of health disguises trends and variations within the population. Any judgement about health standards must be based therefore on a careful analysis of these trends and variations. This introductory chapter provides such an analysis, beginning with the concept of health and its measurement. This is followed by an overview of recent trends, an analysis of the key factors which affect health and illness in the UK, and a discussion of variations between different population groups.

Defining and Measuring Health

Definitions of Health

There are two main ways of defining health: the positive approach, where health is viewed as a capacity or an asset, and the negative approach, which emphasises the absence of specific illnesses, diseases or disorders (Aggleton, 1990, p. 5). The World Health Organisation (WHO) defined health as 'a state of complete physical, mental and social well-being and not merely the absence of disease or infirmity' (WHO, 1946). As well as emphasising health in a positive sense, this definition is significant in stressing mental as well as physical aspects of health, and social as well as individual well-being. It has, however, been criticised for being utopian, though it should perhaps be viewed as an ideal towards which health care and other social actions may be orientated (Twaddle, 1974). In terms of the negative concept of health, an individual is regarded as being healthy when not suffering from a particular illness or disease. The terms 'illness' and 'disease', although often used interchangeably, are different. Disease relates to a biological malfunctioning, diagnosed by doctors, while illness refers both to the personal experience of disease and its wider social implications (Kleinman, 1978). The negative concept of health is closely associated with orthodox medicine, discussed further in Chapter 2, and has predominated.

The Measurement of Health, Disease and Illness

The predominance of the negative concept has had implications for the measurement of health and illness. Rather than indicating standards of health in a positive sense, official statistics have tended to measure how long we live, how we die, and how unhealthy we are. The emphasis has been on life expectancy, mortality (death), morbidity (disease), and the utilisation of diagnostic, treatment and care facilities. These are narrow indicators of health.

However, some indicators can shed light on the health of people in a positive sense. For example, life expectancy and infant mortality statistics have long been used as indicators of population health. Furthermore, 'well-being' is indicated by social surveys of lifestyles which measure 'risk factors' for disease, such as levels of obesity, lack of exercise, and smoking. Also, individual attitudes and experiences of health and illness are increasingly measured. For example, the General Household Survey (GHS) asks individuals about their own attitudes to health, fitness and lifestyles as well as their experiences of ill health and disability. Such surveys serve as indicators of positive health, making it possible to construct a picture of health trends based on people's own judgements. The concept of social well-being can be explored more fully by measuring psychological wellbeing, life satisfaction, and the role of social networks and support. Such surveys are often 'validated' by including explicit criteria established by professionals, or by corroborating subjective experiences with clinical signs identified by a health professional (Bowling, 1997).

Health Trends

The Global Context

Countries such as Britain have been successful in improving health and reducing disease. But some countries, particularly those in the developing world, are still fighting battles which the developed world won long ago. Worldwide, one in every twelve children dies before the age of five from a preventable disease (Unicef, 2002) and these deaths are concentrated in the developing world. For example, Africa's infant mortality rate is over four times that of Europe (WHO, 1999). The average life expectancy at birth in developing countries is two-thirds that of the industrialised nations. The life expectancy for a European male (69) is 20 years longer than for an African (WHO, 1998a). Even so, there are considerable variations between developing countries as well as within them.

The biggest causes of illness and death in the Third World are infectious diseases and those associated with poverty and malnutrition. As the WHO (1995, p. v) has noted, 'Poverty…is the world's deadliest disease.' Two-thirds of deaths in Africa are due to communicable disease, maternal and childbirth conditions or nutritional deficiency, while only a fifth are related to chronic illness (WHO, 1999). However, the latter is becoming more significant as countries industrialise and adopt a consumer culture. Large increases are expected in environmental health problems and diseases related to lifestyle factors. For example, it has been estimated that 70 per cent of the deaths from tobacco by 2025 will be in the Third World (*Independent*, 1997). Increasingly, diseases of poverty and affluence coexist in less developed countries. Added to this is the challenge posed by HIV/AIDS; the vast majority of 34 million people infected by HIV live in sub-Saharan Africa (approximately 25 million) and South East Asia (6 million).

The Industrialised Countries

Compared with the Third World, industrialised countries suffer relatively less from infectious diseases and more from chronic and degenerative diseases. In the nineteenth and early twentieth centuries infectious diseases were far more prevalent in industrialised countries, along with illness due to maternal and childbirth conditions, and malnutrition. Now fewer than 10 per cent of deaths are attributed to these diseases and conditions (WHO, 1999). Chronic disease is now the main cause of morbidity and mortality, accounting for over 80 per cent of deaths in Europe (WHO, 1998a). As in the Third World, broad trends mask a considerable variation in health and illness within and between industrialised countries. Infant mortality rates vary considerably, even among European countries, from under five (per 1000 live births) in France (2000) to over nine in Hungary. Life expectancy at birth also varies significantly, from 67 years in the case of Hungarian males to 76 in Greece and Sweden.

The UK

The main causes of death in the UK, as in other industrialised countries, are cancer and circulatory disease (see Figure 1.1). Compared with other European Union countries, the UK has a lower-than-average mortality rate from cancer for men, but a relatively high female death rate (Eurostat, 2000). In the case of circulatory disease, UK mortality rates are relatively high. Death rates from respiratory disease in the UK are very high by European Union standards, while death rates from external causes, such as accidents, are relatively low.

Evidence from social surveys, such as the GHS, illustrates the importance of chronic illness as a cause of morbidity. In Britain in the year 2001, one-third of men and women reported a long-standing condition. Just under a fifth of the population reported having a *limiting*, long-standing illness. Unsurprisingly,

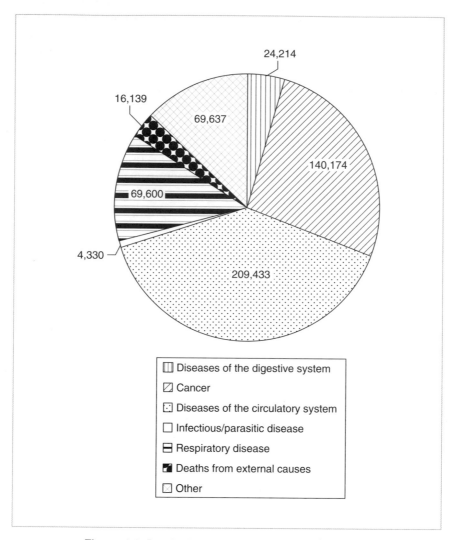

Figure 1.1 Deaths by cause, England and Wales, 2002
Source: ONS Annual Abstract of Statistics 2004 (The Stationery Office, 2004)

elderly people have higher levels of chronic illness and disability: two-thirds of adults aged 75 and over reported having a limiting long-standing illness, disability or infirmity in 2000. However, it is also believed that the elderly tend to under-report chronic illness and disability (Bridgwood et al., 2000). There has been a rise in the level of self-reported long-standing illness in recent years, partly as a result of the ageing population. Nonetheless, all age groups have recorded a rise in self-reported long-standing illness over the last thirty years according to the GHS data.

Other main causes of morbidity and mortality in the UK are accidents (see below) and mental illness. Around one in six adults in Britain have been assessed as having neurotic symptoms (Singleton et al., 2001), including sleep problems, worry and panic. Overall, one in 25 adults have a personality disorder, such as obsessive–compulsive disorders, paranoia or an antisocial personality. Other problems associated with mental health problems include alcohol and drug abuse (see below), suicides and self-injury. Over 4000 people die from suicide each year in the UK. It is more common among men, especially young men and those in unskilled occupations, unemployed people, prisoners, and young women from the Indian subcontinent. Suicide rates are also higher in occupational groups where there is easier access to the means of suicide, including farmers, doctors and other health care professionals and veterinary surgeons. People who misuse alcohol and drugs are also at greater risk of suicide, as are those who have previously harmed themselves.

Factors Determining Health

Several factors have an important bearing on the health of individuals and consequently on overall population health. In this section, the following are examined: health services, biological factors, genetic factors, demographic factors, environment and lifestyle.

Health Services

Good access to high-quality health services is crucial to the maintenance of good health. Research in the USA suggests that curative medicine adds between 44 and 45 months to life expectancy. An additional 18–19 months is added by preventive medicine, such as screening or immunisation (Bunker, Frazier and Mostelle, 1994). Health services must be of sufficient quality and effectiveness to actually improve health. As later chapters will show, health services have lacked a solid evidence base, and in some cases have been delivered in a way that undermines rather than improves health. Moreover, individuals must be able to get access to good-quality services. As will also become clear in later chapters, there are many obstacles which impede access, including financial barriers, geographical factors, and cultural and social class factors. A further factor which impinges on the contribution of health care is the introduction of new technologies (see Exhibit 1.1), which also affects the cost of the health care system.

Exhibit 1.1   New Medical Technologies

New medical technologies are emerging from wider scientific innovations, chiefly in biotechnology and microelectronics. It is impossible here to give anything more than an overview of recent developments and their wider implications (see Wyke, 1996; *British Medical Journal*, 1999).

Diagnostic Instruments

Doctors increasingly use imaging techniques such as MRI (magnetic resonance imaging) which produce detailed cross-sectional images of the body. PET (positron emission tomography) has also been developed to enable closer examination of chemical processes in the brain and in other organs. Other developments include microelectronic instruments for monitoring and investigating signs of disease. Future applications include the development of tiny devices to monitor protein levels in the blood, enabling doctors to determine the severity of heart disease, and 'non-invasive' devices for monitoring glucose levels in people with diabetes. More generally, there has been interest in 'telecare' – systems that routinely monitor individuals for a range of health problems and alert professionals accordingly (see Cross, 2000).

Instruments and Techniques for Treating Disease

Development in fibre optics, microelectronics and microengineering have facilitated improvements in surgical devices. Indeed, keyhole surgery, which involves passing miniature surgical instruments through small holes in the skin, is now routinely practised. Future developments will take the form of sophisticated, remote-computer-controlled instruments for diagnosis and treatment. Already, surgical 'robots' have been used in knee-joint operations, as well as abdominal, urological and oesophageal surgery. Meanwhile, laser techniques have developed rapidly and are now used in the treatment of various diseases and disorders, including tumours and eye surgery, and experimentally in the treatment of heart disease. New-generation laser treatment includes photodynamic therapy, which combines laser treatment with drugs that help to target the laser beams to the tissues that need to be destroyed. There is also much scope for synthetic components that mimic the body's functions, or which correct dysfunctions. The heart 'pacemaker' device is well-known. Future applications include artificial hearts and lungs, and synthetic cartilage.

Information and Communication Technologies

New developments here include the creation of information systems that enable multiple access and contribution to databases (see Exhibit 9.3). Information systems also have an important role in disseminating the latest research and techniques to a wider constituency. Telemedicine, including the transmission of images between health professionals, can improve the speed and quality of diagnosis. It can also produce more efficient working arrangements, such as 'conferencing' between specialists in complex cases.

Genetic Technologies

The mapping of the human genome, coupled with the development of tests for genetic diseases, is perhaps a mixed blessing in the absence of therapies to treat these diseases. However, gene therapies are already being developed and used experimentally (notably for

→

Exhibit 1.1 continued

$\longrightarrow$

cystic fibrosis). Genetic technology is linked with developments in drug therapy. It is likely that in the future advances will be made in pharmacogenetics, enabling drug therapies to be tailored more closely to the individual's genetic characteristics, improving efficacy and reducing adverse effects of therapies.

Drug Therapies

There have been many important developments in drug therapies. Recent examples include drugs for obesity, multiple sclerosis, and brain and breast tumours. Many of these are geared to improving quality of life, as well as saving lives. Genetic engineering offers the prospect of new drugs, making therapies more widely available and possibly cheaper.

Transplantation and New Tissues

Transplantation is no longer a 'new technology'. New drug therapies have improved the efficacy of transplants (especially among high-risk groups), enabling more complex procedures to be undertaken. Future developments may involve the use of animal organs (xeno-transplantation), possibly with genetic modification. Other technologies include growing tissues, including the use of foetal tissue in treatment, notably 'stem cells', which have potential for producing new tissues or new therapies. This is linked to the debate on therapeutic cloning, whereby cells may be taken from an individual and cloned to grow tissues or develop new therapies. In the UK, therapeutic cloning is permitted in connection with research on embryos under 14 days old. Reproductive cloning (i.e. for the purpose of creating a new human being) is illegal.

Developments in technology have adverse as well as positive implications. There are often difficult ethical issues, for example, with regard to the production and use of human tissues. Expensive new technologies may replace effective low-technology interventions. It is important that new technologies work alongside existing cost-effective interventions. Indeed, many low-technology interventions involve personal contact with health professionals and it is important that these relationships are not damaged when new technologies are introduced, otherwise the overall quality of the patients' experience may decline. It has been estimated that new technologies add around 2 per cent to the cost of the NHS (Wanless, 2001). However, the research base for making predictions about the net effect of new technologies on costs is weak (Harrison et al., 1997). Indeed, new technologies offer the prospect of improving cost effectiveness, not only through better quality treatment but by enabling new ways of delivering services that could reduce the overall costs of care (by reducing hospitalisation, for example).

Biological Factors

Biological factors include infectious agents that cause disease. Changes in these factors, such as new or mutated viruses, bacteria and other organisms, may have serious implications for health. Although infectious diseases account for a small proportion of the burden of morbidity and mortality today, they should not be underestimated. Older infectious diseases such as tuberculosis, for example, have become more prevalent in recent years, and are more resistant to treatment. Also, infectious agents have become increasingly resistant to antibiotics, exemplified by the emergence of highly resistant strains of bacteria, such as MRSA. In addition there are relatively new infectious diseases, such as HIV/AIDS and more recently SARS.

Genetic Factors

Genes appear to predispose individuals to particular diseases (Yates, 1996; Appleyard, 2000). Some diseases – such as Huntington's disease – are known as single-gene disorders because a defect in one gene is the key to predisposition. In other cases more than one gene is implicated. For example, breast cancer, where two genes – BRCA1 and BRCA2 – are involved in 80 per cent of 'inherited' cases of breast cancer. A further genetic factor was found in 1999 when researchers identified a possible link between a variant of the apolipoprotein E gene and breast cancer (Hopkins, 1999).

The mapping of the human genome has enhanced the prospects of identifying complex disease genes. Some envisage that in the future it will be possible to conduct genetic tests for many diseases (Mathew, 2001). Optimists believe that genetic screening and treatment based on knowledge of individual genetic characteristics may eventually become a routine part of prevention and early treatment, and will be of great benefit to public health. Others are more cautious, pointing out that early clinical applications are fairly limited (Holtzman, 2001). But even in the absence of genetic therapies, those found to have genetic predisposition could benefit from closer surveillance and, if early signs of the disease emerge, clinical intervention at an earlier stage. Another potential benefit is that individuals may be able to make choices about work and lifestyle that reflect their higher risk. Hence, people with genes associated with cancer may be more willing to accept lifestyle changes that might prevent the disease. However, it is possible that individuals could adopt a fatalistic approach, believing that lifestyle would not affect the final outcome. Moreover, people whose genes do not predispose them to disease might indulge in potentially harmful activities believing themselves to be free of risk.

It is possible that the new genetics could shift attention away from the social, economic and environmental causes of disease which interact with genetic factors in the causation of illness (Holtzman, 2001). Furthermore, knowledge that one is genetically predisposed to disease is likely to place high psychological costs on the individual. There is also concern that the tests might be unreliable predictors of the onset of disease, and that they could encourage an over-zealous approach to treatment. Genetic testing carries a range of other adverse social implications (see Appleyard, 2000; Davison, Macintyre and Davey Smith, 1994). Those with positive tests for cancer could find themselves discriminated against by employers and by financial corporations such as banks and insurance companies. There is also the related question of confidentiality: how will information be handled and who will have access to it? In 2001, the British Government announced a five-year moratorium on the use of genetic-test information by insurance companies amid concern about discrimination. For 'high-value' policies, tests approved by the Government's Genetics and Information Advisory Committee may be used. Currently only one test – for Huntington's Disease – has been authorised. It is also possible that cases could be brought by those claiming discrimination by genetic testing under Human Rights and Data Protection legislation.

Demographic Factors

The nature of health and ill-health varies over an individual's lifetime. There is a life-cycle in operation, with people being prone to certain illnesses at particular times in their lives. Violent death, accidents and injury (both external and self-inflicted) are major causes of death in younger people. Circulatory diseases, cancers and respiratory diseases are the most common causes of death in the older age groups.

Self-reported illness confirms the chronic nature of disease in older age groups. Although total life expectancy has increased, the prevalence of chronic illness and disability in old age remains at a high level, so that for many people additional years of life are plagued with disability (Bone et al., 1995; Dunnell, 1995). The discovery that older people are more likely to die from chronic disease and to have long-standing conditions and disabilities, comes as no surprise. Yet it does raise questions about the implications of an increasing elderly population – a trend which is being faced by most countries (United Nations, 2002). The projected growth of the elderly population in the UK is shown in Figure 1.2. This shows that, following a sharp rise in the elderly population in the 1960s and 1970s, something of a plateau has now been reached. However, there will be a further rise in the proportion of elderly people in the UK in the coming decades, reaching a fifth of the total population by the year 2026. Figure 1.2 also illustrates the growth in the 'very elderly' population over the same period.

The growing proportion of elderly people in society is not a problem in itself. Rather, it is the possible consequences of this growth for health care provision and other social services that has caused anxiety. Elderly people, particularly those over the age of 75, are heavy users of health and social care. The implication is that the growth of the elderly population, all other things being equal, will produce an escalation in the costs of health care: the so-called 'demographic time bomb'.

The rising cost of caring for the elderly is only a problem if society cannot afford it. Yet there is a fear that the growth in the elderly population will not

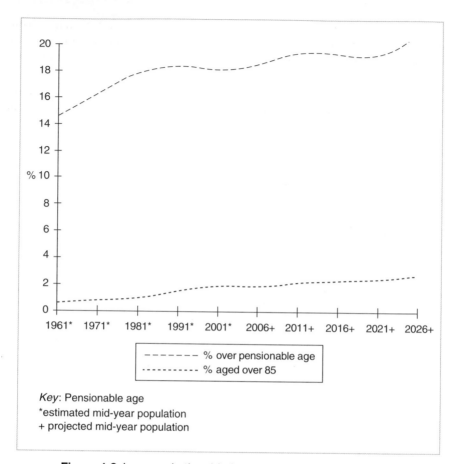

Figure 1.2 Increase in the elderly population, UK, 1961–2026
Source: ONS Annual Abstract of Statistics 2002 (The Stationery Office, 2002)

only add to the cost of care but will prevent society from generating the necessary resources (Johnson, Conrad and Thomson, 1989). In 1961 there were almost six people of working age for every person aged over 65. By the year 2011 this ratio is expected to be around four to one. This implies that the working population will face an increasingly heavy burden of providing the resources necessary for the care of the elderly. However, this gloomy scenario has been challenged. The dependency ratio (that between those of working age and the rest of the population, such as older people and children) is not expected to rise until the second decade of the 21st century (Ermisch, 1990).

Moreover, the cost of the growing elderly population may have been over-estimated (Health Committee, 1999a; Abel-Smith, 1996; Cm 4192, 1999; Wanless, 2001). Wittenberg, Sandhu and Knapp (2002) estimated that long-term care spending needed to grow by 153 per cent in real terms between 2000 and 2031. This represented a 1 per cent increase per year in the costs of social care and a 1.5 per cent increase in health care costs. This appears to be a substantial increase but, providing that the economy continues to grow at a reasonable rate, it is not unsustainable. Indeed, economic growth of 2.25 per cent a year until the middle of next century would mean that spending on long-term care would rise only slightly as a proportion of total national expenditure (Robinson, 2002a). However, it is particularly difficult to predict the impact of the ageing population on health care costs, largely because of uncertainties about the future health status of elderly people, health care costs and the impact of technology. Most health care costs are devoted to people in their last year of life. The predicted rising costs of an ageing population are heavily based on the assumption that more people will survive to the stage at which they will incur high health care costs. A US study (Scitovsky, 1988, cited by Abel-Smith, 1996), however, found that those who die in their eighties consume 20 per cent less in their last year of life than those who die aged 65–79. Another (Graham, Normand and Goodall, 2002) revealed that for those in their last year of life, the average costs of acute care fell with increasing age. For those who survived treatment, however, costs increased with age. The net effect was a small (2 per cent per annum) rise in costs. A further study found that there was a slight increase in time spent in hospital as a result of advancing age at death; in general people deferred rather than increased their overall usage of services (Himsworth and Goldacre, 1999). The implication of these studies is that greater longevity either does not necessarily increase health care costs in the longer term or that this increase is relatively small and manageable (Wanless, 2002; Harrison et al., 1997). A further point is that, in spite of the higher than average levels of disability in old age, elderly people are fitter than is commonly supposed (Jarvis et al., 1996). The vast majority of over-sixties are capable of looking after themselves (and others – the elderly constitute one-third of informal carers). Even among the over-eighties, the majority are fairly mobile. In Britain, for example, researchers found that at age 65 the number of years of life free from limiting, long-standing illness actually increased by around 10 per cent for both men and women between 1981 and 1995 (Kelly and Baker, 2000). Studies in the United States, for example, found that levels of chronic disability among the elderly have declined in recent years, even among the very old (Manton, Stalland and Corder, 1995).

More generally, critics of the demographic-time-bomb thesis view it as an attempt to narrow the foundation of the welfare state, to reduce entitlements and to create new private-welfare markets (Mullan, 2001). There may be something in this. Nonetheless, the growth of the elderly population, coupled with other social changes – in family structures and employment patterns (see Falkingham, 1989) – will test our current health and social care systems. Even if people live healthier lives for longer periods, they will inevitably at some stage require health care and social support. The increase in overall costs may not be as great as alarmist predictions have implied, but, health care systems will still face enormous challenges in accommodating the needs associated with this demographic trend.

The Environment

Accidents

Around 13,000 people die each year from accidents in the UK. Road accidents are a major cause of death and injury. Around 3500 people are killed in road accidents and a further 40,000 seriously injured every year. Over 4000 people are killed and 170,000 seriously injured in domestic accidents, and there are over 500 deaths and almost over 50,000 major injuries associated with work activities.

Although risks will always exist, much can be done to prevent accidents. For example, by altering the environment within which people live and work and by educating individuals about risks. The working environment can pose a wider threat to health over and above the level of illness and premature mortality caused by accidents in the workplace (Watterson, 1994; Snashall, 1996). Occupational diseases, including dermatitis, asthma and deafness, are a significant burden on health services, accounting for 7 per cent of general-practice consultations (McCormick, Fleming and Charlton, 1995). In addition, increasing stress levels in the workplace have been linked to a range of physical and mental health problems (Jenkins, 1993). However, the workplace can provide a setting to promote the health of workers in a positive way, through education and training, rather than simply being a focus for the prevention of occupational injury and illness.

Pollution and contamination

Environmental pollution is linked to major health problems. Air and water pollution can have a significant detrimental effect on the health of the population, particularly upon vulnerable groups such as children and the elderly. Although the impact of environmental pollution is often complex and difficult to measure, efforts have been made to quantify these risks. In a European study, it was found that air pollution caused 6 per cent of total mortality, half of which was attributable to motor traffic (Kunzli et al., 2000). Another problem is toxic waste, which has been linked with birth defects and other health problems by some studies (Fielder et al., 2000; Vrijheid et al., 2002).

Further sources of pollution arise from contamination in the agricultural and food industries. Pesticides, food additives and modern food-production techniques – including the use of antibiotics and growth-promoting drugs – have been blamed for a wide range of health problems (Agriculture Committee, 1998). For example, in the case of BSE and CJD the transmission of infective agents was attributed to changes in food-production methods (The BSE Inquiry, 2000). Concerns about GM foods have fuelled debates about the safety of modern technologies (Toke, 2001).

There has been a sharp growth in food poisoning in the UK over the last two decades. The latest figures show around 100,000 cases a year, though this may be due partly to improved reporting of incidents. Some food-poisoning out-breaks are very serious – notably incidents involving salmonella and *E. Coli 0157* which have led to fatalities and severe disabilities, especially in elderly people and children. The growth of food poisoning has been attributed to food technologies, poor catering standards as well as modern consumption patterns which have seen a rise in 'cook-chill' food, eating out and take-away food. Shortcomings in personal and domestic hygiene among consumers may have also played some part in this trend.

Global threats

Environmental threats to health operate at a global level in many ways. The destruction of the ozone layer is one example, the consequences of which include increased risk of skin cancer and suppression of the immune system. There has also been much discussion in recent years of the impact of climate change – global warming – on our environment. This has several implications for health. Rising temperatures may encourage the spread of infectious diseases. Malaria, for example, is likely to be found in countries experiencing a warmer climate in the future. Other possible health consequences include increased mortality and morbidity from heatwaves (offset by falls in deaths from extremely cold weather), exacerbation of respiratory diseases, an increase in allergic reactions, and health problems associated with disruption to food production and to communities affected by rising sea levels and weather conditions attributed to climate change such as floods, storms, forest fires and droughts (see UK Climate Change Impacts Review Group, 1996; McMichael and Haines, 1997). Global threats to health are usually associated with ecological or environmental disasters but other global factors can be regarded as having significant applications for health. War (including terrorism) has potentially serious implications for health, both directly in the form of casualties and through secondary effects in the form of environmental and ecological destruction, famine and shortages, and disruption of health and welfare services.

Lifestyle Factors

Smoking, poor diet, alcohol and drug abuse and sexual lifestyles all affect health. Although these are within the realms of personal decision-making, it is accepted that the State has a legitimate role in trying to influence them. Arguments arise over the extent to which the State should regulate these choices and how it should do this.

Healthy eating and exercise

Diet has a crucial impact on health (WHO, 1998b). Dietary factors are associated with at least 40 per cent of all cancers (Doll and Peto, 1981), perhaps more

(Austoker, 1994). There appears to be a link between diet and bowel cancer (Royal College of Physicians, 1981), with increased consumption of fruit, vegetables and fibre in the diet generally associated with a reduced risk (Jansen et al., 1999). The link between fibre intake and reduced risk of bowel cancer is less clear, however (see Fuchs et al., 1999).

Diet is recognised as a factor in heart and circulatory disease (COMA, 1994; Key et al., 1996). Researchers have found a link between fibre intake and reduced risk of coronary heart disease (Wolk et al., 1999), while the consumption of fats, particularly saturated fats, has been identified as a risk factor for heart disease (Keys, 1980) – though this has been disputed by others (Atrens, 1994). There has been controversy about the role of cholesterol in heart disease. Although levels of cholesterol in the blood are related to mortality from coronary heart disease across different cultures, there is a wide variation in the mortality rate at each given cholesterol level, implying that other factors may be at work (Verschuren et al., 1995).

High blood pressure, another major risk factor in heart disease and strokes, is related to diet. Excess consumption of salt is associated with higher blood pressure (Elliott et al., 1996). Furthermore, obesity has been identified as a risk factor in heart disease, stroke and cancers – as well as other diseases, such as diabetes (NAO, 2001a; Wilding, 1997; WHO, 1998b). Obesity is defined in terms of Body Mass Index (BMI). This is calculated by dividing the person's body mass in kilograms by their height in metres squared, with a BMI over 30 in England and Wales being classified as obese. Over a fifth of adults in England are currently obese.

The link between obesity and ill health seems straightforward, though there is considerable disagreement about the causes of obesity, and its consequences. Laboratory research suggests that genetic factors may play an important role (Nagle et al., 1999). There are also ecological explanations which suggest that obesity may be a behavioural reaction to abundant supplies of nutrients (Egger and Swinburn, 1997; Hill and Peters, 1998). An alternative view is that the focus on obesity is misplaced. Some argue that it stigmatises individuals (often poor people, women and ethnic minorities who have higher levels of obesity) who are, in effect, blamed for their condition (Orbach, 1978). Classifying people as obese ignores the psychosocial factors that lead people to overeat and underexercise, and may further damage self-esteem. Strategies to combat obesity might also affect other eating disorders by inducing dietary regimes in people already underweight (see Lawrence, 1987).

Some view physical fitness and activity as the most crucial factor (Lee, Blair and Jackson, 1999; Prentice and Jebb, 1995). Thirty-one per cent of the adult population of England is classified as sedentary – not indulging in moderate intensity activity at least 30 minutes per week (this includes heavy gardening or housework, DIY, swimming, cycling, brisk or fast walking – Office for National Statistics, 2000, p. 126). Exercise is also associated with reduced risk for heart disease and stroke and some cancers (Davey Smith et al., 2000; Batty and Thune, 2000). It has also been viewed as effective in preventing osteoporosis, diabetes and mild depression and anxiety (Fentem, 1994), and may also have a role to play in treatment for major depression (Babyak et al., 2000). Exercise has also been associated with improved mental agility in older people (Kramer et al., 1999).

Concern about healthy eating and exercise has focused particularly on children and young people. One survey found that one in five British children ate no fruit in the previous week and that most young people over seven years of age were physically inactive (DoH/FSA, 2000). Another large-scale survey of UK children revealed that obesity ranged from 10 per cent of six-year-olds to 17 per cent of 15-year-olds (Reilly and Dorosty, 1999).

Smoking and health

Smoking-related diseases kill approximately 100,000 people each year and there are at least 24 different causes of death involved including cancer (lung cancer alone kills around 40,000 people a year in the UK) and respiratory disease, strokes and heart disease. Around half of smokers will die from their habit (Doll et al., 1994), and non-smokers may also be at risk (Independent Scientific Committee on Smoking and Health, 1988). There is much concern about passive smoking (He et al., 1999). Smoking is a major cause of morbidity, responsible for more than 225,000 hospital admissions each year (HEA, 1991). Smoking-related diseases are relatively difficult to cure. Lung-cancer survival rates are low – and therefore the most cost-effective strategy is prevention: to persuade people not to smoke and existing smokers to give up. Given the addictive properties of tobacco (Royal College of Physicians, 2000), much emphasis is placed on preventing and deterring smoking among children and young people. However, in 2000, 12 per cent of girl pupils were regular smokers compared with 9 per cent of boy pupils (Boreham and Shaw, 2001), while among the adult population 25 per cent of women and 29 per cent of men were smokers (Walker et al., 2001), compared with 51 per cent and 41 per cent respectively in 1974. Smoking is still more popular among manual than professional groups with a third of women and 44 per cent of men in the unskilled manual group indulging in the habit.

Alcoholic drinks

Alcohol is implicated in a wide range of health and social problems, including accidents (notably road accidents), violent assaults, mental illness, and a range of physical disorders and illnesses. These include 28,000 premature deaths annually in England and Wales from a range of causes including suicide, murder, death from fire, accidents and drownings (Anderson, 1988). Over a quarter of male hospital admissions are alcohol-related (Luke, 1998). There appears to be a broad relationship between the level of alcohol consumption in a society and the level of alcohol-related problems (Edwards, 1994; Colhoun et al., 1997; Her and Rehm, 1998). The doubling of the amount of alcohol consumed per adult in the UK in the postwar period was matched by a similar growth in alcohol problems. Although the overall level of consumption may be problematic in view of this, heavy, 'binge' drinking has been the main focus of concern. In Britain 7.5 per cent of the population (12 per cent of men and 3 per cent of women) have some form of alcohol dependence. Thirty-eight per cent of men and 15 per cent of women engage in 'hazardous drinking' with the highest prevalence among teenagers and young adults (Singleton et al., 2001).

Moderate alcohol consumption may help to reduce the risk of coronary heart disease (Gronback et al., 1995; Rimm et al., 1996), but this benefit appears to be confined to specific groups in the population (postmenopausal women and middle-aged men) and there has been some controversy over whether it is limited to certain types of drink, such as red wine. Meanwhile, other researchers have cast doubt on the protective effect of alcohol (Hart et al., 1999; Law and Wald, 1999).

Concern about drinking among children and young people was heightened in the late 1990s by the marketing of fruit-flavoured alcoholic drinks known as alcopops which were blamed for an increase in teenage drinking and associated drunkenness. In 2000, according to one large-scale survey, 24 per cent of 11–15-year-olds claimed to have consumed an alcoholic drink in the previous week, and there is evidence to suggest that children are drinking larger quantities (Boreham and Shaw, 2001).

Illegal drugs

It is difficult to quantify the health effects of illegal drug-taking, largely because of the huge range of substances involved. Illegal drug-taking is far from being a minority activity. Official estimates put the numbers addicted to drugs at between 100,000 and 200,000 (Cm 3945, 1998). Around a third of the adult population have taken illegal drugs at some time in their life: 6 per cent in the previous month (Ramsey et al., 2001; see also Singleton et al., 2001). The most commonly taken drugs being cannabis and other so-called soft drugs. Fewer than 1 per cent of respondents admit to taking hard drugs such as heroin and cocaine, though there is likely to be some underreporting of this activity. There is particular concern about the scale of drug-taking among the young. Over 40 per cent of teenagers aged under 16 claim to have used drugs (Miller and Plant, 1996), while of the 32 per cent of 15-year-olds who admitted to using drugs, a fifth had done so in the previous month (Boreham and Shaw, 2001).

Although illegal drugs are associated with fatalities, overall mortality is considerably less than that from legal drugs such as alcohol and tobacco; in

1998, 2100 deaths were attributed to drug misuse. Regarding morbidity, illegal drug-taking is linked to a range of problems, often associated with the mode of delivery, such as injections associated with HIV/AIDS infection and hepatitis C. The short-term health consequences of illegal drug-taking include accidents and overdoses, as well as other physical and mental health problems specific to individual drugs. The so-called 'hard' drugs are linked with chronic health problems resulting from long-term use. But soft drugs too are linked with long-term health problems. For example, cannabis has been linked to psychoses, memory impairment, cancer and lung disease (*New Scientist*, 1998).

Sexual health

Although the number of reported cases of sexually transmitted diseases (STDs) has risen during the postwar period, it was the emergence of HIV/AIDS that made it a high-profile issue (Hancock and Carim, 1987). By 2001, over 52,000 cases of HIV/AIDS had been reported in the UK and there were over 12,000 deaths from AIDS over the same period. At present, prevention remains the only effective way of tackling the disease, though drug therapies have led to longer life expectancy and a better quality of life for people with HIV/AIDS. Other STDs also pose serious problems, and are linked with maternal and neonatal illness, infertility and cancers. There have been increases in most STDs in recent years. Cases of herpes and genital warts have increased substantially, while gonorrhoea, chlamydia and syphilis cases more than doubled between 1995 and 2000.

Concerns about sexual health are not confined to unpleasant and harmful diseases. In recent years, teenage pregnancy levels attracted much attention because of worries about abortion rates in this age group and a recognition that most teenage mothers and their children live in relatively deprived circumstances and face greater risks to their health (Social Exclusion Unit, 1999). In England around 90,000 teenagers a year become pregnant, and the teenage birth-rate in the UK is the highest in Western Europe.

Social and Economic Inequalities and Health

According to Graham (2000, p. 3), 'how well and how long one lives is powerfully shaped by one's place in the hierarchies built around occupation, education, and income'. Life expectancy varies considerably between the social classes: on average, men in social classes I and II live for five years longer than those in social classes IV and V (Hattersley, 1997). There are considerable differences in mortality between social classes (see Townsend, Davidson and Whitehead, 1992; Shaw et al., 1999). In the period 1991–3, the standardised mortality rate (SMR) for males aged 20–64 in England and Wales was almost

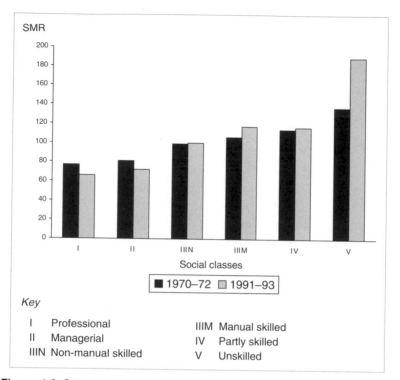

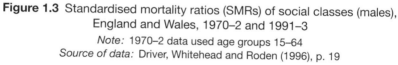

Figure 1.3 Standardised mortality ratios (SMRs) of social classes (males),
England and Wales, 1970–2 and 1991–3
Note: 1970–2 data used age groups 15–64
Source of data: Driver, Whitehead and Roden (1996), p. 19

three times higher for social class V (unskilled manual) than social class I
(professional and managerial) (see Figure 1.3). There are specific inequalities in
mortality from coronary heart disease (see National Heart Forum, 1998) with
the rate in men in social class V being three times that of social class I, while
survival rates for most cancers are superior for higher income categories and
socio-economic groups (see ONS/CRC/London School of Hygiene and
Tropical Medicine, 1999).

Inequalities in morbidity can also be found between the classes. In 2000,
26 per cent of men in professional households reported long-standing illness
compared with 44 per cent in unskilled manual households (Walker et al.,
2001). Around 25 per cent of inequalities in long-term limiting illness in men
(and 20 per cent in women) have been attributed to differences in occupational
class (Borooah, 1999). Among women, obesity and high blood pressure
(Colhoun and Prescott-Clarke, 1996), and poor mental health (Meltzer et al.,
1995) are more common in social classes IV and V than in I and II. Further
evidence of inequalities in health and illness was provided by a study of civil

servants (Marmot et al., 1991) which found that employment grade and salary were strongly related to health status.

Health inequalities can also be found among infants and children (BMA, 1999). The infant mortality rate for social classes I and II was 5 per 1000 in the period 1994–6 compared with 7 per 1000 for social classes IV and V. Accident and injury rates for children also vary considerably by social class. In the mid-1990s pedestrian-injury death-rates for children in social class V were five times higher than in social class I (Roberts and Power, 1996). Not only is poverty damaging to children's health development and educational achievement (Spencer, 1996; Duncan and Brooks Gunn, 1997), but socio-economic factors affecting childhood health subsequently have an impact on adult health status (see Roberts, 1997; van de Mheen, Stronks and Mackenbach, 1998; Curtis et al., 2003). At the other end of the age range, one finds that health inequalities persist into later life (Marmot and Shipley, 1996; Huisman, Kunst and Mackenbach, 2003).

Explaining Health Inequalities

Health inequalities are complex and multifaceted (see Graham, 2000). Statistical evidence of health inequalities does not necessarily mean that they should be regarded as inequitable. Indeed, inequality relates to statistical relationships, whereas inequity implies that a certain distribution is in some way unjust (Kendall, 1998). Moreover, there are several possible explanations for health inequalities, each of which has different implications for policy (see Carr Hill, 1987; BMA, 1995; Klein, 1991). One explanation is that health inequalities are artificially inflated by the use of occupation as a proxy for social class (Illsley, 1986). It is believed that because mortality rates are calculated on the basis of the occupation of the deceased taken from the death certificate, previous occupations that might place the individual in a higher social category are ignored. Furthermore, the changing sizes of social classes could be responsible for exaggerating inequalities. Between 1931 and 1981 social class V shrank by 55 per cent while social class I grew by 217 per cent. Although health inequalities could reflect high mortality within a declining section of society, a number of studies have found that such inequalities remain significant even when changes in the size of social classes are taken into account (see Goldblatt, 1989; Fox, Goldblatt and Jones, 1990; Pamuk, 1985; Davey Smith, Blane and Bartley, 1994).

Another explanation is that social-class differences in health arise from social selection (Stern, 1983; Illsley, 1986). According to this view, health inequalities are caused by healthy people being upwardly mobile, while less healthy people accumulate in social classes IV and V. In other words health inequalities produce social inequalities rather than the other way round. There is evidence that health status influences job selection, particularly in manual occupations, and this should be acknowledged when undertaking comparisons of mortality rates between specific occupations (Goldblatt, Fox and Leon, 1990; Carpenter, 1987). However, studies have confirmed that although social selection has an effect on health inequalities, it is not the primary factor (Donkin, Goldblatt and Lynch, 2002; Chandola et al., 2003; Power, Matthews and Manor, 1996; Hart, Davey Smith and Blane, 1998).

A third explanation focuses on the behaviour of individuals within social classes. Variations in health status are associated with differences in lifestyle between social classes. Hence excessive drinking, smoking and obesity are more common in social classes IV and V than in classes I and II. While this cannot be denied, it is clear that individual choice is one of several factors affecting lifestyle. The social and economic environment within which individuals are located is also important (see also Backett and Davison, 1995). Such factors are important in explaining why certain subgroups continue to pursue lifestyles which carry health risks, such as smoking, for example, and poor nutrition (see James et al., 1997; MAFF, 1998; Dobson et al., 1994).

The fourth explanation is that factors associated with social class are an underlying cause of health inequalities. Some authors argue that occupational class is a useful proxy for a range of socio-economic variables and can provide a powerful explanation of health inequalities (see Townsend, Davidson and Whitehead, 1992). However, others have focused on the specific factors which produce social-class inequalities, such as inequalities in health between geographical areas, deprivation, unemployment, a shortage of good-quality and low-cost housing and income inequalities.

Aside from social class, it is clear that income has an impact on health (Benzeval, Judge and Shouls, 2001). It appears to have a stronger impact than occupation or education, though other indicators such as housing tenure and car ownership are even better indicators of health status. The importance of income is further discussed in the context of income inequality below.

Geographical Factors

One way of exploring the impact of socio-economic factors on health is to look at the inequalities between geographical areas. Research has shown that people living in the worst tenth of areas in Britain are 42 per cent more likely to die before 65 years of age than the average person (Shaw, Dorling and Brimblecombe, 1998). The main factor behind geographical variations in health status appears to be deprivation. The most economically deprived areas tend to be the least healthy (Carstairs and Morris, 1989; Drever and Whitehead, 1995; Charlton, 1996). However, there is evidence that the 'place' or communities where people live has some impact on health inequalities over and above individual characteristics (Curtis et al., 2003; see also MacIntyre, McIver and Soomans, 1993).

Unemployment

Unemployment has a detrimental impact upon health (Bethune, 1996). Even after adjustment for variables such as social class, health status and lifestyle, the relative risk of mortality after five years for middle-aged men who have lost employment has been calculated as double that of those who have remained continuously employed (Morris, Cook and Shaper, 1994). In relation to mental health, unemployed people experience twice the level of neurotic symptoms of those in employment (Meltzer et al., 1995). Differences between employed and unemployed people cannot be explained wholly in terms of previous health or pre-existing circumstances (Moser et al., 1990), though men in manual occupations with limiting long-standing illnesses are more likely to be unemployed than those with similar illnesses in higher socio-economic groups (Bartley and Owen, 1996). Notably, the threat of unemployment and job insecurity carry significant adverse health consequences (Bartley and Owen, 1996; Ferrie et al., 1995; Ferrie et al., 2001).

Housing

Another important indicator of deprivation is housing standards, also closely associated with health. There is a general acknowledgement that 'housing and health are strongly related' (Conway, 1995; BMA, 2003). This has been supported by various studies (Hunt, 1997; Marsh et al., 1999; Wilkinson, 1999). In addition there are links between poor housing and specific health problems, such as overcrowding and psychological stress (Lowry, 1991; Gabe and Williams, 1993). Furthermore, cold and damp housing conditions have been linked to respiratory problems such as asthma and other allergies and infections, particularly among children (Platt, Martin and Hunt, 1989).

In addition, the effect of poor housing probably has an effect over and above the direct impact on specific conditions and illnesses. Greater housing deprivation seems to lead to a greater probability of ill health in general and this impact was likely to be greater among those affected earlier in life (Marsh et al., 1999). Furthermore, the absence of a home undoubtedly has an effect on health status as revealed by surveys of the health of homeless people (see for example, Conway, 1988; Fisher and Collins, 1993; Child Accident Prevention Trust, 1991; Bines, 1994).

The relationship between health and housing, and their 'triangular relationship' with deprivation (see Goodchild, 1998), requires closer scrutiny. In particular, more needs to be known about the impact of housing and anti-poverty strategies on health. As one review has observed, many studies show health gains but studies are often small (Thomson, Petticrew and Morrison, 2001).

Income Inequality and Health

Few informed observers doubt that health status is affected to some extent by social class, deprivation, unemployment and poor housing. More controversially, the *relative income thesis* (Wilkinson, 1996; Lynch and Kaplan, 1997) states that the more equal the income distribution of a particular country, the better its average levels of health will be. These studies showed that income differentials were closely correlated with differences in mortality and life expectancy, while changes in overall material standards had little impact on health standards. Moreover, mortality was found to be lower in societies where income differentials were smaller, even after controlling for average income levels, absolute poverty levels and other socio-economic factors (see also Kennedy, Kawachi and Protherow-Stith, 1996; Wolfson et al., 1999; Ben-Shlomo, White and Marmot, 1996; Stanistreet, Scott-Samuel and Bellis, 1999).

Although the precise causal link between income distribution and health is unclear, a number of potential causes have been suggested. Material inequalities are thought to affect levels of stress-related illness through the perception of social injustice, though more recent work has cast doubt on a direct relationship between stress and vulnerability to disease (Kunst et al., 1998). Another possibility was that inequality could affect social cohesion, through its impact on 'social capital', the networks, norms and trust within communities, whose broader importance for civic culture has been identified by a number of authors including Putnam (2000). Wilkinson (1997) cites research that identifies social trust (as indicated by membership of voluntary groups and levels of trust in the community) as a factor linking income distribution and health (Kawachi et al., 1997; Kawachi and Kennedy, 1997). Meanwhile, a study by Kaplan et al. (1996) found that variations in health outcomes and social indicators were paralleled by the scale of investment in human and social capital. More recently, Rose (2000) found that social capital increased physical and emotional health in Russia, while McCulloch's (2001) study revealed that people in the lowest categories of social capital had increased risk of psychiatric morbidity. Others, while accepting that social networks might well play a role in promoting health, have been more cynical about the impact of social capital and in particular have expressed concern about the lack of clarity surrounding the term (see Muntaner, Lynch and Davey Smith, 2001; Cattell, 2001).

Critics have attacked the relative-income thesis on several grounds. It has been argued that the link between income inequality and overall health standards is tenuous and that health inequalities are more closely related to specific factors, such as absolute poverty and unemployment. Furthermore, it has been claimed that the relation between income inequality and general levels of health is largely a statistical artefact, and that relationships between variables at an aggregate level are wrongly interpreted as applying at the individual level

(Gravelle, 1998). Other critics argue that the relative-income hypothesis is based on flawed measures of income distribution (Judge, 1995).

Further research into comparative health inequalities has cast further doubt on relative-income thesis. Mackenbach et al. (1997) did not find that health inequalities were smaller in countries where egalitarian principles exerted more influence over social and economic policies. Several studies, covering a number of countries (Mellor and Milyo, 2001; Sturm and Gresenz, 2002; Osler et al., 2002; Shibuya, Hashimoto and Yano, 2002), identified individual risk factors (including low levels of income), rather than income inequalities, as the key factors behind health inequalities. However, defenders of the relative-income thesis argued that a shift in relative poverty from elderly people (who have a high death-rate) to younger people (who have a lower death-rate) might have affected these studies (see Lobmayer and Wilkinson, 2000). They also pointed to other studies which demonstrated an association between high levels of inequality and poor mental and physical health (see Kahn et al., 2000).

Other Health Inequalities

Race and Ethnicity

Some ethnic groups have higher mortality rates and poorer health than the rest of the population (see Balarajan and Soni Raleigh, 1995; Harding and Maxwell 1997; Nazroo, 1997; Smaje, 1995; Wild and McKeigue, 1997). For example, people from African, Afro-Caribbean and the Indian communities have higher than average rates of limiting, long-standing illness (Charlton, Wallace and White, 1994; Smaje and Le Grand, 1997). Standardised mortality ratios for all ethnic groups, except Afro-Caribbean people and South-Asian women, are higher than average (Wild and McKeigue, 1997). Neonatal death-rates are generally higher for ethnic groups than for the general population (with the exception of the Bangladeshi community), postneonatal death-rates are lower than average among people of Indian, African and Bangladeshi origin, but above average for Afro-Caribbean and Pakistani communities (see Botting, 1997). In addition, Scottish and Irish migrants living in England have worse than average health (Wild and McKeigue, 1997).

The Asian community has a much higher mortality rate from coronary heart disease than the general population (Wild and McKeigue, 1997). They are also more at risk from other circulatory diseases, as are people born in the Caribbean and in Africa. Certain cancers, such as liver cancer for example, are more common in ethnic groups, though cancer mortality as a whole is lower than in the general population. People originating from the Indian subcontinent have a much higher than average rate of tuberculosis infection, and there is a disproportionately high incidence of diabetes in West Indian and Asian communities. In addition, a small number of diseases are wholly or mainly confined to ethnic populations, including rickets (predominantly affecting people of Asian origin) and sickle-cell anaemia and thalassaemia (affecting people originating from Africa, Asia, the Middle East and the Mediterranean). Finally, there are apparent variations in mental health, as reflected in above-average reported rates of mental illness and admissions to mental hospitals among the Caribbean community (Cochrane and Bal, 1989; Cope, 1989).

There are several explanations for such variations, each carrying different policy implications (see Ahmad, 1993; Smaje, 1995; Nazroo, 1998). Some variation may be due to certain biases arising from inadequate research methods. Criticism has centred on the higher reported rates of mental illness and admissions for Caribbean people, mentioned above, which has been attributed to misdiagnosis and racial stereotyping (see Sashidaran and Francis, 1993). More generally, the methods used to categorise people can produce misleading conclusions. In mortality studies ethnic status is based on country of birth, which is a very crude indicator of ethnicity. Indeed, Nazroo (1997) found that when a more detailed approach to ethnic classification was adopted, certain subgroups did not actually have a higher rate of mortality. For example, in the case of coronary heart disease (CHD) it was found that Pakistani and Bangladeshi people were responsible for the higher rate of Asian mortality, while the Indian community had similar rates as Whites. Furthermore, within the Indian community, Hindus and Sikhs had low rates of CHD mortality while Muslims had relatively high rates.

Although there are methodological problems when measuring the relative health status of ethnic groups, no one seriously believes that the observed variations are entirely artefactual. Indeed, ethnic differences may also be due to cultural or genetic factors. Cultural factors include variations in healthy lifestyles between different ethnic groups, for which there is some evidence (Nazroo, 1997; HEA, 1997). For example, Indian, Pakistani and Bangladeshi men report lower levels of physical exercise than the general population, while Afro-Caribbean and Bangladeshi men report higher rates of smoking. Genetic factors also play a part in health inequalities. As already noted, ethnic groups are known to be vulnerable to a number of diseases and it is possible that genetic scientists may well discover others in the future.

Material explanations relate excess mortality and ill health among ethnic groups to socio-economic disadvantage. There is evidence to suggest that socio-economic class differences are relevant to some ethnic groups: Afro-Caribbean people and the Pakistani and Bangladeshi communities (but not the Indian community) are significantly over-represented in manual households and in lower income groups (Nazroo, 2000). Two-thirds of Pakistani and Bangladeshi households fall into the bottom fifth of the income distribution compared with 19 per cent of white households (Office for National Statistics,

1998, p. 100). Some argue that social class is an inadequate explanation of differences in mortality between ethnic groups and the general population (Harding and Maxwell, 1997). Others have responded by commenting that conventional measures of social class fail to capture the material circumstances of ethnic groups relative to others (see Nazroo, 1997, 1998). Indeed, when alternative measures of socio-economic disadvantage are used (such as car ownership, for example) such factors do correspond to inequalities in health between various ethnic groups. Moreover, other forms of disadvantage might affect ethnic health, including social exclusion and the ecological effects of living in a particularly unhealthy locality (Nazroo, 1998). It is also possible that overt and implicit racism has an effect on mental and physical health (Williams, Lavizzo-Mourey and Warren, 1994). Similarly, institutional race discrimination and insensitivity in service provision (see Kelleher and Hillier, 1996) may affect mortality rates if people from ethnic backgrounds receive inadequate or inappropriate health care (see Nazroo, 1997; Lear et al., 1994) or face difficulties accessing services (Smaje and Le Grand, 1997).

Gender

Important differences in health status exist between men and women (see Hayes and Prior, 2003; Miles, 1991; Doyal, 1995; Annandale and Hunt, 2000). Women live five years longer than men, and death-rates are lower for women compared with men in every age group. However, life expectancy for women in the UK is below the European Union average, while men's life expectancy is slightly above the average. Women have tended to report slightly higher rates of long-standing illness and limiting long-standing illness than men (Walker et al., 2001). Women of all ages report more use of GP and outpatient health services. Men and women differ in their susceptibility to different kinds of illness. For example, disorders and diseases of the reproductive system are more commonly found in women, and women report higher levels of psychiatric morbidity (Singleton et al., 2001; Meltzer et al., 1995). However, in each age group men are more prone to injury and accidental death than women.

Aside from obvious anatomical differences between the sexes, a range of factors explain variations in health status. Socio-economic factors have a differential impact on male and female health: the class gradient for mortality and life expectancy is steeper for men than women (Soni Raleigh and Kiri, 1997; MacIntyre and Hunt, 1997). This is not to say that women are invulnerable to the health effects of socio-economic disadvantage. Indeed, a strong socio-economic gradient exists for psychosocial health: disadvantaged women, and in particular single mothers, have poor levels of psychosocial health (Macran, Clark and Joshi, 1996). This may partly be explained by the difficulties faced by women performing the caring role in the context of financial hardship (Graham, 1993).

The changing role of women in society is also extremely relevant to gender differences in health. Increased female participation in the labour market – often including casual, part-time and relatively low-paid jobs – has uncertain health implications. Although paid work brings in extra income which may improve the quality of life, it can also bring added stress, particularly when coupled with family responsibilities (Doyal, 1995). Paid employment has been associated with more illness for working-class women with children but less illness for middle-class women with the same family responsibilities (Blaxter, 1990, p. 101). But much seems to depend on the aspect of health under consideration and the kind of work undertaken. The association between paid work and better health is less apparent for physical than mental health, and applies less to women in full-time work and those in professional and managerial posts (Bartley, Popay and Plewis, 1992). Interestingly, this study found no relationship between employment status and domestic conditions, suggesting that the impact of paid work in terms of improved income may outweigh any of the negative effects of combining a domestic workload with employment. In general, studies show that employed women have better mental health than those not employed and that some positive effects in terms of physical health can be demonstrated. Even so, the increasing role of women in the workplace brings additional risks and hazards, including stress which could offset the benefits of paid work (Doyal, 1994).

Women's role in society has changed in other ways relevant to their health. Many women have greater financial independence and more freedom of choice than a generation ago. They now participate more in further and higher education, in the professions and in other institutions that were almost exclusively male less than half a century ago. At the same time, women's lifestyles have changed and this too has implications for health. Women are more likely than men to diet and they are more prone to eating disorders (Lawrence, 1987). They are also becoming more similar to men in aspects of health behaviour. Alcohol consumption is increasing in young women and this has been paralleled by an increase in drink-related problems (Ettore, 1997). A quarter of women are smokers, a slightly lower proportion than men (Walker et al., 2001). As noted earlier, among schoolchildren more girls than boys now smoke, raising the prospect that female lung-cancer sufferers could outnumber men in the future. When examining the health variations associated with gender, one should be aware that these interact with cultural and ethnic differences. Many of the changes in female work and lifestyles have not occurred uniformly, and in some ethnic groups there is greater cultural resistance to such trends. Therefore one must take into account the interaction between ethnic background and gender, as well as social class, when evaluating the impact of social change on the health of women.

Men's health is seen as an increasingly important topic. As noted earlier, men are more at risk from certain diseases and conditions than women. Male-specific cancers, such as prostate and testicular cancer are now recognised as major threats to men's health. This has raised questions about 'male disadvantage' in health (Cameron and Bernades, 1998). Indeed, studies have challenged conventional wisdom that men report lower levels of illness. According to the 2000 GHS, within each age group, men are no longer less likely than women to report long-standing illness (Walker et al., 2001). Studies of specific illnesses have found that, apart from psychiatric distress, the 'female excess' of illness is far less apparent and in some cases reversed (MacIntyre, Hunt and Sweeting, 1996). Even in mental health, the belief that women are necessarily more vulnerable to problems has been challenged (Payne, 1996; Hayes and Prior, 2003, ch. 7). The conventional wisdom that, irrespective of morbidity, women are more ready to use health services than men has also come under attack (Hunt et al., 1999; Hayes and Prior, 2003). Moreover, 'masculinity' and in particular men's risk-taking behaviour has also been identified as a key factor in their health and well-being (Sabo and Gordon, 1993). Rather than seeing gender issues in health as being concerned with the neglect of women's health needs, informed observers have recognised that the distinctive needs of both sexes must be taken into account in medical research, service delivery and also in wider social policies (Doyal, 2001; Hayes and Prior, 2003).

Conclusion

Having examined the key health trends, and the factors which lie behind them, one is struck by the magnitude and complexity of the demands placed on health policy-makers and the health care system – even in a comparatively healthy country such as Britain. Another insight resulting from this overview is that many of the factors which affect health lie outside the direct control of health policy-makers, managers and professionals. Indeed, the provision of services is but one of several factors that shape the health of the nation. Finally, the analysis of variations between different social and economic groups in society not only underlines this point, but highlights the scale of the task facing those who wish to improve overall levels of health. For unless these variations and the factors which underpin them are fully addressed, overall improvements in standards of health will become increasingly elusive.

_____ *Further Reading* _____

Bowling, A. (1997) (2nd edn) *Measuring Health – A Review of Quality of Life Measurement Scales* (Buckingham, Open University Press).

Culley, L. and Dyson, S. (eds) (2001) *Ethnicity and Nursing Practice* (Basingstoke, Palgrave).

Doyal, L. (ed.) (1998) *Women and Health Services: An Agenda for Change* (Buckingham, Open University Press).

Graham, H. (ed.) (2000) *Understanding Health Inequalities* (Buckingham, Open University Press).

Nazroo, J. (2002) *Ethnicity, Class and Health* (London, Policy Studies Institute).

Unicef (2002) *We the Children: Meeting the Promises of the World Summit for Children* (Geneva, Unicef).

Wanless, D. (2001) *Securing Our Future Health: Taking a Long Term View – Interim Report* (London, HM Treasury).

Wanless, D. (2003) *Securing Good Health for the Whole Population: Population Health Trends* (London, HM Treasury).

WHO (1999) *The World Health Report: Making a Difference* (Geneva, WHO).

Wilkinson, R. (1996) *Unhealthy Societies – The Affliction of Inequality* (London, Routledge).

Medicine and the Medical Profession

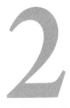

This chapter explores the concept of 'medical hegemony' a domination of health care by medical concepts, expertise and practices. It begins with a discussion of orthodox medicine, followed by an examination of alternative expertise in health care. The medical profession and the roots of its power are then explored in the context of recent challenges to medical hegemony.

Medicine

Medicine is a combination of art and science. It is an art because its practice involves a wide range of skills and judgements. Medicine is also strongly underpinned by scientific methods, principles and disciplines, and it is heavily based on the biomedical model or biomedicine (Engel, 1977). Biomedicine is based on a belief that the foundation for medical practice is scientific experiment, observation and discovery. From this perspective, medicine is the accumulation of a body of scientific knowledge and its subsequent application to the diagnosis and treatment of disease.

The Development of Biomedicine

Important discoveries during the seventeenth and eighteenth centuries laid the foundation for the development of biomedicine. These included the circulation of the blood, the functions of organs, and the impact of external agents on the body. Scientific experimentation gradually became accepted during the nineteenth century as the legitimate source of medical knowledge. Experiments became more sophisticated and important discoveries were made about disease processes. In particular, there were great advances in the understanding of the bacterial causes of disease. Experiments by scientists, such as Louis Pasteur and Robert Koch, led to the identification of the infectious agents which caused major diseases such as cholera and tuberculosis. Medicine increasingly focused on germ theory – the idea that diseases were largely caused by specific infectious agents in the environment.

Medical knowledge of the body's structure and composition also improved during this period. Advances in microscope technology enabled the study of cell biology, facilitating the work of Rudolf Virchow on cellular pathology, the study of cell changes associated with disease. Medical advances arose from a better understanding of body chemistry. The chemical processes that regulated a wide range of the body's activities were revealed, and diseases were attributed to deficiencies in these processes. Particularly important was the identification of the crucial role of hormones and vitamins in the maintenance of health.

Advances in medical knowledge led ultimately to new techniques and interventions, though the path was not always straightforward. Diagnosis benefited from the development of instruments to measure blood pressure, blood flow and heartbeat. Surgery improved with antiseptics, pioneered by Joseph Lister. The emergence of effective anaesthetics not only made surgery more bearable for patients, but gave surgeons extra time to perform operations, facilitating the development of more complex surgical techniques. Furthermore, the increasing institutionalisation of health care in hospitals provided doctors with an environment for observing disease processes and applying new medical technologies.

Meanwhile, the growing knowledge of bacterial causes of disease led to the development of vaccines to prevent these diseases, and so-called 'magic bullets' to cure them. An example of the latter was the discovery of Salvarsan, a treatment for syphilis, by Paul Ehrlich in 1910. This was followed by the development of antibiotics, beginning with the discovery of penicillin by Alexander Fleming in 1928 and its subsequent trial in humans in 1941. The early part of the century also saw attempts to treat diseases caused by hormone deficiencies, such as diabetes, and those caused by vitamin deficiencies, such as rickets.

The postwar period of the twentieth century was a productive time for medical discovery and innovation, with many important therapies being developed, including cortisone (steroids) used to combat a variety of diseases such as arthritis, asthma, eye, skin, liver, kidney and blood disorders, diseases of the digestive system (such as ulcerative colitis), some cancers, and thyroid disorders. As Le Fanu (1999) has noted, this was one of a number of definitive moments in modern medicine, which gave doctors tremendous advantages in treating disease (see Exhibit 2.1). As the twentieth century unfolded, new medical interventions were increasingly based on scientific knowledge and methods. In exploring disease processes, medicine increasingly focused upon specific aetiology, the attribution of disease to specific biological causes and processes. The aim was to reveal the disease process through scientific studies, then to discover how this could be prevented, limited or reversed. Experimentation aimed to isolate the potential causes of disease and reveal possible cures (such as Banting and Best's experiments on dogs that identified the role of insulin in diabetes mellitus). Importantly, this led to the adoption of more sophisticated methods of data collection and statistical analysis to identify relationships between possible causes and symptoms. This

---

Exhibit 2.1 Twelve Definitive Moments of Modern Medicine

1941	Penicillin
1949	Cortisone (steroids)
1950	{ Smoking identified as the cause of lung cancer
	{ Tuberculosis cured with streptomycin and Para-aminosalycylic acid
1952	Copenhagen polio epidemic and the birth of intensive care
1952	Chloropromazine in the treatment of schizophrenia
1955	Open-heart surgery
1961	Charnley's hip replacement
1963	Kidney transplantation
1964	Prevention of strokes
1971	Cure for childhood cancer
1978	First test-tube baby
1984	Helicobacter Pylori as the cause of peptic ulcer

Source: J. Le Fanu (1999) *The Rise and Fall of Modern Medicine*, p. xvii.

---

culminated in the development of the randomised controlled trial (RCT) which was seen as the ultimate test of scientific validity for clinical interventions.

The Features of Biomedicine

Biomedicine concentrates mainly on biological changes which can be defined, measured and isolated. It is directed towards the dysfunction of the organs and tissues of the body rather than the condition of the patient as a whole. Indeed, biomedicine can be regarded as adopting a negative perspective on health (see Chapter 1) because it views health more in terms of the absence of disease than the possession of healthy attributes. Finally, it emphasises the value of advancing technology, both in the diagnosis and treatment of disease. This approach undoubtedly added to both knowledge and understanding of many diseases. It produced improvements in the treatment of patients, which led to gains both in the length and the quality of life. Yet, in spite of these achievements, biomedicine became subjected to considerable criticism. Some argued that it was inappropriate to modern, complex health problems (Inglis, 1981), while others cast doubt on the extent to which the rational scientific principles were actually employed in medical practice (Payer, 1989).

Is Medicine Scientific?

The history of medicine contains many examples where rational scientific principles have been disregarded. One can find cases where good evidence has been contested or simply ignored by other practitioners. Take, for example, the fate of Semmelweiss, a nineteenth-century Viennese obstetrician, who observed that mortality rates from puerperal sepsis (a serious infection affecting mothers following childbirth) was much higher in wards attended by medical students than those where only midwives attended. Guessing that this was due to the cross-contamination of medical students at postmortems (which midwives did not attend), he ordered students to disinfect themselves thoroughly between attending cases. The death-rate dropped dramatically. Yet Semmelweiss's study was received with hostility by the leading lights of the profession, who questioned the validity of his study and scorned his life-saving recommendations (Inglis, 1965). Such a shocking example may be seen as interesting merely for its historical value. But one should not be complacent. One can find examples in the modern context where practice is being conducted either in the absence of scientific knowledge or at variance with it (see Chapter 9). Indeed, Marinker (1994, p. 3), himself a doctor, has written of 'the profound uncertainties and ambiguities in medicine masquerading as facts'.

The biomedical model can be seen as an abstraction which has limited application in practice (Black, 1984). Modern medicine is far more eclectic, taking into account wider influences on health such as lifestyle and emotional factors (Brewin, 1985). According to Tudor-Hart (1981), doctors are increasingly concerned about health promotion, the environment and public health, and as a result are more likely to intervene at a social and political level in order to promote health in a broader and more positive sense. However, other doctors are critical about social models of health, seeing them as a distraction from the real task of improving care and treatment for patients (Le Fanu, 1999; Fitzpatrick, 2001).

Certainly, the biomedical model does not describe the approach of every medical practitioner in all situations. It applies perhaps less to general practitioners and community-based doctors than to their hospital colleagues. Moreover, the biomedical model cannot be entirely insulated from the culture in which it is being applied. Doctors are influenced by non-medical models of health (Gaines, 1979). Both medical and lay models are shaped to some extent by the culture in which they operate (Helman, 1990; Herzlich and Pierret, 1985).

The extent to which the identification of disease is influenced by culture was explored in a comparative study of medicine and health in West Germany, France, Britain and the USA (Payer, 1989). The study found that the choice of diagnoses and treatments was not a scientific process, for two main reasons. First, most consultations were about health problems – such as fatigue or anxiety, for example – for which there are no scientific solutions. Secondly, cultural factors, which vary from nation to nation, had a great impact on the treatment of disease and upon the diagnosis of illness. Hence blood pressure considered high in the USA was likely to be seen as normal in the UK. While low blood pressure, considered to be a problem by German doctors, was not so regarded by their British and American counterparts.

Subjectivity

Medicine may not be as scientific as doctors claim. It has been pointed out that doctors do not agree about the meaning of the term 'disease' (Campbell, Scadding and Roberts, 1979). As Smith (2002) has noted, the concept of non-disease is therefore equally slippery, and raises questions about whether particular conditions, such as baldness, big ears and cellulite, are actually diseases. Confusion within the medical profession surrounding the concept of disease, and variations in its application, means that medicine is far more subjective than is commonly supposed.

Diseases are essentially deviations from normality. Yet, except in extreme cases, deviations from normality are inherently ambiguous (Twaddle, 1974), and require interpretation, which is in turn influenced by cultural and social factors. Kennedy (1981) claimed that doctors make two sets of judgements when diagnosing patients. Firstly, they must assess whether the patient's problem or condition represents a deviation from what would be considered normal. Secondly, they have to make a value judgement about the deviation itself, and whether this constitutes a disease.

Obesity, for example, is seen as a major health problem and is linked to a range of serious medical conditions (see Chapter 1). It is defined objectively – in terms of a Body Mass Index. Yet the extent to which an individual's body weight is judged to deviate excessively from the norm cannot be divorced from cultural values and expectations. Dutch doctors, for example, were found to be more likely to diagnose obesity than their British counterparts (Payer, 1989). This is not to deny the link between obesity and chronic illness, rather that its status as a medical condition is strongly influenced by social and cultural values and this may also apply to other conditions with an overt social dimension.

Difficulties in Applying the Biomedical Model

Biomedicine is challenged by conditions that are difficult or impossible to diagnose. Signs and symptoms may be highly ambiguous. Furthermore, many illnesses do not have objective symptoms or signs and this can lead to disputes about whether disease is present at all. Such controversy has surrounded myalgic encephalomyelitis (ME), an illness with influenza-like symptoms followed by chronic physical and mental fatigue. ME sufferers are in no doubt that they are ill, but doctors have been reluctant to accept their condition as a genuine illness, largely because there is no objective test for the condition (see Exhibit 2.2). Additional problems arise where diseases have multiple causes. Here the existence of the disease may not be in doubt, but its causes may be disputed. Many cancers, for example, result from the interaction of several factors relating to the individual and the environment. This creates scope for interpretations and subjectivity, which can only partly be addressed by scientific analysis. Modern medicine, however, remains strongly wedded to the guiding principles of the biomedical model. This is confirmed by the re-emphasis on evidence-based medicine (see Chapter 9). It is also reflected in the failure of alternative models to displace this orthodoxy.

Exhibit 2.2 Myalgic Encephalomyelitis and Chronic Fatigue Syndrome

ME is a syndrome which involves chronic physical and mental fatigue. Other symptoms include vertigo, ringing in the ears, blurred vision, muscle spasms, memory impairment, excessive sweating and an inability to concentrate. The commonest age at which the disease begins is early twenties to mid-forties. The illness can be long term, with a significant minority suffering permanent disability.

Those suffering from ME have difficulty in obtaining the social support and understanding which the sick normally expect. They also claim that many doctors cannot offer much help in the way of advice, care or treatment, with some being less than sympathetic to sufferers, believing they are simply neurotic. The medical profession has been reluctant to acknowledge ME as a genuine illness, opinion being strongly influenced by a study of an outbreak at the Royal Free Hospital in 1955 which identified the incident as a form of mass hysteria. One of the main difficulties in obtaining recognition for ME is that there is no clear test to confirm diagnosis, although some research has identified the presence of a virus in a minority of sufferers.

However, a combination of media coverage, pressure from patients and, increasingly, pressure from some doctors (some of whom have suffered from the illness) prompted a more considered response from the medical profession. In 1996 a working party from the Royal Colleges of General Practitioners, Physicians and Psychiatrists examined the evidence regarding ME. It concluded that chronic fatigue syndrome (CFS), deemed a more appropriate term for the symptoms of ME, deserved to be taken seriously. The working party noted that although psychological and social factors were present in many cases, the illness should not be regarded as a psychiatric illness (Mulube, 1996). Government also began to take a more sympathetic line. In 2002, the Chief Medical Officer for England endorsed the view of an independent working group that CFS/ME is a chronic illness and that health and social care professionals should recognise it as such (DoH, 2001a).

Other Medical Models: Public Health Medicine

Public health has been defined as 'the science and art of preventing disease, prolonging life, and promoting health through the organised efforts of society' (Cm 289, 1988). McKeown's work (1979), the definitive statement of the revitalised public health perspective, argued that modern medicine focuses primarily upon the disease process within the individual and ignores the wider social, economic and environmental factors relevant to health.

Much of McKeown's argument was based on historical evidence that challenges the conventional view of the contribution of modern medicine. Diseases such as measles, whooping cough and tuberculosis were in decline before the introduction of immunisation and effective medical treatment. McKeown identified better nutrition and rising standards of living as the key factors in the reduction of morbidity and mortality, rather than medical intervention. Improvements in health have also been attributed to better hygiene during the Victorian era (Wohl, 1984). McKeown pointed out that the major causes of ill health and death – cancer, heart disease and circulatory disease – were largely due to individual behaviour and the environment. Orthodox medicine was viewed as providing an inappropriate response to these problems because it was reactive, waiting for illness to happen, and required conclusive evidence of a specific disease process. Modern health problems – as suggested earlier – frequently involve a complex combination of factors, and action is often needed to protect and promote health when evidence is less than complete (McKeown, 1979).

While many of McKeown's conclusions have been supported by others (Bynum, 1994; Fuchs, 1974; McKinlay, 1979; Powles, 1973), some have challenged aspects of his thesis. Szreter (1988) accepted that modern medicine cannot be credited with the decline in mortality over the past century, but disputed that rising nutritional and living standards were the main reasons for falling mortality rates. He argued that the medical profession played a key role in improvement of health through its involvement in the Victorian public health movement, and by promoting local preventive measures, including the establishment of community health services. Sagan (1987), while sharing McKeown's cynicism about the impact of medical care, rejected the argument that public health measures or nutrition were primarily responsible for declining mortality. Sagan identified the reduction in family size and modern parenting behaviour as the main reasons for the improvements in health and identified the social-support function of the family unit as being particularly significant in the maintenance of mental and physical health. Finally, McKeown's thesis was attacked for not appreciating fully the contribution of modern medicine. The Victorian period brought important innovations, such as chloroform anaesthesia and antiseptics, but more importantly it laid the foundations for later discoveries and made possible the development of new forms of treatment which were effective. Le Fanu (1999, p. 320) pointed out flaws in McKeown's arguments. For example, the falling rate of TB deaths (which, as McKeown correctly observed, preceded important medical interventions such as streptomycin) was likely to have been influenced by the practice of treating patients in sanatoria. Although treatment was limited, sufferers were placed in an isolated environment, reducing opportunities for spreading infection.

In addition, many of the subsequent improvements in medical treatment not only saved lives but improved the quality of life for many. Improvements in quality of life do not always show up in mortality and morbidity indicators. Hip replacements are a commonly cited example (Morris, 1980). Furthermore, as shown in the previous chapter, medical care does add significantly to life expectancy.

In the nineteenth century the public health model provided a rationale for such interventions as sanitary improvements, housing reforms and vaccination.

For most of the twentieth century it was very much a junior partner to the biomedical model. In the last three decades, however, there has been a revival of interest in public health and the impact of environment and lifestyle on health. These led to the introduction of health strategies directed at tackling some of the main causes of illness and death in the UK and in many other countries (see Chapter 13).

Alternative Medicine

The main forms of alternative medicine are shown in Exhibit 2.3 (see Micozzi, 1995; Saks, 2003; Sharma, 1995; Kelner et al., 2000; House of Lords, 2000). The distinguishing feature of alternative therapies is their marginal standing in relation to the medical establishment and the health care system, rather than any common approach. Some therapies have similar features to biomedical approaches. Osteopathy and chiropractic, for example, are aimed at correcting the body's mechanical functions, just as (by different methods and using different theories) the biomedical approach has tended to emphasise physical dysfunction. Homoeopathy uses drugs aimed at specific disorders, though it takes a different view of the causal processes at work, while many plants used in herbalism have been exploited by orthodox medicine.

Most alternative therapies are interventionist – they involve treatment for specific disorders. They are often focused on the individual, though some take into account relevant environmental factors in a more systematic and comprehensive way. Alternative therapies are not necessarily in competition with conventional medicine. Patients using them do not necessarily lose confidence in orthodox medicine. Moreover, some doctors also practise alternative therapies. Even those who do not practise alternative therapies acknowledge their contribution and, as will become clear in a moment, there has been growing support in recent years for a more integrated approach.

Exhibit 2.3 Alternative and Complementary Medicine

Acupuncture

This practice, developed in ancient China, is based on the theory that there is a connection between body organs and body surface. Acupuncture involves using needles to stimulate acupuncture points under the skin in an attempt to influence the related organs. It is claimed that acupuncture has a more general effect in promoting relaxation and relieving pain.

Homoeopathy

This is a system of medicine based on the principle that agents which produce certain signs and symptoms in healthy people cure the same signs and symptoms of disease. The more

→

Exhibit 2.3 continued

→

a drug is diluted, the more potent it will be as a cure. Furthermore, the treatment given will be tailored to the individual, rather than to the characteristics of the disease as is generally the case in mainstream biomedicine.

Chiropractic

This is a manipulative therapy designed to maintain the spinal column in a good state of health without the use of drugs. The therapy is aimed at dealing with specific disorders such as back and neck pain, headaches and other disorders of the nervous system.

Osteopathy

This is similar to chiropractic in that it involves the manipulation of the spine in order to remedy disease and dysfunction of the musculo-skeletal system. However, osteopaths' manipulative techniques are based on different theories of the causes of illness from those adopted by chiropractors.

Herbal Medicine

This is the use of plants and herbs to deal with specific illnesses and to maintain health. A related therapy – aromatherapy – involves body massage using oils extracted from plants.

Hypnotherapy

The inducement of trance has been used to combat a variety of psychological disorders such as anxiety, phobias and insomnia. Hypnotherapy is sometimes used by individuals who are trying to change unhealthy lifestyles such as smoking. Hypnotherapy has also been used in the treatment of conditions with physical symptoms where there may be an underlying psychological cause.

Reflexology

This therapy is based on a belief that different areas of the feet are internally linked to other parts of the body. Manifestations of illness are treated by massaging the relevant area of the foot which corresponds to the parts of the body affected.

Aromatherapy

This therapy uses oils extracted from aromatic plants to enhance health. These essential oils are believed to have subtle positive effects on the mind and emotions, as well as on physical ailments. The therapy is aimed at the whole person, and involves the application of oils by massage, bathing, compresses and inhalation.

Nonetheless, alternative therapies have in the past been viewed with considerably hostility by the orthodox medical establishment (see Saks, 1995). For example, a British Medical Association (BMA) working-party report of the 1980s strongly criticised the lack of a rational scientific base for many of the alternative therapies and firmly rejected the theories which underpinned them (BMA, 1986). The BMA position has since shifted. In 1993 it produced a further report which was far more positive about the role of alternative medicine while continuing to stress the importance of evaluation and the need for statutory regulation of alternative practitioners (BMA, 1993).

Alternative therapies have already begun to move in this direction. Some therapists now operate under the auspices of a national regulatory body, licensed by the State. The General Osteopathic Council (GOC), created by legislation in 1993, regulates professional standards, ethics, discipline and qualifications for these practitioners. The GOC also maintains a register of practitioners and from 2000 only those included on the register will be legally permitted to call themselves osteopaths. Chiropractors have since followed osteopaths in securing statutory regulation. Meanwhile, other therapies have systems of voluntary regulation of varying degrees of formality. To respond to criticism about efficacy, alternative therapies are increasingly seeking ways of demonstrating this. For example, one study found a greater improvement among patients with low back pain who were treated by chiropractors compared with those receiving conventional out-patient management in hospital (Meade et al., 1995). However, studies of the impact of alternative therapies are often challenged because – often for practical reasons – they do not adopt the randomised controlled trial (RCT) method of evaluation favoured by conventional medical researchers (see Chapter 3).

Alternative therapies continue to flourish. Surveys reveal a high level of public interest in alternative therapies. A House of Lords enquiry (2000, p. 12, p. 24) into alternative therapies reported that 20 per cent of the population had used these therapies in the previous 12 months and that satisfaction levels were generally high. The most popular therapies were herbal remedies (which has been used by 34 per cent) and aromatherapy (21 per cent) followed by homeopathy and acupuncture (17 per cent and 14 per cent respectively).

In the UK alternative medicine was boosted by the changes in the way NHS services were funded. Under GP fundholding (see Chapter 10) there was an incentive to refer patients to alternative therapists because of their relatively low cost and increasing popularity. In the mid-1990s around 45 per cent of GPs commissioned or provided alternative therapies (Thomas, Nicholl and Coleman, 1995). In addition, over two-thirds of health authorities commissioned these therapies (Adams, J., 1995). Surveys have indicated that patients would like to see alternative therapies available on the NHS, though in practice there are significant barriers to availability (see Low, 2001). The popularity of alternative medicine and its growing use alongside orthodox treatment have produced pressures to establish closer links with alternative medicine. Indeed, many now believe alternative medicine is a misleading term, preferring instead 'complementary and alternative medicine' (CAM). There does seems to be a growing accommodation between orthodox medicine and CAM, which some have identified as evidence of a new medical pluralism (Cant and Sharma, 1999). However, as these authors argue, though there is evidence of a change of attitudes, it is important not to exaggerate the degree to which these therapies have been incorporated into the medical mainstream. Some therapies are more acceptable to orthodox practitioners than others, notably those that are amenable to scientific methods of evaluation. Even where CAM is accepted, it is generally on the terms set by orthodox medicine. As Cant and Sharma put it, 'the persuasiveness of the biomedical model in judging other providers remains relatively intact' (1999, p. 186).

Lay Models of Health and Illness

Lay views of health are notoriously complex and have a certain independence (Fitzpatrick, 1984; Williams and Calnan, 1996; Calnan, 1987; Helman, 1990). Moreover, while orthodox medicine has supremacy in the realm of formal health care, lay health beliefs, knowledge and behaviour have an enormous impact on health care in practice, particularly as only a minority of symptoms ever come to the attention of doctors and other health care professionals (Scambler, Scambler and Craig, 1981).

Health beliefs may influence the decision to seek treatment. If individuals do not perceive themselves to be ill, their symptoms are unlikely to be presented to doctors. As a result, their illness will probably remain hidden and the condition will not come to the attention of the doctor (Mechanic, 1961; Robinson, 1971). Even if the individual sees a doctor and is diagnosed as having a particular disease, this does not guarantee that the patient will agree with the diagnosis. Neither does it ensure that he or she will comply with the prescribed course of treatment (Ley, 1982; Thompson, 1984).

The medical profession can circumvent this by surveillance methods, such as screening programmes, which can be used to detect the early signs of disease. Another strategy is compulsory treatment, which has been used in the treatment of mental illness. Lay perspectives, though influenced by medical perspectives, are shaped by deeper cultural and ideological influences within society (see Calnan, 1987). In recent years calls to place the patient at the centre of health care have added weight to the legitimacy of the 'lay perspective' (Coulter, 2002; Williamson, 2000). This has been evident in growing acknowledgement of the importance of partnership and self-management in care, particularly with regard to chronic illness where the patient has been recognised as an expert in his or her own right (see Exhibit 12.2).

The Medical Profession

Medicine as a Profession

There is much disagreement between sociologists over the term 'profession' (see Johnson, 1972; Wilding, 1982). However, most would agree that medicine has the key features commonly associated with a profession, primarily the application of a body of expertise, knowledge and skills. It operates within a framework of licensing, where only those sufficiently qualified can practise legitimately following a considerable period of approved education and training (see Exhibit 2.4). There is a long-standing system of self-regulation in medicine, though this system has been under pressure in recent years. Furthermore, as with other professions, those who practise medicine tend to be drawn from upper-middle-class backgrounds. Finally, medicine has been organised by a range of self-governing institutions which take responsibility for education, licensing, the maintenance of standards and the representation of interests.

Exhibit 2.4 Medical Education and Training

Undergraduate medical education is provided by the university medical schools. Currently, having successfully completed the course, students obtain provisional registration from the General Medical Council (GMC) for their pre-registration year working as a house officer in a hospital setting, leading to full registration. Specialisation then takes place as doctors choose which branch of the profession they will follow: hospital medicine or general practice (some may later choose to specialise in public health medicine). Trainee GPs undertake a three-year course which includes working in hospitals and attachment to a training practice. Doctors specialising in hospital or public health medicine proceed through a succession of training posts with a view to securing the post of consultant. However, this system is to change. Government has proposed a foundation programme for trainee doctors and is exploring ways of reducing the length of specialist training.

Several bodies have a role in setting and monitoring standards in this field, including the GMC, the Royal Colleges, and the Quality Assurance Agency for Higher Education (which regulates universities and colleges of higher education). Despite this regulatory framework, concern about the quality of medical education has continued (see Goodfellow and Claydon, 2001) and the core curriculum for medical students is currently being revised. With regard to postgraduate medical training, a new body, the Postgraduate Medical Education and Training Board, has been established to set, maintain and monitor standards.

Postgraduate medical training had already been changed following the Calman report (DoH, 1993), prompted by the European Union's criticism of specialist medical registration in the UK. The Calman report proposed a reduction in the length and an increase in the intensity of the postgraduate training period from an average of twelve years to seven. It also recommended the creation of a unified training grade for higher specialist training, the Specialist Registrar Grade. Calman also called for a new Certificate of Completion of Specialist Training (CCST), defining the end-point of specialist training and making the holder eligible for a consultant appointment. Meanwhile, a 'New Deal' for junior doctors was agreed which set targets for reducing their hours of work. The New Deal limited junior doctors' hours to 83 a week by April 1993, and 72 by the end of 1994 (no more than 56 of which should be spent actually working). A further review of the New Deal in 1998 sought to clarify working arrangements (with regard to rest periods, for example) and put in place new monitoring arrangements. However, in reality many junior doctors continued to work longer than these limits, with over a third claiming to exceed the 56-hour week (Hall, 1999). From April 2003 trusts that fail to comply with the New Deal could be sued for breach of contract. Furthermore, a new European Directive will reduce junior-doctor hours to 58 per week from 2004, 56 hours

→

Exhibit 2.4 continued

$\longrightarrow$

by 2007 and 48 hours by 2009. New provisions for rest time due to be implemented from 2004 will, in effect, reduce time spent on call. Despite the expansion in medical training places and the proposed shorter training period for some new consultants, these pressures are likely to prompt significant changes in working practices within the NHS.

Important changes have taken place in the organisation of clinical education and training. Workforce Development Confederations (WDCs), which consist of employers and other stakeholders (health authorities, NHS trusts, primary care trusts, higher education institutions, medical schools, postgraduate deans, local authorities) are responsible for identifying training and education needs across the entire workforce. They are expected to work with all the professional groups to ensure adequate numbers of trained staff. They work with postgraduate deans on the management and delivery of postgraduate medical and dental education. They also commission training from trusts.

Efforts have been made to strengthen continuing professional development (CPD). This is closely connected with a number of agendas: revalidation – which means that doctors have to prove that they have the necessary knowledge and skills to continue to work effectively; lifelong learning – that all staff including doctors are willing to continue their learning experience throughout their careers; and leadership training, which requires clinical staff to learn new skills that enhance their effectiveness as professionals (see DoH, 2000a, 2000b). It is also relevant to plans to improve the quality of care (see Chapter 9). The GMC and the Royal Colleges have a major interest in CPD, largely because of revalidation, as do the Workforce Development Confederations, which draw up local investment plans across the range of professional groups. Furthermore, the new NHS University is expected to play a major role in developing postgraduate and continuing education and training (DoH, 2001b). It may address some of the concerns about the haphazard nature of CPD and doubts about its cost-effectiveness (Brown et al., 2002). It is expected that in future CPD delivered across professions will become much more common. At the same time there are efforts to promote integrated curricula for professionals at pre-registration stage, to enable them to share learning experiences. This approach is seen as a more efficient way of delivering education and training, and as a way of breaking down professional barriers in the delivery of care.

According to Freidson (1988, p. xv), 'it is useful to think of a profession as an occupation which has assumed a dominant position in a division of labour so that it gains control over the determination of the substance of its own work'. Over the years the medical profession successfully monopolised important areas of work and was able to insulate itself from external interference. Within health care, medical knowledge has been the dominant form of expertise with doctors enjoying superior status relative to other professional groups. The medical profession has adopted two approaches: exclusion and incorporation (see Seale, Pattison and Davey, 2001). The way in which alternative therapists have successfully been excluded in the past by the orthodox medical profession has already been noted. Now, with regard to some alternative therapies, the medical profession has tried to accommodate and incorporate them. The incorporation strategy has already been employed with regard to most other health care professions, which act for the most part under medical direction and instruction.

The common characteristic of these professions is their limited autonomy and weak political organisation and leverage. Nurses, for example, have much less control over health care than doctors (Salvage, 1985). Much of their workload is routine and, according to nurses themselves, their contribution to the care of patients is not maximised (see Exhibit 2.5). Politically, nurses have been less well-organised than the medical profession (Hayward and Fee, 1992; Hart, 2004). Tension between the medical and nursing professions, which occurs within the everyday working environment (Walby and Greenwell, 1994), has tended to be implicit rather than overt. Where there has been open conflict between the nursing profession on the one hand and the medical profession on the other, the latter has invariably dominated. An often-cited example is the struggle between doctors and midwives over childbirth and maternity care (Donnison, 1988).

According to Armstrong (1990), the status of nursing and other health professions improved during the twentieth century, through registration, education, self-discipline and licensing. Although these groups achieved professional recognition, the core of medical power was not eroded, due in no small measure to the ability of the medical profession to shape the development of other health professions (Larkin, 1983). The rising status of nursing and other health professions, reflected in improvements in education, training and research, facilitated the transfer of routine medical tasks, but did not undermine the doctor's dominant position within the division of labour in health care.

Exhibit 2.5 Nursing: Power and Professional Status

The history of nursing in Britain has often been presented as one of 'thwarted aspiration' (Nottingham and O'Neill, 2000). The conventional view is that the nursing profession developed under an umbrella of medical protection (Salter, 1998) but at a price: the 'handmaiden' role of nurses became enshrined both in practice and within managerial and political processes. The subservient role of nursing was also bound up with gender relations, not simply because most nurses were women and most doctors male, but because nursing itself was constructed as an extension of (women's) domestic labour and the caring role within the family (Gamarnikow, 1978; Davies, 1995). Until relatively recently, medical hegemony appeared self-evident both in everyday practice, with regard to health service management, and at the policy level (Keen and Malby, 1992). However, over the last two decades nurses have sought to strengthen their claims for professional status and extend their role within health care (see also Chapter 9).

According to Witz (1992), the nursing profession adopted a dual-closure strategy comprising of *exclusion* – the denial of professional status to those not meeting certain criteria – and *usurpation* – extending their remit to include work currently undertaken by doctors. The former strategy emphasised a scientific approach to nursing knowledge, focusing upon research, evidence-based practice, and high-quality professional education and training, with a stronger academic element. This was embodied in education and training reforms known as 'Project 2000', where apprentice-style training for nurses was replaced by pre-registration courses based in higher education institutions (HEIs). Trainee nurses were regarded as students and, as such, less subject to the routine demands of the NHS. The new courses were taught at

→

Exhibit 2.5 continued

→

degree and diploma level, and operated under standards set by the nurses' professional bodies and higher education regulatory agencies. However, concern about the lack of clinical skills of newly qualified nurses prompted changes (see UKCC, 1999; DoH, 1999a). Attempts were made to increase and improve clinical placements. Clearer standards were also set, outlining the skills expected of trainees. Nurse cadet schemes were introduced to re-create an apprentice-style, non-academic route into nursing. Furthermore, changes in the commissioning of education and training (see Exhibit 2.4) have tied HEIs more closely to the needs of the NHS as identified by employers.

There has been a greater emphasis on self-regulation and standard-setting by nursing bodies in recent years (DoH, 1999a). The former UK Central Council for Nursing, Midwifery and Health Visiting (UKCC), which maintained a register of qualified persons and handled complaints, drew up a code of professional practice and specific guidelines for professional practice (UKCC, 1992a, 1992b, 1996). It also introduced a requirement that those on the register must renew their registration every three years by demonstrating that they have undertaken Post-Registration Education and Practice – a form of continuing professional development. Subsequently the UKCC (and the National Nursing Boards, which were responsible for quality assurance in nursing and midwifery education) was replaced by the Nursing and Midwifery Council (NMC) in 2002. This body now has the remit for the regulation of nurses, midwives and health visitors, and maintains a register of qualified persons, sets standards for education and training (implemented by separate authorities in Scotland, Wales and Northern Ireland), practice and conduct. It also considers allegations of misconduct or unfitness to practice which, if upheld, can result in a range of sanctions.

Attempts have been made to clarify the nursing role and set explicit standards of care. *Essence of Care* (DoH, 2001c) set out the key elements of nursing care, along with benchmarks of best practice, in several areas: principles of self care, personal and oral hygiene, nutrition, continence and bladder/bowel care, pressure ulcers, safety of clients with mental health needs, record-keeping, communication, and privacy and dignity. Meanwhile the Chief Nursing Officer for England set out ten key roles for nurses: the ordering of diagnostic investigations; making and receiving referrals direct to other professions including therapists; admitting and discharging patients for specified conditions within agreed protocols; managing the patient case-load for some conditions; running certain clinics; prescribing medicines and treatments; carrying out resuscitation; performing minor surgery and outpatients procedures; triage; and taking the lead in how health services are organised and delivered.

This followed on from earlier attempts by the nursing profession to clarify their expertise. The so-called 'new nursing' represented an attempt to shift nursing from a task-based model to one based on patients' needs (Fatchett, 1998, p. 123). It located the key expertise of the nurse in the understanding of these highly specific needs. It also emphasised the importance of the nursing process, along with systematic evaluation of the impact of care. Elsewhere, nurses' claims to a specific expertise became embodied in models that gave nurses a key role in the management of care, such as Nursing Development Units, where nursing staff led the management of patient care (Pearson, Punton and Durant, 1992; Salvage and Wright, 1995; Malby, 1996).

Nurses increasingly undertake roles which in the past were done by doctors, especially junior doctors. Though driven primarily by a need to reduce juniors' workload rather than by the demands of nurses (Read and Graves, 1994), this created new opportunities, and nurses took on clinical roles in relation to assessment and treatment (Kendrick, Weir and Rosser, 1995). In some cases this led to the creation of new roles, such as nurse practitioners, who have a

→

Exhibit 2.5 continued

→

greater degree of autonomy and can examine patients, prescribe drugs, order tests and treat minor injuries. Studies of their role have shown that, compared with doctors, they provide an equivalent quality of care and greater levels of patient satisfaction (Horrocks, Anderson and Salisbury, 2002). Clinical nurse specialists possess specific expertise in relation to certain conditions or procedures, and some are permitted to undertake minor surgery. There are a range of other specialist nursing roles including clinical educators, practice-development nurses and research nurses. In the field of primary care, new services such as Walk-in Clinics and NHS Direct are staffed by nurses, and some of the pilot schemes in primary care are led by them (see Chapter 10). Nurses in the community now perform a wider range of tasks, have a key role in assessment and co-ordination of care and have prescribing powers, while practice nurses have taken on a greater role in relation to health promotion (Broadbent, 1998). Nurses are seen as key players in the improvement of quality of care. The modern matrons, announced in the NHS Plan, are responsible for improvements in the patient environment, and are charged with strengthening clinical leadership. More generally, leadership development and training has been actively encouraged by both government and the nursing professional bodies. Meanwhile, the new post of nurse consultant has been created to improve clinical leadership and develop expert nursing practice.

Critics argue that the nurses' professional project has been divisive, and has led to the creation of two types of nurse: a small elite which undertakes higher level tasks and leadership or managerial roles, and a larger, less-skilled workforce undertaking basic care. There are fears that this is moving nursing away from its 'core business', the provision of care, which could be devalued by being left in the hands of a less qualified and 'non-professional' workforce (Miers, 1999, p. 91). Moreover, as these staff take on roles formerly undertaken by qualified nurses, and do so in a way which lies outside their control, this could undermine the security of the nursing profession and further encourage replacement by task-based support workers, such as health care assistants (Health Services Management Unit, 1996). It is argued that, despite the claims of nurses for professional practice, in reality doctors still control their work (Salter, 1998). They are only permitted to occupy roles which doctors allow them to perform, and operate under protocols, through accreditation or under conditions controlled by the medical profession. Moreover, as long as doctors have overall accountability for patient care they will be reluctant to relinquish oversight. However, others have observed that there is a confusion of accountability (Doyal, Dowling and Cameron, 1998) and that those taking on of new roles may expose themselves to greater personal liability when things go wrong (Dowling et al., 1996). Indeed, nurses performing new roles may require additional indemnity insurance to protect themselves from ruinous litigation. Finally, from a feminist perspective it is argued that by seeking professional status through processes of exclusion and usurpation, nurses are in fact adopting a male-dominated definition of professionalism based on competition, control, detachment, scientific method and autonomy, rather than on a new professionalism based on feminine values of co-operation, caring, attachment and reflection (Traynor, 1999).

Doctors, Patients and the Public

Another aspect of medical hegemony is found in the doctor–patient relationship. Most observers have emphasised the power of the former (see Byrne and Long, 1976; Tuckett et al., 1985), though this relationship does vary according to the type of illness. In chronic illness there appear to be more opportunities for patients to participate in decision-making (Szasz and Hollender, 1956). Moreover, as already noted, lay views can influence practice and doctors cannot divorce themselves entirely from broader cultural influences.

Nevertheless, doctors have tended to dominate the relationship, especially in the UK where patients have traditionally been passive and deferential. This may be due to the long history of charitable health care, which placed most patients in a dependent position or to the class system, with (working-class) patients dutifully respecting their (upper-middle-class) practitioners. A further possibility is that the absence of a health care market in the UK in the post-Second-World-War period inhibited the kind of health care consumerism found in the United States. The passivity of the patient may also have been reinforced by the British 'stiff upper lip' and reluctance to complain. Compounding this was the paternalistic welfare state, which gave service users little information or choice.

Patients are now less passive. As already noted, there has been a greater emphasis on patient-centred care and partnership in the management of illness. Patients are more willing to complain and seek redress. They desire more information and increasingly use sources other than their doctor, such as the Internet. In addition, reforms have been introduced, aimed at strengthening public and patient involvement in health and improving complaints processes. These are discussed further in Chapter 12.

Finally, a series of major scandals in the NHS during the late 1990s – paediatric heart surgery at the Bristol Royal Infirmary, organ retention at Alder Hey hospital in Liverpool, and the case of Dr Harold Shipman – threatened public confidence in the profession (see Chapter 9). Nonetheless, the medical profession has continued to enjoy high social status. Public-opinion surveys point to a high degree of satisfaction with the work of doctors and high levels of trust in the profession. In March 2000, following Shipman's conviction, 87 per cent of the public stated that they would generally expect doctors to tell the truth (*British Medical Journal*, 2000). A year later this had risen to 89 per cent (*Health Service Journal*, 2001). Compared with other professions, medicine continues to enjoy a high level of public confidence and support.

Explaining Medical Hegemony

Four factors underpin the hegemony of the medical profession: its social status; its role in legitimising health and illness; the clinical autonomy of doctors, and the political organisation and leverage of the profession. These factors will now be examined in the context of changes which, some suggest, indicate important challenges to medical hegemony.

Social Composition

The social status of the medical profession can be attributed in part to the social background of its members. There are three common beliefs about the composition of the medical profession: firstly, that it is male-dominated; secondly, that most doctors come from 'medical families', where at least one parent has a medical background, and, thirdly, that it is largely restricted to those from upper-middle-class backgrounds.

Just under 40 per cent of doctors in England are female (DoH, 2002a), while women are in a minority in the higher clinical grades – just under a quarter of consultants are female. Women are particularly under-represented in the more prestigious specialities, such as surgery, where they constitute only one in twenty consultants. They are strongly represented in general practice (where over 30 per cent are women, a third of these working part-time), paediatrics, and accident and emergency medicine. Women have made greater inroads into hospital medicine, the proportion of female hospital doctors more than doubling over the past 20 years. Currently a third of hospital doctors are women. Furthermore, the proportion of women studying medicine has more than doubled over the same period. Over half of new medical students are now female.

Turning to the second point, it is not true to say that most doctors come from 'medical families', though a considerable proportion do. Allen (1994) discovered that 16 per cent had followed either one or both parents into the profession. The same study confirmed that doctors were drawn mainly from the upper middle classes. At the time of application to medical school, three-quarters had fathers whose occupation placed them in social classes I or II. This proportion has not varied significantly in recent years. Medicine is still to a large extent socially exclusive, though it is possible for people from working-class backgrounds to break into the profession. Indeed, the proportion of newly-qualified female doctors coming from skilled-manual-worker family backgrounds has increased in recent years. The Blair Government has explicitly tried to address the class differential in medicine. The creation of new places at medical schools was accompanied by efforts to make medicine more attractive to candidates from middle- and lower-income families, including new courses to support entrants from these backgrounds.

Legitimation of Health and Illness

Medical knowledge is regarded as an important source of power (Foucault, 1973; Turner, 1987). Doctors have the power to define and redefine the social meaning of various conditions and states. According to Parsons (1951), the function of medicine in legitimising illness is particularly important. Parsons regarded illness as a form of social deviance that could undermine the social system. It therefore had to be controlled, the instrument of control being the medical profession. Hence, doctors certify who is ill and who is not. The genuinely ill (as certified by the medical profession) are absolved of responsibility to fulfil social obligations, while those whose sickness is not legitimised are labelled as malingerers and subjected to social disapproval and sanction. In this way the extent of deviance is controlled through the 'sick role', and social order is preserved.

Parsons' analysis has been challenged on a number of grounds (see Turner, 1987). It has been argued that exemption from social obligations varies according to particular types of illness and with the social position of sufferers. Even when an illness is recognised by the medical profession as being genuine, sufferers may continue to be stigmatised if their condition is seen as a continuing threat to the social order (Goffman, 1968). Hence the consequences of social disapproval are not confined to malingerers. Indeed, individuals suffering from genuine illnesses may be deprived of privileges and rights. Mentally-ill people, for example, may be deprived of their liberty while individuals diagnosed as being HIV-positive may be discriminated against in the markets for jobs and housing. Moreover, the assumption that the sick role removes responsibility from the individual is in some circumstances incorrect. For example, drug addicts and alcoholics are often blamed for their particular illnesses.

In spite of these flaws, Parsons' focus on the function of medicine in legitimising illness provided at least a partial explanation of the role of the medical profession in modern societies. It also stimulated others to explore further and clarify this important role. Further work in this field sought to reach a deeper understanding of the role of the professions, including medicine. Johnson (1995), adopting a Foucauldian perspective (Foucault, 1979) and building on work by Starr and Immergut (1987), Larson (1977) and Abbott (1988), perceived the professions as socio-technical devices through which the means and ends of government are articulated. Hence in the realm of health care the medical profession can be seen as a resource of governing. In other words its expertise, technologies, practical activities and social authority can make modern, complex societies amenable to governing by, for example, overseeing established definitions of illness.

Clinical Autonomy and Self-Regulation

Clinical autonomy is seen as an important symbol of medical power and status, though it is more than this, giving doctors an advantage over both patients and other health professionals in clinical settings. Doctors are resistant to direction in clinical matters. As professionals they believe in their own judgement to guide diagnosis and treatment. Yet there is often disagreement on what constitutes a clinical decision. Williams (1988) has noted the difficulties in distinguishing between clinical and other factors such as the availability and use of resources. Doctors agree that clinical decisions cannot be taken in a vacuum, detached from personal, moral, ethical, legal and economic constraints (Hoffenberg, 1987). Johnson (1995) too points out that autonomy of technique is not determined solely by doctors themselves but is the product of a discourse involving doctors, officials and the public.

Doctors resent interference in matters concerning the admission and treatment of patients. Even peer review (the monitoring of medical work by the profession itself in an attempt to maintain and promote good practice) continues to be viewed with suspicion by some doctors and the prospect of supervision and direction being undertaken by people with a non-medical background is anathema to them. In addition to clinical autonomy, the medical profession treasures the power of self-regulation. In the UK the main body responsible for regulating the profession is the General Medical Council (GMC). It sets out standards of practice (GMC, 2001), maintains a register of doctors, regulates the fitness of doctors to practise, and investigates complaints about doctors from the public, the police, the NHS and other doctors. It also has an important role in relation to medical education (see Exhibit 2.4). The GMC, established by the 1858 Medical Act, has for most of its life been dominated by doctors and, in particular, the interests of the medical elite. Over the last few decades, however, the GMC has been forced to be more responsive both to the profession and to public opinion. This culminated in a number of reforms aimed at increasing lay involvement, strengthening the accountability of the GMC to the public, and improving the effectiveness of medical self-regulation within a broader statutory framework of health professional regulation (Salter, 1999; see also Chapter 9).

According to some, doctors suffered greater blows to their autonomy in recent years compared with other professions such as the legal profession (Brazier et al., 1993). Certainly, the fortunes of the medical profession compare adversely with predominantly private-sector professions in an era when the public sector has been under attack (Perkin, 1989), though doctors arguably suffered less than many other public-sector professions in this period (Deakin, 1991). There has also been an increasing use of NHS disciplinary procedures to remove and suspend doctors from their posts, which undermines the tradition of self-regulation. Managers have a greater say over appointments of hospital medical staff and extra pay given to consultants. Furthermore, employment contracts of hospital medical staff are now more specific and consultants have to agree 'job plans' with trust management and will be subjected to annual appraisal (see Chapter 9). Meanwhile, in general practice there has been an attempt to influence medical practioners' work through changes in contracts, incentive payments and the introduction of salaried GPs (see Chapter 10).

Doctors in the UK have been subjected to a barrage of reforms designed to make them more accountable and to provide more information about the quality and effectiveness of services they provide (Moore, 1995; Davies, 2000). These included management changes, such as the introduction of general management, and the creation of clinical directorates to manage medical activity (see Chapter 9). The work of doctors has come under greater scrutiny with the introduction of medical audit, clinical governance, clinical performance indicators, and new national bodies to scrutinise performance, such as the Commission for Health Improvement (CHI) and now the Commission for Healthcare Audit and Inspection (CHAI). Another development has been the creation of bodies to issue guidance on standards of treatment, such as the National Institute for

Clinical Excellence, and the National Service Frameworks. The introduction of commissioning and service agreements placed greater attention on the effectiveness of medical work by highlighting the relationship between resources and outcomes. Finally, the consumerist agenda has brought a series of reforms which doctors believe has challenged their autonomy and self-regulation. These include changes to complaints processes, such as the extension of the Health Ombudsman's powers to cover clinical complaints, as well as the specification of patient rights and standards of service they can expect.

Political Power, Politics and the State

As Salter (2000, p. 5) has observed, 'the power of the medical profession is based on its unique access to, and regulation of, a body of knowledge that is highly valued by both society and state'. The growing state involvement in health care during the twentieth century (see Chapter 4) placed great emphasis on an effective working relationship between the state and the medical profession (see Moran, 1999; Salter, 1999). The result was an implicit concordat or compact between the state and the profession under which, according to Salter (1998, p. 98), 'the medical profession gained money, status and the power to protect and regulate its privileges; the state gained a health care system to protect and regulate its populace'. This happened not only in the context of the NHS, but in other health care systems too (see Moran, 1999), although the exact nature of these arrangements varied considerably.

The compact has clear advantages for both sides. Government was absolved of day-to-day responsibility for managing professional activity and of blame for tough decisions about the allocation of care and treatment. The doctors retained professional status, economic security and considerable autonomy, while retaining supremacy in the division of labour in health care. Closer relations with the state also brought the institutions of medical representation into closer contact with government (Klein, 1990).

During the postwar period the medical profession maintained its preeminence largely through its political leverage (Moran and Wood, 1992; Moran, 1999) and the strength of its professional bodies and institutions. The role of the GMC in relation to education and regulation has already been discussed. The other principal medical organisations are the British Medical Association (BMA) and the Royal Colleges of Medicine (see Watkins, 1987).

The British Medical Association (BMA)

The BMA is the main representative organisation for British doctors. Over three-quarters of practising doctors are members, and it has a long-established reputation as an effective pressure group (Bartrip, 1996; Grey-Turner and Sutherland, 1982). The BMA lobbies on public health issues, such as smoking and road safety, but most of its activity is concerned with sectional issues such as doctors' pay and conditions of work. The craft committees, which operate under the auspices of the BMA, are recognised by the Department of Health as negotiating bodies acting on behalf of each branch of the profession: hospital consultants and specialists, junior doctors, doctors specialising in public and community health, general practitioners and academic medicine.

During the postwar period, the BMA was regarded as a powerful group, accepted by the government and possessing extensive political contacts. Over the years it has enjoyed the privilege of being consulted by government on a wide range of health policy matters. However, the BMA's relationship with the Conservative governments of the 1980s and 1990s was less than harmonious. The BMA openly opposed a range of government policies, such as the NHS internal market. Moreover, when introducing these policies the Conservative government often failed to consult the BMA to the same extent as in the past, especially during the Thatcher government's period of office (see Baggott and McGregor-Riley, 1999). Even when discussions took place, its advice was frequently ignored (see Lee-Potter, 1997; Timmins, 1995).

These developments must be seen in perspective. Hostility between government and the profession has broken out on a number of occasions in the postwar period. During a contractual dispute in 1965 general practitioners threatened mass resignation from the NHS. In the 1970s there was an enormous dispute between the government and the medical profession over the phasing-out of pay beds in the NHS. Klein and Day (1992) argue that the disputes of the 1980s were of a different order from those of the 1960s and 1970s. Yet they also point out that they are not unprecedented. Similar structural upheavals in health care took place in 1911 (the introduction of National Health Insurance) and again in 1945 (the creation of the NHS). In both cases, the government of the day confronted the profession and introduced structural change in spite of opposition. Klein and Day also note that the period following such reforms has tended to be more constructive, with the government working once again with the profession in an atmosphere of co-operation.

Under New Labour, relations between the BMA and government initially improved. However, amid continuing concerns about doctors' workload, the centralisation of health policy, and the scale of reform, criticism began to re-emerge. At one point Prime Minister Blair indicated that the BMA was one of the 'forces of conservatism' inhibiting public-service reform, which led to a rift between the association and the government. At the time of writing, the situation is more difficult to interpret. The government has responded to criticism by increasing NHS funding, but is insistent that all the professions including doctors must co-operate in the process of reform which accompanies this.

The Royal Colleges of Medicine

The responsibilities of the Royal Colleges (such as the Royal College of Physicians, the Royal College of Surgeons, and so on) include the accreditation and training of specialists (see Exhibit 2.4) and the promotion of good practice – they undertake audits and publish guidelines on best practice. They are also important politically: they are consulted by government on a wide range of health issues concerning the medical specialities and medicine in general. But they tend to operate in an informal way and usually operate with a much lower public profile than the BMA. Nonetheless, they are in regular contact with the Department of Health, putting forward their views on a range of issues, and are represented on important official committees.

The Royal Colleges have raised their public profile over the years. In the 1960s, for example, the Royal College of Physicians began to publicise the health dangers of tobacco and called for action to reduce smoking. Along with the Royal Colleges of Psychiatrists and General Practitioners, it has called for action on alcohol abuse. In the 1980s, three Royal College presidents became further involved in public controversy, this time over the funding of the NHS when they went public with their criticism of the Thatcher government's handling of the NHS. Audit and good-practice guidelines published by the Colleges have also attracted media attention and stimulated public debate – the Royal College of Psychiatrists' (1995) study of suicides and homicides by mentally ill people, for example.

In recent years, there has been considerable criticism of the Royal Colleges. They are regarded as ancient, wealthy and noble institutions, in need of modernisation. They are seen as male-dominated, but this may be less of a problem as more women qualify as specialists and as the Colleges set out plans to increase female membership. However, the Colleges differ considerably (some are relatively new: for example, the Royal College of GPs was formed in 1952 while the Royal College of Physicians was founded in 1518). Nonetheless, they tend to be depicted as shadowy bodies or 'cosy clubs', that exist primarily to protect professional interests rather than to maintain professional standards. Consequently, recent scandals have given critics plenty of ammunition. Much of this criticism has been acknowledged by the Colleges' leadership who fear they may be marginalised as new systems of audit, training and regulation develop.

Although still a force to be reckoned with, the medical profession does not perhaps enjoy the unrivalled supremacy that it once had. Other political-interest groups, representing patients, other professionals and organisational interests in the NHS (e.g. trusts), are much more closely involved in the policy process today (see, for example, Allsop, Baggott and Jones, 2002). Moreover, the profession's political relationship with the state has been weakened by the crumbling of support for the original compact between the medical profession and the state, not only in the UK but in other countries too. Democratic (public expectations and demands for transparency) and economic (cost containment and technological change) pressures have made it untenable (Salter, 1996; Moran, 1999). This has led to calls for a new, explicit compact that reflects the requirements of the modern age, spelling out the rights and responsibilities of the medical profession, the public and the profession. According to Salter (2000), a rebalancing of the original concordat is needed. This requires a new set of power relations within the medical profession committed to reform and which fulfils a number of basic conditions including the development of a common discourse, public credibility and accountability, public involvement, coherence and non-duplication. It should also cover all aspects of medical work including the creation and transmission (not just the application of) knowledge. Edwards, Kornacki and Silversin (2002) argue that a new compact must be based on a re-evaluation of the relationship between doctors and health care organisations, the state and the public. On a practical level this might mean greater involvement of doctors in developing service standards in return for compliance. They also suggest a more mature debate with the public about the limits of health care and about medicine itself, particularly its uncertainties. Finally, in this context Ham and Alberti (2002) have also called for a new compact setting out patients' rights and responsibilities; more effective accountability; the provision of adequate resources and training; emphasis on partnership with patients; support for effective care; and a recognition of the importance of stewardship: government must facilitate the above by encouraging public debate in an attempt to move away from the blame culture.

Medical Power in Decline?

Given that the foundations of medical hegemony have been challenged, it is legitimate to ask whether the power of the medical profession is declining. From the doctors' own perspective there is clearly much concern about their standing and authority both within the NHS and in wider society. There appears to be declining morale among doctors across all specialities and this is not a problem confined to the UK (Smith, 2001; Le Fanu, 1999; Edwards, Kornacki and Silversin, 2002). This is attributed not simply to workload and pay, but to changes in patients' expectations, and perceptions that health service reforms have eroded medical autonomy.

The challenge to the medical profession appears to be fairly universal (Hartley, 2002; Godt, 1987; Freddi and Bjorkman, 1989; Moran and Wood, 1992; Wilsford, 1991; Harrison and Ahmad, 2000; Salter 2000). Indeed, in some countries, notably the USA, the challenge has been perhaps even greater, with some claiming that medical autonomy has been seriously eroded (Armstrong, 1990; Ginzberg, 1990; McKinlay, 1988). Alford (1975), in attempting to make sense of power relations in the US health care system, devised a model of structural interests with wider significance in the debate about medical power. According to Alford, the health care system comprises three structural interests. The dominant interest is the *professional* monopoly of the medical profession. The subsidiary interest is that of the *corporate rationalisers*. These are the politicians and managers of health care (and, in the American context, the private funders of health care). These interests seek to challenge the professional monopoly by introducing planning and cost control, with the aim of limiting medical autonomy. As spending on health increases, these challenging interests become more influential. Finally, there is the *community interest*. This is the repressed interest, which lacks coherence and a power base and as a result, exerts little influence over health care.

North (1995) has reapplied Alford's model to the present-day NHS. She notes that the original classification of interests is not always appropriate. For example GP-led commissioning bodies are a combination of professional monopolist and corporate rationaliser. Even so, she observes that the values of the corporate rationaliser are becoming ever more influential. Although professional monopolists – such as hospital consultants – remain powerful, they are increasingly subject to the discipline and ethos of the corporate rationalisers. These issues are discussed further in later chapters. Others, however, emphasise that medicine still draws on many sources of power to prevent or divert pressures for change (Coburn, 1992). Indeed, observers of US health care indicate that the medical profession can, when under pressure, retain sufficient professional power to enable it to dominate, if not control, the health sector and that, at the very least, reports of its decline are exaggerated (Bjorkman, 1989; Mechanic, 1991).

Indeed, it is difficult to evaluate the impact of change upon the medical profession. As Elston (1991, p. 61) has observed, 'too often different theories about the present and future status of medicine seize on one aspect of change and draw general conclusions about overall rise or fall, ignoring other, countervailing tendencies'. A great deal depends upon how medical domination has been conceived in the past. The focus on the technical autonomy of the profession is only one of several aspects that need to be considered (see Light, 1991). Moreover, as Johnson (1995) argues, the benchmarks of medical autonomy and state intervention taken in isolation provide a narrow basis for evaluating the power of the profession. One should instead look at the role of the medical profession in the broader context of the state and with regard to the institutionalisation of expertise. According to this perspective, it is not inevitable that increasing restrictions on aspects of medical autonomy will undermine the profession. Autonomy may well be strengthened if the profession's expertise continues to be valued. However, it should be noted that Johnson himself argued that professionalism as an institutional form might be undermined by the emergent expertise in appraisal and performance-monitoring.

Others also note that the impact of recent changes on medical autonomy and power is complex. Harrison (1999) observed a redistribution of authority within the profession: from consultants to GPs in the light of the growing acknowledgement of the contribution of primary care; from rank-and-file doctors to those holding managements posts and to doctors that set standards of practice for others to implement. This redistribution is seen by some as a way of keeping external control at bay (Freidson, 1988). Indeed, as Annandale (1998) and Salter (1996) have both observed, restricting the autonomy of doctors does not necessarily weaken the profession as a whole.

Conclusion

During the twentieth century the medical profession consolidated its dominant position within the health care system. Recently, medical hegemony has been under pressure on several fronts. Orthodox medicine has been criticised, and complementary therapies have become popular. Nursing and paramedical professions have striven for higher status, while orthodox medicine's 'poor relation', the public health approach, has experienced a revival. There has been a greater acknowledgement of lay perspectives on health and illness. Moreover, during the 1980s medical organisations began to lose influence over important policy developments and their relationship with government became strained. Doctors voiced fears that their independence and autonomy were at risk because of government reforms.

However, these developments, and the challenges they pose for the profession, must be seen in relation to the pre-existing medical hegemony and within the broader context of the modern state. Despite the dire predictions, those factors which underpin the power of orthodox medicine remain. As a result, 'the acquiescence to medical ways of thinking', which Walby and Greenwell (1994, p. 74) rightly identified as the basis of medical authority, persists. Consequently, the medical profession continues to exert a powerful influence within the health care system.

_____*Further Reading*_____

Annandale, E. (1998) *The Sociology of Health and Medicine. A Critical Introduction* (Cambridge, Polity Press, in association with Blackwell Publishers).

Davies, C. (1995) *Gender and the Professional Predicament in Nursing* (Buckingham, Open University Press).

Fitzpatrick, M. (2001) *The Tyranny of Health: Doctors and the Regulation of Lifestyle* (London, Routledge).

Hart, C. (2004) *Nurses and Politics: The Impact of Power and Practice* (London, Palgrave).

Inglis, B. (1965) *A History of Medicine* (London, Weidenfeld and Nicolson).

Le Fanu, J. (1999) *The Rise and Fall of Modern Medicine* (London, Abacus).

Payer, L. (1989) *Medicine and Culture* (London, Gollancz).

Saks, M. (2003) *Orthodox and Alternative Medicine: Politics, Professionalisation and Health Care* (London, Continuum).

Critical Perspectives on Health Care

3

Medicine faces challenges on a number of fronts: from alternative practitioners, from other health care professionals and from lay people. To these one may add a number of broader critical perspectives of health care, discussed in this chapter. These are divided into three categories: New Right, managerialist and rational–economic critiques; Marxist, socialist, communitarian and Third Way perspectives; and feminism, Green critiques and the medicalisation thesis. Together these have provided a wide range of ideas for health care reforms.

New Right, Managerialist and Rational–Economic Critiques

In recent decades there has been a powerful critique of the way health care is managed and, in particular, how resources are used. This led to a sharper focus upon the efficiency and effectiveness of health care systems, the measurement of health outcomes, and closer monitoring of the performance of health professions and agencies against explicit criteria. Many, though not all, who adopt this perspective emphasise the virtues of competition and markets, and the need to view service users as consumers (see Chapter 12). Many also look to the private sector as a source of ideas for reform, and as a participant in reform programmes. These ideas are not confined to health care but have been applied across the public sector in the UK. Within the health sector, they have been articulated by people from a variety of backgrounds: not just economists, accountants, business people and right-wing politicians, but also health professionals, health service managers and patients.

The New Right

The New Right political philosophy has been particularly influential in liberal democracies since the late 1970s. It is a broad set of ideas that combines conservative ideas about the authoritarian state, with a radical agenda for increasing the role of markets and reducing state bureaucracy. There are many different sources of these ideas, principally the neo-liberal schools of thought, such as the Austrian School associated with Hayek (1944), the Chicago School, of which Milton Friedman (1962) is perhaps the best known, and the Virginia School associated with Niskanen (1971), among others. Although these writers adopt different approaches, they share a faith in the capitalist system. They argue that business and commerce should have greater freedom, that individuals should be recognised as consumers, that markets should be encouraged and be as free as possible from restrictions, and that the state should be reduced in size and scope. The New Right perspective upholds the importance of private ownership and endorses lower taxation. It supports high levels of personal responsibility and encourages self-help and voluntarism. Its commitment to individual freedom is tempered by a recognition that strong government is required to maintain social order and protect property rights, indicating tensions within the philosophy. Indeed, as Gamble (1994, p. 23) has noted, the New Right does not signify either a unified movement or a coherent doctrine. Nonetheless, this has not prevented these ideas from exerting a strong influence over political actors in recent decades.

For the most part, New Right ideas have been applied generically across the whole range of public services. Given the high level of state involvement in health care in most countries, these ideas have had important implications for this sector. There have also been specific critiques of health care from a New Right perspective (see Green, 1990; Gladstone, 1992; Butler and Pirie, 1988). In particular, a greater role for private enterprise – in both funding and provision of health services – was advocated as a means of challenging state dominance in this field. This argument was used to justify policies such as privatisation and the contracting-out of health services (see Chapter 6). Moreover, even where it was acknowledged that public authorities should retain a major role in the funding and provision of services, New Right ideas were drawn on to justify the introduction of competitive pressures through internal, or quasi-markets, in the health sector (see Chapter 5).

Managerialism

Coinciding with the ascendancy of the New Right were other ideas, often labelled as 'managerialism' or the 'new public management' (see Pollitt, 1993a; Horton and Farnham, 1999; Ferlie et al., 1996; Clarke and Newman, 1997). Many of these ideas had been around for some time, and the rise of the New Right amplified their appeal. As with the New Right, managerialism has not been specific to the health sector but has been applied across the public sector, and it is an international phenomenon.

The essence of the managerialist approach was captured by Osborne and Gaebler (1992) who outlined ten principles for public-services reform in a US context: competition, empowerment of communities, a focus on outcomes, orientation to particular goals, customer-focused services, preventive rather than reactive intervention, entrepreneurial government, decentralisation, market orientation, and multisectoral action where government should 'steer' rather than 'row'. Despite their appeal to reformers, there were clear tensions between some of these principles, notably the impact of greater competition and decentralisation on government's ability to 'steer'.

In the British context, managerialism embodied the following ideas:

1 A willingness to consider alternative forms of public service provision, even where the state retained overall responsibility for policy and funding.
2 A focus upon partnerships between the public, the private and the voluntary sector in the delivery of services.
3 An emphasis upon competition, with the introduction of internal markets within the public sector as well as external competition from the private sector.
4 A strong belief in the principles and practices of private sector management. The writings of management 'gurus', focusing on continuous improvement in quality (see, for example, Peters and Waterman, 1982) were particularly influential here.
5 A desire to introduce systems of performance management, notably for professional work, where previously there had been considerable autonomy and discretion. This was associated with what Michael Power (1994) called the 'audit explosion', where trust and traditional forms of accountability were replaced with formal systems of target-setting and performance assessment. This was consistent with neo-Taylorist 'scientific management' that emphasised central direction, performance-monitoring, and the creation of incentives and disincentives to attain key productivity targets (Taylor, 1911; Pollitt, 1993a; Hadley and Clough, 1996).
6 Managerialism placed great emphasis on the service user as a customer or consumer, implying greater choice and responsiveness in public services.
7 There was great emphasis on cultural change and the need to introduce what Clarke and Newman (1997) have labelled a 'tyranny of transformation' in public services.

These managerialist ideas added impetus to those already developing within health care and in the wider public sector. For example, back in the 1970s improvements in effectiveness and efficiency of health care were actively being discussed, and managerialist approaches were able to build on these ideas. In the 1980s, ministers drew explicitly on the advice of businessmen when formulating and implementing health care reform (see Chapters 5 and 9).

Efficiency and Effectiveness

Before we examine these ideas further, it is important to establish what is meant by efficiency and effectiveness in the health care context. At its simplest, an effective procedure is one that produces a desirable health outcome, such as the successful recovery of a patient following an operation. In reality, judgements about effectiveness are rarely so simple because there is often disagreement over what is a desirable outcome and whether it has in fact been achieved. According to some, the medical profession tends to judge the effectiveness of a treatment too much in terms of its success in saving lives (Kennedy, 1981; Illich, 1975). However, it is increasingly recognised that the effectiveness of treatment which saves lives but which severely reduces the quality of life is highly questionable, if not unethical (GMC, 2002).

Efficiency can be distinguished from effectiveness. In simple terms, efficiency is achieved where output is maximised from a given input of resources though, in reality, the concept is far more complex (Culyer, 1991). There are at least four types of efficiency in relation to health care, shown in Exhibit 3.1.

Exhibit 3.1 Types of Efficiency

1 Providing only services that are effective (i.e. where there is clear evidence that patients enjoy better health as a result of care).
2 Providing effective services at minimum cost.
3 Concentrating resources on effective services, provided at minimum cost, that offer the most benefits in terms of health.
4 Providing a mix of effective services at minimum cost and on such a scale that the benefits to society of providing more services are outweighed by the additional costs.

Source: A. Culyer (1991) 'The Promise of a Reformed NHS: An Economist's Angle', *British Medical Journal*

It is possible for a medical procedure to be effective but not efficient. Patients may be cured following medical intervention, but at an unjustifiably high cost relative to the benefits of the treatment. Or there may be an alternative treatment which is at least as effective but can be provided at a lower cost. From an economic point of view it is not sufficient that health care be effective: it must also be efficient.

Inefficiency in Health Care

Cochrane (1971), a strong advocate of evaluation in medicine, identified four main aspects of inefficiency in health care: the use of ineffective therapies; the inappropriate use of effective therapies; the inappropriate use of health care settings; and incorrect lengths of stay in treatment facilities.

Later in this chapter, discussion of Illich's (1975) concept of clinical iatrogenesis raises questions about harmful treatments and practices. Yet there are therapies which, although not positively harmful to patients, are simply ineffective and represent a waste of resources. To prevent this, Cochrane urged the use of the Randomised Controlled Trial (RCT). The RCT randomly allocates patients to one of two groups. The first receives the treatment being evaluated. The second (the control group) is either given a placebo (in the case of a drug trial, for example, a pill without an active ingredient) or is left untreated or given an alternative treatment. The outcomes for the two groups are then compared. RCTs provide the basis for recent efforts to promote evidence-based medicine (see Chapter 9). However, there are problems associated with their use, the most important of which are ethical. For example, it is difficult to justify entering patients in a trial if, as a result, they will be refused treatment likely to improve their health or save their lives. Indeed, doctors are reluctant to evaluate by RCT when there are already indications that the treatment will be effective, when there is no alternative treatment available, or where the known side-effects of treatment are minimal.

Other criticisms of RCTs is that they discriminate unfairly against some interventions, notably public health interventions and alternative therapies which are difficult if not impossible to evaluate by RCT. According to Britton et al. (1999), RCTs may underestimate the benefits of public health interventions (because the trials tend to attract people who already have a healthy lifestyle). Treatment trials, on the other hand, tend to attract sicker people, exaggerating the impact of these interventions. Another point is that it may be inappropriate to generalise from a randomised trial if sections of the population (notably children, the elderly and ethnic minorities) are under-reported, which is often the case. In addition, as Black (1996) argues, there are situations where RCTs may be inappropriate: where infrequent yet serious adverse outcomes occur as a result of treatment (such as extreme adverse reactions to a drug); when evaluating inventions designed to prevent comparatively rare events (such as cot death, for example); when the outcomes of intervention are in the distant future, and, finally, where the effectiveness of the intervention depends heavily upon the patient's active participation (undermined by the random allocation to treatment under RCT).

Inappropriate Use of Effective Therapies

There is evidence that some medical services have been overproduced and over-supplied. Diagnostic tests, such as X-rays, are a common target for criticism (Audit Commission, 1995a). A tendency to overdiagnose illness has also been observed. A classic study in the USA during the 1930s revealed that doctors tended to recommend tonsillectomies in about half the children they examined, even where they had been previously diagnosed as not requiring the operation (Bakwin, 1945). More recent studies also reveal a tendency to recommend unnecessary treatment. In the US, one study found that the proportion of coronary artery bypass surgery undertaken deemed either 'inappropriate' or 'equivocal' varied between 23 per cent and 63 per cent (Winslow et al., 1988). In the UK, a study in the Trent region found that almost half of coronary angiography and bypass surgery was performed for inappropriate or equivocal reasons (Gray et al., 1990). Further studies have since found evidence of inappropriate/equivocal interventions in this field (Leape et al., 2000), while others have indicated that *underuse* of certain procedures, including coronary revascularisation, is associated with adverse outcomes (Hemingway et al., 2001).

Appropriateness is difficult to define. However, it is increasingly accepted that it must be related to the capacity of patients to benefit from treatment as well as the risks involved in treatment. Hence a small benefit from a particular treatment may not be worth the risk of harm, even if this is also relatively low (see Davey Smith and Egger, 1994). Moreover, questions may be raised about the necessity for treatment, even if it is deemed appropriate. According to Kahan et al. (1994 – cited by Muir Gray, 2001, p. 235), there are four criteria for identifying necessary interventions: the procedure must be appropriate (the benefits should sufficiently outweigh the risks); it would be improper not to recommend the service; there is a reasonable chance it will benefit the patient; and the benefit to the patient is not small.

Suspicion about inappropriate intervention has been fuelled by the considerable variation in diagnosis and treatment which exists between countries. For example, Caesarean sections show considerable variation ranging from just under 22 per cent of deliveries in England, Wales and Northern Ireland to around 12 per cent in Sweden (Royal College of Obstetricians and Gynaecologists et al., 2002). There are also variations in the management of illness, particularly with regard to average lengths of stay in hospital. In 1996 the average in-patient stay in the UK was 9.8 days, compared with 7.2 days in Denmark, 32.5 days in Holland and 15.8 days in Australia (OECD, 2001). The accuracy of comparative studies can be challenged on methodological grounds. It is particularly difficult to establish how variations in patient stays, for example, are related to the prevalence and severity of illness in the general population. The pitfalls of international comparisons should always be remembered when interpreting such data. One should also take note of variation in surgical rates within countries as well as between them.

Nevertheless, there are several possible explanations of why doctors might overprovide medical services, and why this might vary between countries. Some doctors may simply prefer intervention to inaction (Illich, 1975; Kennedy, 1981). According to Payer (1989), this interventionist philosophy is more deeply ingrained in some countries (such as the USA) than in others (for example, the UK). Other factors may reinforce this culture: doctors may overprovide services if they fear the consequences of litigation. Failure to intervene may be construed as negligence and it is easier to prove medical negligence than incompetence or malpractice. Legal factors may partly explain the variation between countries.

Litigation by patients is more common and generally more successful in the USA than in the UK, though British patients are becoming increasingly litigious. Over-provision may also reflect patients' demands and expectations in a broader sense. Doctors feel that they are increasingly expected to 'do something' by the patient and that such pressure is partly, at least, responsible for 'inappropriate' or 'equivocal' referrals and treatment. The system of remunerating doctors may also encourage oversupply. In the USA, most doctors traditionally received a fee for each service. In an attempt to restrain health care spending, the Americans have introduced tighter regulation of fees and new forms of health care provision. Meanwhile, in the UK, as we shall see in later chapters, there have been several attempts in recent years to tie doctors' performance more closely to remuneration.

Other Aspects of Inefficiency

Cochrane (1971) believed that medical treatment was often given in inappropriate settings and that this could be unnecessarily expensive. He argued that certain conditions could be treated more efficiently outside hospital, perhaps in the GP's surgery, or at home. Cochrane also pointed out that patients were often kept in hospital for much longer periods than necessary, further adding to costs. It is widely believed that costs can be reduced by reorganising health care so that patients spend less time in hospital and more time in community settings. The expansion of day surgery, made possible by new surgical techniques, is an important development in this respect, as are changes in both primary and intermediate care discussed in later chapters. However, it should be noted that other significant costs may be incurred in caring for patients outside hospital. Good primary or intermediate care is not a cheap option, though it may be more cost-effective. Furthermore, as more of the cost may fall upon the family or on social services in these settings, it is important to acknowledge this when calculating the balance of costs and the benefits of transferring care from hospital into the community (see Chapter 11).

Calculating Cost-Effectiveness

Economists have devised techniques to measure cost-effectiveness of health care. One technique, the Quality Adjusted Life Year (QALY), has attracted considerable attention (Williams, 1985; Carr-Hill, 1991; Drummond et al., 1997). The benefits of health care, measured in QALYs, are calculated from estimates of the length and quality of a patient's life following treatment. The costs of treatment are then expressed in terms of a cost per QALY (see Exhibit 3.2). The QALY can be used to compare the relative cost-effectiveness of different treatments for the same illness. More controversially, the technique can be used as a rationing tool, facilitating the expansion of treatment of certain illnesses (those that achieve QALYs at a lower cost) at the expense of others (those that achieve QALYs at high cost).

There is strong opposition from health care professions to the use of cost–benefit criteria in this way. Doctors claim that QALYs undermine their clinical judgement (Smith, 1987). Williams (1988) denies this, arguing that the technique is intended only to improve accountability for the use of resources. Loewy (1980) has criticised the ethics of QALYs, commenting that optimisation of survival and not optimisation of cost-effectiveness is the only ethical rule to follow. Others have attacked QALYs for their discriminatory impact on vulnerable groups, such as the disabled and the elderly (Jones and Higgs, 1990), for whom the benefits of treatment (in terms of survival and externally-assessed quality of life) are lower.

The calculations themselves are rather crude. Reducing the quality of life to a single index is problematic, as individuals differ widely in their judgements. Other, more patient-sensitive measures have been devised (Carr-Hill and Morris, 1991). But these raise further problems of comparability between treatments and across different groups of patients (Cairns, 1996). Other technical problems can be found in the calculation of the health care costs. Many costs, including those that fall on families, social services and the wider community, are difficult to establish and are either underestimated or omitted from the calculations.

Exhibit 3.2 QALYs (Quality Adjusted Life Years)

QALYs can be used to compare the relative benefits of different forms of care and treatment. Each year which the patient is expected to survive following a course of treatment is weighted by a factor reflecting quality of life. The quality of life weighting relates to various dimensions of disability and distress (which can be converted into a single index – see Rosser and Watts, 1972; Rosser and Kind, 1978; Drummond et al., 1997). Once the number of QALYs generated by each treatment is calculated, it is then possible to compare the relative costs in order to find out which treatment has the lowest cost per QALY. A simple worked example is shown below:

Treatment A

Cost = £10,000 per patient
Life expectancy after treatment = 20 years
Quality of life: (Rosser's Index: No Distress; Slight Social Disability) = 0.990

Treatment B

Cost = £5000 per patient
Life expectancy = 18 years
Quality of life: (Rosser's Index: Mild Distress; Slight Social Disability) = 0.986

$\longrightarrow$

Exhibit 3.2 continued

$\longrightarrow$

Treatment A

QALY = Life expectancy × Quality of life = 20 × 0.990 = 19.8
Cost per QALY = 10,000/19.8 = £505 per QALY

Treatment B

QALY = Life expectancy × Quality of life = 18 × 0.986 = 17.748
Cost per QALY = 5000/17.748 = £282 per QALY

In the light of this simple calculation, Treatment B appears to be more cost-effective than Treatment A. In practice, however, other factors such as 'discount rates' are also included to reflect different preferences with regard to time.

The application of QALYs to health care decision-making in the UK has been fairly limited and mainly confined to raising questions, or identifying the parameters of debate about resource decisions rather than as a solution to problems of resource allocation. It is one of several methods that can be used. Another is the DALY (Disability Adjusted Life Year), which gives different states of health a disability rating (Murray and Lopez, 1996). There have been similar criticisms of this technique; that the combination of information about quality and length of life into a single index is problematic; that the index discriminates against the elderly and places less value on the lives of disabled people, and that it cannot capture subjective valuations of life and illness states (see Arnesen and Nord, 1999).

A Confluence of Ideas?

The greater emphasis on efficiency and effectiveness within health care, and the development of evaluation tools, provided a bedrock on which the broader ideologies of managerialism and the New Right could build. Most people broadly support the promotion of greater efficiency in health care, evaluation of effectiveness, prioritisation on the basis of need, better management, a focus on improving service quality and a greater emphasis upon financial, professional and political accountability. Yet there is a great deal of suspicion about the way these ideas have been applied in practice. In particular there is concern that they provide a justification for systems of performance management which focus only on what is measurable. This reduces the whole exercise to a numbers game (see Boyle, 2000), undervaluing intangibles that cannot be measured, or can only be measured with great difficulty (such as professional goodwill). Secondly, it is argued that reforms inspired by these ideas have led to a loss of accountability and trust. As Onora O'Neill (2002) pointed out in her 2002 Reith lectures, the introduction of managerial systems in the public sector and the increased regulation of public-sector professionals appears to have damaged rather than improved public accountability and trust. Thirdly, the emphasis on better management and improved efficiency is seen as part of an agenda by which politicians are seeking to limit the rights of individuals to welfare services, including the NHS. It is argued that managerialism facilitates a 'core' service mentality leading to greater rationing and targeting of services, leaving users to pay directly for services that are considered 'extra-contractual' (see Clarke and Newman, 1997). Finally, the managerialist perspective is seen by some as a strategy for professional advancement by economists, auditors, accountants and other business and management-related occupations. Indeed, health economists in particular have been characterised as imperialists seeking to colonise the minds of health care practitioners (Ashmore, Mulkay and Pinch, 1989). Along with other professional groups, such as accountants, management consultants and NHS general managers, they have been seen as challenging the existing medically-dominated structure of professional power within health care. These issues are further discussed in Chapter 9.

Socialism, Communitarianism and 'The Third Way'

From an orthodox Marxist perspective, contemporary health care can be analysed in terms of the class structure of capitalist societies, the search for profits, and the role of the state in ensuring both capitalist domination and capital accumulation (see Navarro, 1978; Doyal, 1979). Other socialist perspectives, examined in this section, share many of the concerns of the Marxists and propose similar (though less radical) solutions. Finally, some aspects of the collectivist ideas of Marxism and Socialism appear in communitarian and 'Third Way' approaches to public policy.

Marxists identify a powerful tendency for capitalists to exploit workers in an attempt to increase profits and accumulate more capital. Marx himself identified three main consequences of this process: inequality, as the material conditions of the workers declined relative to the capitalists; crisis, as the capitalist system found it more difficult to continue exploiting labour in the long term; and conflict between the classes, leading ultimately to socialised control of the means of production (Marx and Engels, 1976). The consequences of the unbridled capitalist system were evident during the period in which Marx was writing. Poverty and material deprivation were widespread, and the conditions endured by the working classes were a breeding ground for disease. Although the wealthy were not immune, the poor suffered disproportionately (Smith, 1979). In addition, there were wide inequalities in the standards of health care received by the different social classes (Abel-Smith, 1964). However, Marxists did overlook that self-interest could provide a springboard for employer initiatives to promote the health of their employees, including the funding and provision of health services. They also ignored voluntary and charitable efforts in the health field, some of which were initiated, sponsored and supported by profit-making organisations and others by labour organisations.

Moreover, since the death of Marx, capitalist states have responded to the social problems and economic tensions of capitalism in ways he did not foresee: intervening in the economy to moderate economic crises; replacing capitalist production with public ownership in many areas; and creating welfare states to cushion the impact of capitalism. Neo-Marxists, seeking to apply Marx's philosophy in the modern context, argue that, in spite of these changes, the system is essentially the same: the state primarily remains a defender of capitalism, not a guardian of social welfare. It is this general principle which guides their analysis of health care in capitalist states.

Inequalities, Class and Capitalism

In Chapter 1 a number of significant socio-economic inequalities in health and illness were identified. Marxists attribute these to material inequalities generated by capitalism. Although there is much consensus that material conditions are important factors in health and that specific conditions such as poor housing and unemployment are risk factors for ill health, it is not clear to what extent health inequalities are directly, exclusively or wholly a product of capitalism. Indeed, health and social inequalities vary considerably between capitalist countries, and persisted in communist countries throughout the postwar period.

Marxists also pointed out that, even in state health systems, health care will be unequally allocated, though the greater the reliance on private enterprise, the greater the inequality. This was reflected in the 'inverse care law', observed within the NHS, which posits an inverse relationship between needs and the availability of medical care (Tudor-Hart, 1971). As we shall see in a later chapter, it has been found that poorer areas tend to have worse health services. There are also acknowledged problems faced by some social groups in gaining access to care. However, equity is a complex concept and can be interpreted in different ways (Pereira, 1993; Whitehead, 1994), leaving much scope for debate about the extent of inequity in access to health care (see Chapter 8).

Marxists believe that the health care system is a microcosm of capitalist society. The upper and upper-middle classes are in a position to decide on key questions of resource allocation and the organisation of care. Furthermore, Marxists identify a class bias in the NHS, with upper and middle classes (and increasingly, in recent years, business people) dominating health authorities. They further believe that the medical profession, as the most socially exclusive group in health care, is part of the general conspiracy. As we shall see in Chapter 7, health authority membership is far from representative of society. But to equate socio-economic class with support for capitalism is too crude. Many health authority members, even those drawn from upper-middle backgrounds, have strenuously opposed moves to commercialise the NHS. Similarly, the fact that doctors are drawn from higher social classes does not necessarily make them allies of business. On the contrary, British doctors have been broadly support- ive of the NHS, though they have been opposed to certain models of state own- ership. One should note that the internal market – the most explicit attempt to introduce capitalist values into socialised medicine – was strongly opposed by most doctors and health professionals, though some aspects (notably GP fundholding) did appeal to some sectors of the medical profession (see Chapter 5).

Profits and Capital Accumulation

Marxists accept that state health care has to some extent moderated the health problems generated by the capitalist system, but has been unable to counteract them. They further point out that state health services allow some scope for pri- vate enterprise, which has never been totally eradicated even in state health care systems. For example, when the NHS was created, consultants retained the right to treat private patients and GPs secured their status as independent con- tractors. The profit motive has also survived in many areas vital to health care, such as the supply of medical equipment, pharmaceuticals, hospital building and construction: the so-called medical–industrial complex (McKinlay, 1979; Moran, 1999).

In recent years, private-sector involvement in UK health care has increased substantially, with the contracting out of ancillary services and the growth of private health care. Policies such as the Private Finance Initiative offer further opportunities for private corporations (see Chapter 6). Moreover, the intro- duction of business-style management processes and market mechanisms into health care has placed emphasis upon commercial motives and judgements. This mirrors developments elsewhere. Even in the US, for example, where the private sector has traditionally had a larger role, observers talk of a corporate transformation in health care led by investor-owned 'for-profit' enterprises (Relman, 1980; Salmon, 1995).

Marxists argue that state health services assist capital accumulation in other ways. They make more palatable the problems which arise from capitalist pro- duction. Industrial pollution, accidents and injuries and stress-related illness are seen by Marxists as consequences of the relentless quest for profits. Health prob- lems associated with consumption of commercially-produced goods such as alcohol, tobacco and junk food can be viewed in a similar way. Marxists believe that the people are fooled into thinking that 'what is politically and collectively caused can be individually and therapeutically cured' (Navarro, 1978, p. 92).

Individuals who suffer ill health can obtain treatment from state-financed health services in such a way that public awareness of the root causes of illness is obscured. Protest is thereby neutralised, allowing capitalists to continue making their profits at the expense of public health. Yet the creation of state health services did not reduce public protest nor the need for public health campaigns. Governments in capitalist states have been persuaded to take action against pollution, accidents at work, alcohol and tobacco and so on, even where this has offended vested interests. Commercial organisations have formidable lobbying powers to prevent this, but they are not invulnerable (see Baggott, 2000).

There are a number of other ways in which health services are seen as assisting profit-making and capital accumulation. Modern capitalism needs high-quality labour in order to thrive. Marxists argue that the productivity of labour can be maintained by protecting the health of key workers (skilled and technical workers). Moreover, the quantity of labour available to capitalists can be increased when necessary by relieving people of at least some of their caring duties. At the same time, health services become the dumping ground for the 'economically unproductive' (the mentally and physically ill and the infirm elderly) who cannot be 'used' by the capitalist production process. This process now appears to be operating in reverse. A major strand of policy in recent years has been to reduce state responsibilities for health and health care. Informal carers increasingly shoulder the burden of looking after the sick and the elderly. Successive governments have also encouraged self-care and individual spending on health care. Marxists explain these trends by arguing that capitalism has entered a further phase (O'Connor, 1973; Offe, 1984). This has taken the form of an initial crisis, the main features of which are rising tax burdens, high inflation, trade-union militancy and a stifling of capitalist activity. In response, the state has adopted policies to curb welfare expenditure and to encourage private enterprise, leading to a reinvigoration of capitalism, but at the cost of greater social conflict and inequality.

The Contribution of the Marxist Approach

The main contribution of the Marxist perspective, rather like the public health approach discussed in Chapter 2, lies in its focus upon the social and economic roots of ill health. The Marxist emphasis on inequalities in health care also reminds us that we should never assume that access to health care will always be fair, even in state systems. Marxists help to explain the motives of private health care providers. This is particularly important in view of the expansion of private care and private-sector management practices in the NHS. Finally, they shed light on why commercial activities harmful to health may be tolerated by governments.

There are, however, a number of criticisms. The Marxist critique of the NHS fails to recognise its contribution to the improvement of health care across the social spectrum. Furthermore, as we have seen, the Marxist approach to class relations in the NHS is flawed, and its assertion of class inequalities in access to health care are too crude. Another criticism is that Marxists are short of specific recommendations for improving health care. Marxists point out that health and health care will only improve significantly when the general social and economic organisation of society is changed: when capitalism itself is superseded. However, as already noted, health and health care inequalities persisted under communism and these countries had a poor record on industrial pollution, alcohol and tobacco-related problems and other public health problems linked with industrialisation.

Other Socialist Approaches

The declining appeal of Marxism, not least within the British Labour Party, does not mean that it is a redundant perspective. However, there are other socialist perspectives which, though sharing some of the concerns of the Marxists, take a more pragmatic approach to reform. Socialism is a broad church, but one can identify three principles that are particularly important in relation to health with which most socialists would agree: first, a concern for humanity – society must protect the weak and vulnerable; secondly, a belief that capitalism is often inefficient, particularly where the provision of collective goods is concerned; thirdly, that the state, through taxation, public spending and direct service provision, is a key instrument for improving social welfare.

These principles, applied to health care, underpin a range of policies: the creation of state health services, initiatives to redress health inequities and assistance for vulnerable groups (Carrier and Kendall, 1990; Tudor-Hart, 1994; Widgery, 1988). Perhaps it is a testament to the power of these principles that, in spite of the dominance of New Right and managerialist ideologies in government over recent decades, they still determine the parameters of health policy debate. But it would be foolish to argue that nothing has changed; indeed, socialism itself has changed. While retaining their humanitarian concern, many socialists have begun to question whether or not the state can deliver the gains in efficiency and equity in health care and in other public services. This is connected with the development of political ideas on the left, notably the adoption of communitarian ideas and the development of the Third Way.

Communitarianism and the Third Way

The rise of the New Right and managerialist ideas forced many socialists to rethink their philosophy. This process was particularly important for the leaders of socialist parties such as the British Labour Party. During a period when they lost four consecutive general elections, the Labour leadership began to explore ways of extending their electoral appeal while retaining their socialist credentials. The electorate was perceived to be more middle-class and consumerist, and more cynical about state intervention, even though public support for the welfare state and the NHS remained high.

Senior Labour politicians were attracted by communitarian ideas (see Tam, 1998). Communitarians (not to be confused with communists, who adopt a strictly Marxist approach) emphasise the importance of community values to sustain civic society (see, for example, MacIntyre, 1981). These ideas were articulated by the American sociologist Etzioni (1993) who argued that the rights of individuals must be balanced by responsibilities to the wider community, the ultimate goal being to create inclusive communities with shared values. Etzioni acknowledged that the state has a crucial role to play in maintaining strong communities and civic values. Its functions in relation to education, welfare and the criminal justice system are viewed as particularly important because they can be used to reinforce civic values (such as respect for others' property, participating in community life, equal opportunities, and so on). However, communitarians accept that the state cannot and should not do everything. They point out that much can be done through self help and voluntarism, with citizens themselves acting responsibly, identifying social problems and helping to overcome them (see Atkinson, 1994).

Communitarianism appeals across the political spectrum, and has attracted considerable attention from those on the political right who now wish to emphasise the importance of civic values within a neoliberal context (see Gray, 1993). According to Driver and Martell (1997), there are several different forms of communitarianism. They argue that the dominant form, adopted by 'New' Labour, promotes conservative values, focuses on individuals, is more conditional (i.e. emphasises responsibilities as a condition for having rights) and seeks to prescribe values rather than allow them to develop from the bottom up. This squares with the broader critique of the dominant form of communitarianism: that it is authoritarian, patriarchal, moralistic and tends to blame the individual for society's ills (see, for example, Campbell, 1995).

Because of the variety of interpretations, applying communitarian ideas to the health sector is not straightforward. On the one hand, communitarian ideas are likely to favour universal and inclusive health care systems because of their role in building social solidarity, mutual support and positive, caring values. However, they tend to endorse greater individual responsibility in the use of such services, including greater individual responsibility for one's own health. Communitarians also endorse self-help and voluntary health provision, particularly as a source of service innovation. Communitarian ideas can also be used to justify more private funding of health care, such as charges and insurance coverage for those who can afford to cover themselves for health risks. At the very least they legitimate additional co-payments by patients to cover non-health care elements of hospitalisation or residential care.

Another set of ideas, closely associated with New Labour and its reform programme, is the Third Way (see Giddens, 1998; Finlayson, 1999; Driver and Martell, 2002). This too is an amalgam of ideas, and does not fit easily into any single ideological pigeonhole. It derives from some of the New Right and managerialist ideas described earlier, mixed with elements of socialist and communitarian thought. Interpretations of the Third Way vary, and it is very much an unfolding project with ideas being shaped as reforms are implemented. However, its main principles can be described as follows:

- What counts is what works: policy should be guided by what is effective rather than ideological prescriptions.

- Society should be inclusive, with all citizens seen as stakeholders (see also Hutton, 1996).

- Voluntary activity should be encouraged by the state.

- Equality of opportunity rather than equality of outcome is the key social objective.

- Governing institutions must be responsive to people's preferences and must engage more with the public. There must be greater decentralisation and democracy.

- Governing institutions and processes must be reconfigured in order to tackle complex problems. In particular, traditional ways of governing and institutions must be reformed.

- The political and economic power of the private sector must be harnessed for the collective good.

- The state itself must be entrepreneurial in finding new opportunities for wealth creation and in problem-solving with regard to social problems.

In the UK context, these ideas manifested themselves in the Blair Government's modernisation project which emphasises sweeping changes in public services. In the context of health care, this project has legitimised changes in NHS organisation and service delivery, closer relationships between public and private sectors, 'joined-up government', stronger professional regulation, and systems of user involvement. These policy developments will be explored in some depth throughout the remainder of this book. However, as with other reformist ideas, one should bear in mind that internal tensions exist between Third Way principles. As a result, some have been given greater weight than others, and this balance has varied between different policy areas. Although there is considerable disagreement over where the balance lies, critics have argued that in general the Third Way has been much closer to the New Right and managerial approaches mentioned earlier than to traditional notions of collectivism and social justice associated with socialism (Harrison, 2001).

Feminism, Green Critiques and the Medicalisation Thesis

Feminism

As Annandale has observed (1998, p. 63), it is possible at a general level only to talk of a feminist vision, and there are in fact many different 'feminisms' (see also Miers, 2000). Nonetheless, these perspectives have in common an understanding that patriarchy – the male domination of society – privileges men by taking the male body as 'normal' and constructing the female body as 'deficient' and therefore associated with illness. Within the context of health care, they explore how gender shapes the division of labour in health care, how women's health problems are socially constructed, and the consequent impact on women's health (see Wilkinson and Kitzinger, 1994; Doyal, 1995; Miles, 1991; Doyal, 1998; Hayes and Prior, 2003).

In traditional societies, women were invariably cast in the role of healer. As societies developed, the healing role became professionalised (Leeson and Gray, 1978). Where women were allowed to undertake health care roles, they were subservient to the male-dominated medical profession. This continued even where female health care roles became professionalised, as illustrated, for example, by the 1902 Midwives Act (Donnison, 1988). This Act established state regulation of the midwifery profession and was the product of a protracted battle between doctors and midwives over who should control childbirth. It introduced a number of safeguards to protect the doctors' role and limit that of midwives. During the latter part of the nineteenth century, nurses also successfully pressed for professional recognition, but on terms acceptable to the doctors (Abel-Smith, 1960).

The professionalisation of nursing and midwifery enhanced the social status of these occupations but did not challenge the power of the medical profession, which remained hostile to women even after allowing them into its ranks. Even today women are still under-represented in the medical profession, particularly in the prestigious specialties and at the highest echelons (see Chapter 2). Women have made considerable progress in the professions allied to medicine – physiotherapy, occupational therapy, radiography, dietetics, speech therapy and so on – but these, like nursing and midwifery, invariably play a supporting role to medicine. However, one area of progress has been in management, where women make up just under half of senior managers. It is argued that women's health care roles place them in a subservient position. Nursing and other non-medical health professions are predominantly female. Other health occupations are also composed mainly of women. Seventy per cent of ancillary workers in the NHS are female, as are over four-fifths of clerical workers.

How can subservience and exploitation of women within the health care system be explained? According to Davies (1995), in the context of the nursing professions, it is not simply a result of poor political organisation. The answer lies in the gendering of social institutions – health care delivery is deeply affected by cultural codes of gender in which masculinity is associated with achievement and activity, and femininity with the caring role. Nursing, and other health occupations predominantly undertaken by females, stand for these gendered characteristics. This devalues their role and places them at a distance from real policy debates. Witz (1992, 1994) similarly notes that the 'problem' of nursing is a problem of gender. Nursing is, therefore, seen as 'women's work', which (wrongly) devalues both the task undertaken and the person undertaking it. Professionalisation has been seen as one way in which nursing can improve its status (see Exhibit 2.5), but, as Davies has observed, professionalism is itself gendered and dominated by a masculine paradigm, and a more effective approach might be to move beyond this and establish a new and distinctive form of professionalism based on values such as interdependence, cooperation, facilitation and the reflective use of experience and expertise, rather than the control of knowledge (see also Miers, 2000).

It is further argued that male domination of medicine and health care leads to a failure to understand women's health care needs. There is some evidence (discussed in more detail in Chapter 8) that health services discriminate against women; that compared with men they have difficulty gaining access to certain services and, when they do, the quality of service is poorer. There is also a belief that the health care system, and doctors in particular, take a rather peculiar view of women's health, which focuses very strongly on their reproductive role. This is often seen as a legacy from the past, especially the Victorian period when the health of women was defined by male doctors very much in terms of reproduction. Many social and psychological problems experienced by women were therefore identified as 'hysteria' and attributed to disorders of the sexual organs. Some women were subjected to surgical 'cures' such as the removal of the sexual and reproductive organs (Dally, 1991; Daly, 1979, pp. 225–8).

It is argued that this preoccupation with female gynaecological problems continues today. Doyal (1979, 1995) argues that doctors still hold a narrow view of female health problems, shaped by the belief that men are normal and women abnormal in respect of intellect, emotion and physical functioning. Abnormalities in women are still associated with their reproductive role. It is argued that doctors assume that motherhood and the maternal instinct is the main driving force in women's lives, and that a denial of this instinct causes depression and other health problems. They are also believed to view women as prone to neuroses and emotionally unbalanced (Miles, 1991).

Some complain that the medical profession fails to take into account the particular needs of women and actually places them in a position where they can be exploited and even abused (Jenkins, 1985; Roberts, 1992; Foster, 1995). A commonly cited example is childbirth (Oakley, 1980, 1984; Kitzinger, 1994) where it is argued that women have lost control of the birth process, that it has become medicalised and treated like an illness. This process has been assisted by the use of technology. Most births still take place in controlled conditions in hospital, the seat of medical power and technology, and Caesarean sections have risen. The effectiveness and efficiency of this technology has been challenged and there are suspicions that its main function is that of control. However, the picture is complicated by the fact that for many women the choice of a Caesarean section is viewed positively (Amu, Rajendran and Bolaji, 1998; Patterson-Brown, 1998).

Women have expressed feelings of powerlessness in the field of gynaecology. Some radical feminists see gynaecology as a means of controlling women's bodies, and consider that interventions, rather than improving health, lead to the unnecessary degradation and mutilation of women (Daly, 1979). While this may be disputed, doctors have in the past often failed to heed women's concerns about treatment. For example, in relation to breast cancer it is recognised that radical mastectomy (the removal of the breast) can have a devastating psychological impact on women and there have been well-founded criticisms, not just of the inappropriate use of such techniques but of the absence of counselling facilities and the failure to explain beforehand the risks and benefits of the operation (Batt, 1994). However, feminist writers have also pointed out that the whole experience of breast cancer is influenced by the cultural emphasis on breasts as objects of male sexual interest (Wilkinson and Kitzinger, 1994), and that treatment emphasises 'cosmetic' factors at the expense of women's health. Indeed it has been argued that breast-conserving surgery may not necessarily be in the long-term interest of the woman, and the increased use of this therapy may not be appropriate (Nattinger et al., 2000). Meanwhile, attention is distracted away from potential underlying causes of breast cancer in the environment (Batt, 1994; Wilkinson and Kitzinger, 1994). Similarly, in relation to cervical-cancer screening, it has been pointed out that the pain, discomfort and embarrassment that women endure is too easily dismissed (Milburn and MacAskill, 1994) and that the principal aim of this technology is primarily the surveillance and control of women's bodies by the medical profession (McKie, 1995). Similar arguments have been voiced by critics of mass breast-cancer screening (Hann, 1996).

Feminist Solutions

Feminists blame failures of the health care system on wider social processes of male domination. The overall solution proposed is to change society by improving the status of women (though the different 'feminisms' disagree on how this should be achieved). On a practical level, within health care, the position of women could be strengthened through greater participation in medicine. There has been a considerable increase in the proportion of women training as doctors (see Chapter 2). However, this will not guarantee that women will stay in medicine, or that they will rise to the highest echelons. Flexible career-development programmes may help more women to move up the ladder, but other obstacles – such as the allegedly male-dominated culture of some medical specialties – will persist until the proportion of women at senior levels begins to increase significantly. Women may also benefit by shifting the balance in health care away from doctors and towards those professions where women predominate. This could be secured through greater professional autonomy for midwives, nurses and professions allied to medicine, though, following Davies (1995) above, a more effective approach would be to challenge the masculine paradigm of professionalism that currently predominates and to encourage all health care practitioners to become more interdependent, facilitative and co-operative.

Women are also likely to benefit from moves which give them more choice in health care (though these choices may be shaped by wider social factors and the quality of information – as with regard to Caesarean sections and breast-conserving surgery above). Particular services designed to cater for their specific needs, such as Well Woman Clinics, have been seen as a proactive development, though some see them as increasing 'surveillance' (Foster, 1995). None the less, self-help groups offer women a greater opportunity to make decisions about their health (Phillips and Rakusen, 1989). Furthermore, women's health lobby groups represent an important political force with the potential to shape health services (Doyal, 1995; Foster, 1995). However, there is no systematic way of involving women's groups in policy and planning processes at national or local level in the UK, though some other countries have established consultative mechanisms (for example, New Zealand) or a policy process for women's health (Australia) (see Doyal, 1998). A further area of possible action relates to research. It has been argued that medical research downplays the importance of women's perspectives and that, as a result, the diversity and specificity of women's health needs are not fully revealed (Doyal, 1998). This is believed to occur because medical research is strongly influenced by male perspectives. A possible solution to this is to divert resources into women-centred research projects.

Although attempts to improve the role and status of women in health care must be applauded, it is important to realise that some changes may not provide clear benefits for all women. It is possible that benefits will accrue to women in the higher social classes, who are more articulate, more vociferous and highly motivated to do something about the problems they experience. This raises the possibility of the emergence of a two-tier system of care, to the disadvantage, perhaps, of working-class women or those from minority ethnic backgrounds. It must be noted though that the concept of universality of women's experiences has much less attraction for feminists today and, as a result, the variations in the health experiences of women – relating to ethnic background, social class, disability and so on are – increasingly recognised (Doyal, 1995; Graham, 1993).

It is also ironic, as noted in Chapter 1, that many of the illnesses from which women now suffer increasingly have arisen from the adoption of male lifestyles. Many women nowadays are also expected to combine the traditional role of mother/housekeeper with that of worker, which for some is stressful and possibly harmful to their overall health (though the evidence is mixed – see Chapter 1). The health consequences of a changing role for women are, therefore, far from straightforward.

Green Perspectives

Green perspectives adopt an ecological model of health (Hancock, 1985; Pietroni, 1991). They place an emphasis on the complex and multiple sources of illness arising from the environment. Mankind's interaction with the natural environment is seen as a crucial relationship in the production of health and illness. According to Greens, major health problems – such as food poisoning, cancers and heart disease – are linked to the food-production system and environmental pollution. Moreover, the social and economic structure of industrial societies is seen as a major source of ill health in the form of stress-related illness induced by working conditions, lifestyles and poverty.

Greens have much in common with socialist perspectives and public health approaches. They argue strongly for a precautionary approach based on the assessment of risks and emphasise collective solutions to address the root causes of illness. This may take the form of action at the global level, such as international treaties to limit pollution and global warming. They also advocate small-scale local solutions, believing that this can promote community participation in relation to both environmental problems and solutions. At the same time, local action can aggregate into a major impact nationally and internationally. But Greens are not so naïve as to think that this will happen in the absence of a supportive framework at a higher political level.

Greens are cynical about the preoccupation with technological innovation in health care and the power of scientific systems of health expertise. They believe that environmental solutions are often more cost-effective than complex technological solutions, but they recognise that the latter are supported by a powerful political network comprising scientific expertise, government and corporate interests. Nonetheless, they continue to criticise the technological imperative and argue that resources should be diverted to identifying and preventing problems rooted in the environment. Furthermore, Greens generally support low-technology interventions and endorse complementary and alternative therapies.

Iatrogenesis: Illich's Thesis

It is one thing to argue that contemporary health care is inefficient, insensitive or misdirected; to argue that the medical establishment is a direct threat to health is far more radical. Yet this is precisely the argument advanced by Illich (1975) in his examination of the nature and extent of iatrogenesis – illness caused by medicine. Illich identifies three dimensions of iatrogenesis: clinical, social and cultural, and each will now be examined in turn.

Clinical iatrogenesis

Clinical iatrogenesis occurs when illness is caused by diagnosis or treatment undertaken by medical practitioners. Illich begins by claiming that the successes of modern medicine are overrated. In accordance with those who support the public health approach, he observes that better housing, better nutrition and an improved environment were more effective in reducing mortality and morbidity. He then goes on to argue that a number of aspects of medical treatment are actually useless and ineffective, while others are positively dangerous. He identifies several types of clinical iatrogenesis: diagnostic errors, accidents during the course of treatment, and the side-effects of treatment. There is evidence of clinical iatrogenesis in health services, and this is further discussed in Chapter 9.

Social and cultural iatrogenesis

Turning from clinical to social iatrogenesis, Illich argues that health is undermined by the impact of medical organisation on social life. Illness is created as more and more social and individual problems are labelled as medical problems (see also Zola, 1975). Illich argues that this process of medicalisation is harmful because it gives the medical profession enormous power to judge others. As individual conditions and experiences are defined as illnesses, they fall within the judgement and control of the medical profession. Social iatrogenesis is therefore a kind of medical imperialism, with doctors identifying illness in ever more aspects of an individual's life. A further reason why Illich believes medicalisation to be harmful is that it moves the focus away from activities which deal more effectively with the problems faced by society and the individual. It also stifles lay initiatives which might otherwise arise to tackle these problems.

The third type of iatrogenesis identified by Illich is cultural. Medicine seeks to alleviate pain. Most people would agree that this is a noble aim. However, Illich argues that pain is an important part of human experience. To overcome suffering, to cope with pain, to face and accept death are not necessarily negative experiences. By denying these experiences and turning them into technical matters, medicine therefore undermines the individual's personal capacities. Moreover, because most pain and suffering in industrial society is man-made, there are wider implications. Illich argues that the alleviation of pain and suffering leads to the neutralisation of political forces which might otherwise arise to prevent the underlying causes of illness.

Illich's solutions

Attempts to assert political control over medicine and therefore redirect health care are doomed to failure, according to Illich. Moves to increase consumer control of health care and to impose a more rational organisation of health care will, in his view, be ineffective in reducing medical power and may actually worsen the situation. He argues against a public health approach because it implies that individuals are presumed ill until proved otherwise, and because medical influence will spread to other areas of social and economic life, leading to more social iatrogenesis.

Illich does accept that health and health care may be improved by focusing on equity, which in turn raises questions about the social and economic causes of illness. But he goes on to argue that iatrogenesis will not be checked if the concern with equity is confined to matters of health service provision. The only real solution, therefore, is to limit the scope of professional monopolies and to extend personal responsibility for health. In his own words, 'that society which can reduce professional intervention to the minimum will provide the best conditions for health' (Illich, 1975, p. 274).

Challenges to Illich

Illich's thesis arises out of a more general critique of industrialisation, institutionalisation and professional power in modern societies. His arguments have not gone unchallenged (see Horrobin, 1977). Doctors argue that much clinical iatrogenesis is an inevitable consequence of the advancement of medical science. According to this view, the frontiers of knowledge can only be moved forward by attempting new treatments, some of which may prove initially to be harmful to the patient. This is the price of long-term success. The failure to try new therapies, doctors argue, would have kept medicine in the Dark Ages.

A further counter-argument is that much clinical iatrogenesis is the result of patient ignorance. For example, the failure to follow medical advice properly, particularly for medicines, is a well-known source of adverse reactions. From this viewpoint, clinical iatrogenesis may be reduced through doctors educating patients and communicating with them more effectively, increasing rather than reducing the scope of professional responsibility. Another point is that Illich ignores the positive aspects of medicine. Though iatrogenesis has to be recognised and reduced, modern medicine has contributed to improvements in health, particularly by improving the quality of life for many sufferers. Illich's thesis can therefore be criticised as being polemical and unbalanced in that he does not appear to accept that modern medicine has any redeeming features.

Illich is criticised for being utopian. The processes of industrialisation, institutionalisation and professionalisation, which are the main causes of the problems he identifies, cannot simply be rolled back. It could be argued that professionalism combined with self-regulation and peer review are the most effective safeguards against malpractice in an industrialised society, given the complex division of labour and the diversity of knowledge and expertise. It may be more fruitful to reform the professions rather than undermine or bypass them. The introduction of systems of incident reporting, inspections and audit, discussed in later chapters, may be less radical but might provide a more practical way of reducing clinical iatrogenesis.

Conclusion

The various critiques explored in this chapter, along with alternative perspectives on health discussed previously, have highlighted a range of problems and issues facing modern health care systems. These include a lack of accountability in health care, the dominant role of orthodox medicine and the medical profession, the lack of responsiveness to users and consumers, the need to evaluate the quality and cost-effectiveness of health care, the problems of health inequalities, and the need to tackle the wider social, economic and environmental causes of ill health. All health care systems in the developed world are confronting these issues and developing their own particular response to them.

Critical perspectives on health care have provided a wealth of ideas for would-be reformers of the health care system. Some of the ideas and arguments may be regarded as extreme – certainly to defenders of the status quo. Some are flawed and have attracted justified criticism. But this has not stopped them from shaping debates about the future of health care, nor has it prevented policy-makers from drawing on these ideas when reforming health care policies and programmes, as will become clear in subsequent chapters.

_____ *Further Reading* _____

Carrier, J. and Kendall, I. (1990) *Socialism and the NHS* (Aldershot, Avebury).

Doyal, L. (1995) *What Makes Women Sick?* (London, Macmillan).

Driver, S. and Martell, L. (2002) *Blair's Britain* (Cambridge, Polity Press).

Ferlie, E., Pettigrew, A., Ashburner, L. and Fitzgerald, L. (1996) *The New Public Management in Action* (Oxford, Oxford University Press).

Horton, S. and Farnham, D. (1999) *Public Management Britain* (Basingstoke, Palgrave Macmillan).

Illich, I. (1975) *Limits to Medicine* (Harmondsworth, Penguin).

Mooney, G. (1994) *Key Issues in Health Economics* (Hemel Hempstead, Harvester Wheatsheaf).

Power, M. (1994) *The Audit Explosion* (London, Demos).

Tudor-Hart, J. (1971) 'The Inverse Care Law', *Lancet*, 27 February, 405–12.

The Evolution of the British Health Care System

An understanding of how the British health care system evolved is necessary to place contemporary developments in context. The chapter begins by looking at the system of health care which existed before the NHS. This is followed by an examination of how and why the NHS was created. Finally, the experience of the NHS in the post-Second-World-War period up to the Royal Commission's inquiry in the late 1970s is explored.

The Health Care System before the NHS

Before the NHS, Britain's health care system was a rather disorganised and complex mixture of private and public services (Webster, 1988; Abel-Smith, 1964). The private sector consisted of voluntary hospitals, private general practitioners, and other voluntary and commercial organisations. The public sector comprised municipal hospitals and community health services run by local government. In addition, local government was responsible for sanitary and environmental health services and health-related services such as housing.

General Practice

Prior to the creation of the NHS, general practitioners (GPs) were private practitioners who charged a fee for their services. In Victorian times the fear of being unable to pay these fees led to the development of club practice. The more affluent sections of the working class would subscribe to friendly societies who, in turn, hired the services of GPs on behalf of their members. Club practice covered around a third of the working class by the end of the nineteenth century (Honigsbaum, 1990). However, these schemes tended to exclude those not in work, such as the unemployed, married women, children and the elderly. Meanwhile, doctors became increasingly worried about lay interference in medical practice, and the poor remuneration evident in some club practices.

In 1911 the Liberal government introduced its own plans for general practice in the form of the National Insurance Act. This led to the provision of sickness benefits, free GP services and free drugs for the employed working class. Employers, workers and the government each contributed to the compulsory scheme. The scheme was administered by local insurance committees, which included the representatives of approved societies (friendly societies and industrial insurance offices and trade unions), local authorities and GPs (Honigsbaum, 1979).

The government's initial plans angered the British Medical Association (BMA). The BMA believed that remuneration for GPs was inadequate. It feared that GPs would be subject to the same kind of interference experienced under the club-practice system. This fear was understandable, given that approved societies had a majority on the insurance committees which adminis-tered the scheme. The government did make several compromises, such as removing the power of insurance committees over doctors' remuneration, and establishing the principle that patients would be free to choose their doctor. These concessions – coupled with the fear of an alternative scenario; a state medical service employing salaried GPs – won the day (Brand, 1965).

By the outbreak of the Second World War, 43 per cent of the population were covered by the National Health Insurance (NHI) scheme, and 90 per cent of GPs participated in it (Webster, 1988, p. 11). Although the scheme was a land-mark in state intervention in health care, it only applied to the services of GPs, not specialist hospital services (except for the treatment of tuberculosis). Moreover, the scheme excluded the unemployed, and dependants such as married women and children (see Jeffreys, 1998).

The Private Sector: Voluntary Hospitals

The voluntary hospitals were established by philanthropy or by public subscription. Most were created in the eighteenth and nineteenth centuries, although some were older, having been founded in the early Middle Ages. Many voluntary hospitals, however, were of more recent origin: of those exist-ing in 1938 over a third had been founded after 1911 (Webster, 1988, p. 2). Traditionally, voluntary hospitals gave care free of charge, reflecting the chari-table motives behind their foundation. When originally founded their prestige was such that doctors often waived their fee for the privilege of being associated with them. The doctors would make a living by treating the rich, whose con-tributions supported the hospital. The wealthy were treated at home while hos-pitals catered mainly for the less well-off who could not afford to pay for treatment. Yet admission to these hospitals was quite selective: the very poor and those with infectious diseases were frequently denied access (Abel-Smith, 1964). By the outbreak of the Second World War in 1939, the voluntary hospitals had changed considerably. Only about a third of their income now came from charitable contributions. They began to charge patients for services to a much greater extent. Patients, in turn, took out health insurance plans to cover these payments. Voluntary hospitals continued to face financial problems, despite efforts to raise funds. Yet they retained their prestigious status, and continued to make a major contribution to health care. In 1938 one in three patients still received treatment in a voluntary hospital.

Other Voluntary Organisations

The health care system before the NHS involved an array of other voluntary health care organisations. As well as running hospitals, voluntary organisations provided community health services. They increasingly worked in partnership with local authorities in fields such as child welfare, maternity, aftercare, district nursing, and the care of mentally ill and physically disabled people.

The Public Sector: Local Authority Health Services

Even before the creation of the NHS, the public sector had the largest share of hospital-based care. On the eve of the Second World War, two-thirds of patients were being treated in local authority hospitals. Local government operated a considerable and diverse network of hospitals. These included isolation hospitals for infectious diseases, hospitals specialising in the treatment of tuberculosis, maternity hospitals and mental hospitals. From 1875 onwards local government had the power to run general hospitals, but few authorities actually did so.

The local authorities also inherited a hospital service which grew out of the nineteenth-century system of relief known as the Poor Law (Hodgkinson, 1967). This notorious system, introduced by the Poor Law Amendment Act (1834), effectively institutionalised poverty. Local Poor Law authorities established workhouses where relief was given on the principle of 'less eligibility' in an attempt to discourage the poor from seeking help. This system, despite its defects and inhumanity, actually exposed a high level of illness among the workhouse inmates. This had two important consequences. First, it led to the development of publicly-funded health services in the form of Poor Law infirmaries, which developed later into separate institutions for the 'sick poor'. In addition, the poor were eligible for free GP services, following a means test. Secondly, the recognition of the cost of the 'sick poor' led to a series of inquiries into the environmental (but not the economic) causes of their condition, such as Edwin Chadwick's famous report on the sanitary condition of the labouring population (Chadwick, 1842). These inquiries led in turn to the development of public health legislation, beginning with the Public Health Act of 1848 which gave localities the power to promote a healthier environment.

Although public health legislation was introduced at national level, it was down to local government to implement the statutes, enforce the regulations and develop public health services. Local health committees were set up to administer this process. Local medical officers of health (MOHs) were also appointed to act as guardians of public health. Gradually, local authorities began to provide a wide range of health-related services. These included water supply, sanitation, food and hygiene inspection, and pollution control. Their role later extended to housing as well as personal and community health services such as school health services, midwifery, community nursing and child-welfare clinics (see Baggott, 2000, ch. 2).

This system of public health administration grew up separately from the Poor Law hospital network; the latter came under the responsibility of the Poor Law Boards until their abolition in 1929. After this date most of the former Poor Law hospitals became municipal hospitals under the control of local public health authorities. However, many chronically ill people continued to reside in institutions under the control of the public assistance system. As Webster (1988, p. 5) has pointed out, around 40 per cent of residents in Poor Law institutions in England and Wales in 1939 were classified as 'sick'.

On a number of occasions suggestions were made to integrate health services and local-authority hospital, community and environmental health services. In 1909 members of the Royal Commission on the Poor Laws produced a dissenting minority report which argued for a unified state health service run by local authorities (Cd 4499, 1909). This report, which was considered too radical at the time, also sought to establish the principle of free health care for the poor as a right, though it fell far short of recommending a comprehensive state health service available to all and free at point of delivery, an idea widely accepted a few decades later.

The Acceptance of a Comprehensive State Health System

Criticism of the British health care system began to accumulate after the First World War. Health care was fragmented into hospital, community and public health services. There was little co-ordination of health care to tackle the complex needs of vulnerable groups such as children and the elderly. Moreover, access to health care was limited for many of these groups. The growth of health insurance and charging for hospital services meant that, for many, health care depended on ability to pay. Furthermore, access to high-quality health care varied throughout the country and was apparently unrelated to the level of need (Political and Economic Planning, 1937). According to some, the mismatch between geographical need and availability has been exaggerated (Powell, 1992). Nevertheless, it was widely believed at the time that some form of national planning was required to relate the need for services more closely to availability.

A series of reports in the 1920s and 1930s exposed the problems of the health services and charted future paths for reform. The Dawson report of 1920 argued for the integration of preventive and curative medicine under a single health authority which would co-ordinate a network of local hospitals and health centres. The report stated that the provision of the best medical care should be available to all, but did not elaborate on the question of how this would be financed (Cmd 693, 1920). A further contribution to the debate was made by the Royal Commission on National Health Insurance, which reported in 1926 against a background of concern about access to specialist medical services. It urged the approved societies which operated the NHI scheme to pool their surplus resources to fund such care. It also indicated that the long-term future lay in direct funding of health care by the state (Cmd 2596, 1926).

The failure of the health care system to cater for those requiring specialist care was a further concern in the BMA report of 1929 (BMA, 1929). This report argued that NHI should be expanded to cover specialist services provided by the hospitals. It suggested that the scheme should be extended to the families of insured workers. But the BMA plan was not fully comprehensive: it intended to exclude the wealthier classes from the scheme; it also side-stepped the crucial issue of how the higher cost of the extended service would be funded.

The interwar period, with high rates of unemployment, created conditions that undermined the operation of NHI. In 1932 alone, 200,000 workers lost their right to benefits under the National Health Insurance scheme because of unemployment. There was also growing criticism of the insurance companies in relation to the system of health insurance, mainly from trade unions and GPs (Honigsbaum, 1989). It is often thought that the Second World War, which led to a dramatic expansion in government intervention in health services, was a major reason behind the creation of the NHS. The government created an Emergency Hospital Service (EHS) to co-ordinate the patchwork quilt of public hospitals and voluntary hospitals. The task of organising the EHS, according to Abel-Smith (1964, p. 440), 'brought home to all concerned the failings of Britain's hospital system'. The experience of the EHS was no doubt useful in showing how the state could co-ordinate the health care system. But it is generally accepted that the irrationality and inadequacy of the British health care system was evident long before the scheme was created. There was a general consensus about the need for a more comprehensive health service well before hostilities began.

The Creation of a National Health Service

Towards a Comprehensive Health System

In the years before the Second World War, the government considered the integration of existing health services. In 1936 the Minister of Health asked his

Chief Medical Officer (CMO) to report on the feasibility of a comprehensive health care system. The CMO recommended that local authorities should provide the basis for any comprehensive scheme, and the Ministry of Health began to develop policy ideas along these lines. Its plans included transferring responsibility for NHI to local authorities and extending coverage of this scheme to dependants (see Klein, 1983, ch. 1). These long-term plans were halted by the need to address short-term emergencies, the first being a financial crisis that hit many voluntary hospitals, including the London teaching hospitals, in 1938. The second was the outbreak of war, which led to the creation of the EHS, discussed above.

During the war, the idea of a comprehensive health service became bound up with the broader aim of reconstructing Britain. A major landmark was the ministerial announcement of October 1941, which set out the government's intention to create a comprehensive hospital service after the war. It was not clear at this stage that the service would be free. Moreover, there was no question at this stage of voluntary hospitals being taken into public ownership, though it was expected that they would co-operate closely with local authorities to produce a more coherent pattern of hospital provision.

Meanwhile, the medical profession was formulating its own plans for a new health service. In 1940 the BMA established a Medical Planning Commission to consider the future development of medical services. The Commission produced an interim report two years later which set out many features which were eventually incorporated in the NHS (BMA, 1942). These included the regionalisation of hospital administration, a prohibition of full-time salaried service for GPs, and the remuneration of GPs mainly by a capitation fee (a fixed payment for every patient registered with them). The Commission supported an extension of NHI to pay for hospital and community health services, but did not reach clear conclusions about the coverage of the new scheme. Later, however, the BMA endorsed a scheme which provided for the whole community (Grey-Turner and Sutherland, 1982, p. 38).

Then came the Beveridge report (Cmd 6404, 1942). In setting out a broad framework for the postwar welfare state, Beveridge supported the idea of a comprehensive health service available to all. The final version of the report left open the precise financial and organisational details of the service. However, it was these detailed matters which produced the most controversy.

Organising the New Health Service

Despite the broad agreement on the need for a comprehensive health service, there were widely differing opinions surrounding the organisational and financial principles of such a service. The Ministry of Health favoured a municipally-controlled health service, as set out in a confidential memorandum of 1943 named (after the Minister of Health) the Brown Plan. This would have given local authorities the responsibility for organising services and sought to bring both general practitioners and the voluntary hospitals under local government. The GPs were not happy with this proposal – they had long been suspicious of local authority services (Jeffreys, 1998; Lewis, 1986). Their discontent was shared, for different reasons, by a number of local authorities depressed by the prospect of running such an expensive new service. The voluntary hospitals were also unhappy, fearing the loss of independence implied by the prospect of central government funding being channelled through the local authorities. In short, the Brown Plan pleased no one.

The government offered a compromise. A White Paper containing revised proposals was eventually published in 1944 (Cmd 6502, 1944). Under this scheme, health services would be comprehensive and free at the point of delivery, and GPs would come under the control of a Central Medical Board. They would not be directly under the influence of local government except where they worked in health centres run by local authorities. GPs working in such health centres would be salaried, as would new entrants to the profession, while other GPs could be salaried if they wished. Private practice was permissible and the right to buy and sell practices was retained, though some restrictions would be imposed on these activities. Finally, the hospital service was to be operated by joint local authority boards responsible for controlling municipal hospitals and co-ordinating the activities of the hospital network in the area.

The doctors, fearing a loss of autonomy, rejected the White Paper. Their lobbying was effective in that all the major proposals were dropped, including the establishment of the Central Medical Board. The government agreed that the responsibility for GP services would remain with local committees on which the GPs would have a majority. The local authorities' control over doctors working in health centres was eroded to the point that their function was largely that of landlord. The provision that doctors working in health centres would be salaried was also dropped.

The local authorities also obtained concessions. The joint boards that would have taken control of municipal hospitals were subsequently confined to a local planning role, leaving control in the hands of individual local authorities. This made it politically possible to allow medical representation on these boards, a move which had been strongly resisted by local authorities as long as the boards had control over municipal hospitals. In addition, expert regional planning bodies were proposed. This was mainly to satisfy the demands of the voluntary hospitals, in particular the more prestigious teaching hospitals, which had lobbied for a regional tier to advise on planning and developing specialised medical services.

A further White Paper embodying the revised proposals was planned, but meanwhile Labour had left the coalition government. This second White Paper was suppressed before the 1945 election and, as a result of the Conservative

Party's defeat at the polls, was never published. Even so, some of its proposals reappeared in the Labour government's plans, namely the regional structure and the separate local administration of GP and hospital services, discussed below.

Bevan's Plan

The 1945 General Election produced a clear victory for the Labour Party. Clement Attlee, the new Prime Minister, appointed Aneurin Bevan as Minister for Health, giving him the task of rescuing the plans for a new health service. Despite the support within his own party for a comprehensive health service based on local authority control, Bevan opted for nationalisation of the entire hospital sector within a tripartite system of provision.

This option was chosen not on ideological but on practical grounds. As Honigsbaum (1989, p. 95) correctly notes, 'far from being a dogmatic socialist, Bevan proved to be a pragmatic reformer'. Yet there was considerable opposition to his plan. Bevan was challenged by his Cabinet colleague Herbert Morrison, a staunch defender of local government interests who argued against the nationalisation of the municipal hospitals. Bevan won this battle, but local authorities continued to have a significant role in health care through their provision of community services, personal social services and public health functions (Timmins, 1995, pp. 116–18).

The other main source of opposition to Bevan's plan came from the medical profession, particularly the GPs, whose views were forcefully put by the BMA. Many GPs were alarmed not only about the principle of nationalisation, but also about proposals to ban the sale of practices and to control the geographical distribution of new entrants to general practice. Their biggest fear, however, was the prospect of a salaried medical service. To win their support, Bevan permitted GPs to remain as independent contractors. They would be allowed to provide services to NHS patients on the basis of a contract negotiated between the Ministry of Health and the profession's representatives, and would be paid mainly by capitation payments. A part-time salary element for all GPs was included in Bevan's original plan, though this was later restricted to new GPs for a limited period only. As a further concession, which was instrumental in securing the co-operation of the profession, Bevan agreed to a ban on full-time salaried medical services.

The interests of the GPs as independent contractors were also protected by the creation of a separate administrative branch. It was agreed that GP contracts, and those of dentists, pharmacists and opticians, would be administered by executive councils. These bodies would consist of part-time appointees nominated by the Minister of Health, the local authorities and the independent contractor professions themselves, with the last of these groups providing half the members.

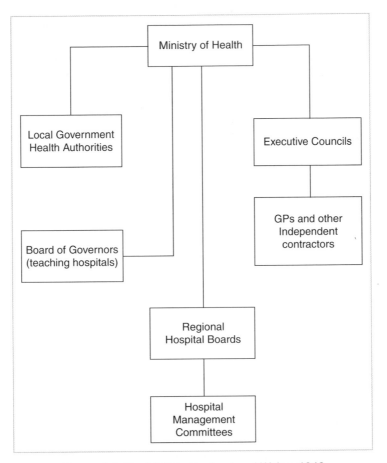

Figure 4.1 The NHS in England and Wales, 1948

The local authorities and the executive councils formed two parts of the tripartite structure (see Figure 4.1). The third part was the hospital service which, with the exception of the English teaching hospitals (see below), had a two-tier structure. The top tier consisted of Regional Hospital Boards (RHBs) responsible for the overall planning, co-ordination and supervision of hospital services within a large area. The RHBs were appointed by the Minister of Health after consultation with local authorities and the medical profession. The second tier, responsible for the actual running of the local hospital service, consisted of Hospital Management Committees (HMCs), whose members were appointed by the RHB, following consultation with local authorities, the medical profession and voluntary associations.

The prestigious teaching hospitals in England were each administered by a board of governors appointed by and accountable to the Minister of Health. Though they themselves did not regard their position as being privileged, the treatment given to the elite hospitals was seen by the rest of the hospital sector as favourable. This appears to have been part of a strategy by Bevan to buy off the medical elite – the top consultants – who worked in these hospitals. The consultants were also courted with generous salaries, merit awards, the retention of pay beds within NHS hospitals, and the option of combining private practice with NHS work. The strategy was apparently successful in promoting the support of the consultants. Hence the famous comment attributed to Bevan that he 'stuffed their mouths with gold' (cited by Timmins, 1995, p. 115).

Aside from these concessions, the consultants tended to take a more favourable view of the NHS than their colleagues in general practice. Many consultants believed that a comprehensive state health system would produce a more efficient and technically advanced service. The GPs, on the other hand, were more concerned about threats to their independence. These differences were reflected in the divisions between the BMA, a stout defender of GPs' interests (and strongly opposed to Bevan's initial plan), and the Royal Colleges, representing the consultants' views, which were more supportive of the government's plans. Indeed, the BMA only agreed to advise its members to join the NHS at the 'eleventh hour', following a series of concessions from Bevan and several ballots of its membership. Senior members of the Royal Colleges – such as Lord Moran, the President of the Royal College of Physicians – were active behind the scenes in building support for the NHS and in promoting a compromise between Bevan and the GPs (Webster, 1988, p. 116).

Aneurin Bevan is popularly remembered as the father of the NHS. Yet, as Honigsbaum (1989, p. 217) has observed, 'Bevan had the good fortune to spearhead a movement that already had force.' Yet one should not belittle his contribution. Bevan's vision, skill and strategy made possible the political settlement that allowed the NHS to emerge. Moreover, this generated an organisational structure which, though flawed, was to last almost thirty years.

The Experience of the NHS: 1948–79

The NHS provided a comprehensive system of health care, available to all, which was not based on the ability to pay at the point of delivery. The fact that the service was national raised the possibility that a high standard of health care could become available to all. The bringing together of a range of services under the direct responsibility of the Ministry of Health created the potential for a more coherent, planned and integrated health care system. Finally, the funding mechanism for the new service – based on taxation (with a contribution from National Insurance funds) – meant that spending on the NHS would be under the watchful eye of the Treasury. This arrangement ensured that the NHS became one of the most cost-effective health care systems in the world.

The NHS became a popular institution. For the generation that lived under the previous system, it represented a major achievement. It was similarly popular with the generation that grew up with the welfare state. However, despite its popularity, the NHS has faced a number of problems during its lifetime and has not always tackled these successfully (Webster, 1988, 1996). By the late 1970s the situation became so serious that even the considerable achievements of the NHS appeared to be under threat. The NHS came to be widely perceived as in a constant state of crisis (Haywood and Alaszewski, 1980). This impression continued throughout the 1980s and into the 1990s (see Chapter 5). Some of the difficulties facing the NHS were evident from its earliest days, and arose from its original organisational structure and financial framework. Others were new, reflecting fresh challenges and rising expectations of the service. Another set of problems was caused, at least in part, by botched attempts to reform and reorganise the service, while others were due to changes in the wider political and economic environment.

Problems with the Structure of the NHS

As noted earlier, the original structure of the NHS in England and Wales was tripartite, comprising the family practitioner services (GPs, dentists, pharmacists and opticians) administered by executive councils, local authority community health services (such as community-based nursing and midwifery), personal social services and public health, and the nationalised hospital service.

It was soon evident that the original NHS structure was flawed. The major problems were overlap, duplication and lack of co-ordination between the three parts of the structure (Ministry of Health, 1959, 1963; BMA, 1962; Allsop, 1984, pp. 50–2). During the 1960s the structure came under increasing pressure, leading ultimately to government proposals to reorganise the service (Ministry of Health, 1968; DHSS, 1970). After some deliberation, and two changes of government, new proposals were brought forward (DHSS, 1971; Cmnd 5055, 1972) and a reorganisation eventually implemented in 1974. Separate reorganisations were implemented in Scotland, Wales and Northern Ireland (see Exhibit 4.1).

The new structure in England embodied three tiers of health service management below the Department of Health and Social Security (DHSS) (which had succeeded the Ministry of Health in 1968) at regional, area and district level. New health authorities, responsible for planning and development of services were established at regional and area level. Like the RHBs and HMCs which preceded them, these bodies were ultimately accountable to ministers and appointed under their authority.

The reorganisation did not solve the structural problems of the service. The family practitioner services supplied by GPs, dentists, pharmacists and opticians

---

Exhibit 4.1 The NHS Outside England (1948–79)

Different NHS organisational structures were established in Scotland from the outset. The Scottish NHS was the responsibility of the Secretary of State for Scotland. Although the Scottish health services were organised according to the same tripartite principle found in England and Wales, there were some differences; for example, the Scottish teaching hospitals did not have their own separate governing structures, and the ambulance service came under the hospital service rather than the local authority health services. The Scottish NHS was reorganised in 1974, but again there were differences from England and Wales. This involved the creation of health boards administering health services formerly organised under the tripartite system: hospital, community health and family practitioner services. Another feature of this new organisation was the creation of a Common Service Agency providing support services to the central administration and health boards.

In Northern Ireland, the NHS had developed in a different way, largely as a result of the province's self-governing arrangements (suspended in 1972 as a result of the 'troubles' and recently resurrected in a different form). The NHS in Northern Ireland was reorganised in 1973. Responsibility for health care (including hospital and community health services) and social services was given to Health and Social Service Boards covering four geographical areas. Under each board was a district, responsible for planning, managing and co-ordinating health and social services. A Central Services Agency undertook some functions undertaken by the new family practitioner committees created in England and Wales (such as payments to family practitioners) as well as other NHS support services.

In Wales, the seventies brought a measure of administrative devolution for the NHS. The Secretary of State for Wales acquired the responsibility for the NHS in Wales from 1974. The reorganisation of the NHS in the same year highlighted other differences, notably the absence of a regional tier. As in Scotland and Northern Ireland, Wales had a similar body for common services (the Welsh Health Technical Services Organisation, later renamed the Common Services Agency).

Sources: R. Levitt, A. Wall and J. Appleby *The Reorganised National Health Service*, ch. 6; C. Webster *Health Services since the War, Volume I.*

---

were not fully integrated. They remained separate, under new family practitioner committees (FPCs) which replaced the former executive councils. The NHS became responsible for community health services, transferred from local government. But the latter retained responsibility for environmental health services and social care. So there remained three separate agencies involved in the provision of state health care. Tripartism proved remarkably resilient (see Figure 4.2).

The new NHS structure was criticised for having surplus tiers of management and requiring too many administrators. New systems of planning and management which accompanied these organisational changes were similarly criticised. These were held responsible for slow decision-making and a lack of accountability. Yet the search for an 'organisational fix' (Klein, 1983, p. 90) continued. Despite the problems associated with the reorganisation, policy-makers still placed their faith in structural reform (McLachlan, 1990) giving rise to a further reorganisation in 1982 (see Chapter 6).

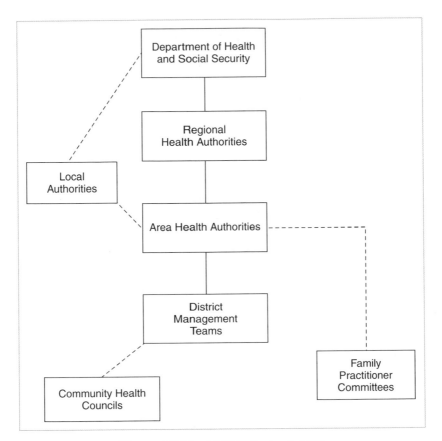

Figure 4.2 The NHS in England, 1974

Accountability, Control and Planning

The problems of the NHS were more than just structural. It became clear that there was a fundamental contradiction at the heart of the NHS with respect to the powers and responsibilities of Health Ministers. Health Ministers had full responsibility for health policy, but had little direct control over the activities of the NHS. It was well-known that power over service developments was concentrated at local level; in the hands of doctors who were not accountable to ministers for their actions or for the resources they used. At the end of the day the medical profession had an effective veto power over the implementation of policies. But health authorities, responsible to and appointed by ministers (yet drawn in part from local government and the health professions), could not be relied upon to implement policies designed by central government (Haywood and Alaszewski, 1980; Elcock and Haywood, 1980).

Government nevertheless attempted to influence service developments through the health authorities. Instead of clarifying the goals of the service, it preferred to emphasise the importance of specific service developments. This began with the Hospital Plan of 1962 (Cmnd 1604, 1962), which, although closely associated with the then Minister of Health, Enoch Powell, was already in motion before his arrival (Webster, 1996, p. 102). This was essentially a plan for capital expenditure in the hospital sector, though it did set out norms for the provision of beds for various medical specialities. The Hospital Plan has been seen as an important landmark in the history of the NHS, and of the British welfare state (Lowe, 1997). As Mohan (2002) has observed, it followed 13 years of limited achievements and represented an important symbolic commitment to plan future services on a rational basis – with regard to needs. Its shortcomings have also been widely acknowledged (see Mohan, 2002). The bed 'norms' were a crude benchmark of need, and reflected a more general technical problem – the lack of good information about service needs and standards. The Plan served to underline the dominance of the hospital sector and, (despite the publication of a community health services plan the following year, Cmnd 1973, 1963) did nothing to redress the imbalance between hospital and community services or to promote their integration. Finally, the plan was vulnerable to cost pressures and economic circumstances. As a result, capital spending did not accelerate as planned.

A more elaborate planning process for the NHS was introduced in 1976. Ministers explicitly set out their priorities, emphasising the so-called 'Cinderella services' (services for the elderly, the mentally ill and the mentally and physically disabled), primary care and preventive medicine (DHSS, 1976a, 1977). This guidance was filtered down to the lowest tiers of the NHS, which formulated their own plans within this framework. These plans were then passed back up the structure to enable the DHSS to monitor the consistency of the local and national plans and the overall development of services. The planning process was persuasive rather than directive. Health authorities (and the medical profession at local level) were thus able to resist a dramatic shift in priorities. The planning process was also criticised as being too cumbersome, and involving too many advisory and planning bodies. This prolonged the planning process, confused the setting of objectives and inhibited the achievement of new priorities.

Funding, Efficiency and Resource Allocation

Since its creation, the resourcing of the NHS has been a constant issue of debate. The NHS had hardly begun its life before it was faced by a financial crisis (Webster, 1988). In the 1950s the Conservative government, worried about the resources consumed by the service, established the Guillebaud inquiry into the NHS. The report of this inquiry (Cmnd 9663, 1956) was unexpectedly favourable, concluding that spending on the NHS was not as extravagant as some had suggested, and that in many respects it provided good value for money. The Guillebaud report also pointed out that there were deficiencies in some services and that this required more spending rather than less.

The Guillebaud report strengthened the case of those who argued for greater NHS expenditure. It also seemed to settle publicly the issue of how the NHS should be funded. One of the major controversies of the immediate postwar period surrounded the issue of how resources should be raised. The Labour Government's decision in 1951 to introduce patient charges for spectacles and dentures – which led to the resignation of Bevan and other ministers – was followed by the Conservative government's introduction of prescription charges. But, throughout the fifties and sixties, alternative funding mechanisms were actively being considered by Government 'behind closed doors' (see Webster, 1996). Ideas included support for a contribution-based funding system – a form of state health insurance – for consultation fees when visiting a GP and for additional charges for food and accommodation while in hospital. These, however, were rejected by government before they could be turned into concrete policy proposals. Nonetheless, these issues arose again and again in subsequent decades (see Chapter 6).

During the 1960s health expenditure continued to grow – though it had to compete with other social policy priorities such as education, for example, and did not always succeed (see Webster, 1996, pp. 188–9). Then, in the 1970s, government attempted to exert a much tighter control over public expenditure in view of the deepening economic crisis. The NHS, like many other public services, faced financial restraint. This in turn focused even greater attention on the need for greater efficiency in order to maximise the use of existing resources.

At the same time, it also became evident that something had to be done about the distribution of resources. As Webster (1996, p. 28) has observed, many of the 'notorious inequalities' which had discredited the prewar system of health services had been imported into the NHS. Ministers attempted to redirect resources to 'neglected' groups, such as the elderly, in line with their priorities. Also there was an increasing emphasis on geographical inequalities in health service funding. In the 1970s the highest-spending NHS regions spent around two-thirds more per head than the lowest-spending regions (Griffiths, 1971). In an attempt to iron out these inequalities, and to ensure that health authorities received a budget more appropriate to the health needs they faced, the Labour government introduced the RAWP (Resource Allocation Working Party) formula in 1977 (Mays and Bevan, 1987).

RAWP sought to allocate resources on the basis of a formula reflecting each region's relative health care needs. First, an assessment of relative need was established based on indicators of illness, such as regional population size and structure, standardised mortality ratios for specific conditions, and so on. Secondly, a target level of funding for each region was calculated by dividing the resources available by the estimate of relative need. Thirdly, in view of the likely disruption caused by changing the funding system immediately, budgets were allocated in such a way as to move the regions towards their target funding levels. Hence, over a number of years, those regions below their target received a greater increase in their resources than those regions over target.

Scotland, Northern Ireland and Wales had their own equivalents of RAWP which similarly sought to relate budgets to indicators of need. Yet while the case for a more rational allocation system was widely accepted, there was much concern about the operation of these schemes in practice (Goldacre and Harris, 1980; Radical Statistics Health Group, 1977). This centred mainly on the accuracy of the indicators of need within the redistributive formula. There was particular criticism of the use of standardised mortality ratios. Many observers regarded morbidity data as being a better indicator of the need for health services, while others argued that indicators of deprivation provided a better measure given the relationship between poverty and ill health.

The formula was also attacked for failing to account for the different costs facing each region (and each district therein). Some modifications were made to the formula to reflect the higher costs of delivering services in London, teaching hospitals, supra-regional specialties (provided for the benefit of populations in more than one region), and cross-boundary flows (the treatment of patients from another region). Despite these changes, RAWP was still regarded by many as a rather blunt instrument which in times of financial stringency could have serious effects on services in those districts which lost out in the redistributive process.

There was also the related question of health inequalities and the access to health services. The NHS had been created as a free service, though charges were subsequently imposed. Yet despite the removal of most of the financial barriers to care, social class differences in health status persisted. It was also alleged that the provision of health services favoured the middle classes, and that working-class people faced problems of access to services. The Labour government of the 1970s responded to increasing concern by setting up a working party under Sir Douglas Black, to examine health inequalities (see Chapter 13). Related to this was an acknowledgement that the NHS was divorced from many of the factors that influenced health and had little impact on social, economic and environmental factors. This was remedied to a limited extent by a greater emphasis on health promotion and prevention from the 1970s onwards (Baggott, 2000).

Primary and Community Health Services

Throughout the postwar period, at least up until the 1980s, the primary care sector was regarded as a relatively neglected area, with considerable scope for improvement (Marks, 1988; Taylor, 1988). But the sector was not given priority

(Stowe, 1989). Politicians realised that building a new hospital was far more popular than extending primary care services. This mentality reinforced decisions about resources, with the hospital sector increasing its share of the NHS budget up to the 1980s.

The reasons for this relative neglect are not difficult to discover. At the time the NHS was created, the status of those working in primary care was much lower than that of their colleagues in the hospital sector, as reflected, for example, in the relationship between hospital consultants and GPs. In addition, professionals working in the hospital sector tended to have more political influence than those in primary care. The differences in status and political influence persisted to a considerable extent over the postwar period. A further problem for the primary care services was their lack of visibility. With the possible exception of the family doctor service, the public never seemed to regard them with the same kind of importance as hospital services. This continues to some extent today, posing particular problems for those seeking to adjust the balance between primary and secondary care (see Chapter 10).

Differences in prestige, political influence and political visibility provide only a partial explanation of why primary care was neglected by policy makers. To some extent, central government did not have the means to forge new directions in primary care. Until 1974 community health services were largely in the hands of the local authorities, and central government faced considerable difficulties in developing a national vision for these highly fragmented local services. Furthermore, primary care services provided by the NHS structure were delivered largely by independent contractors: GPs, dentists, pharmacists and opticians. Beyond altering these contracts, government could not compel the professions to support particular policy initiatives. Even when contracts were altered, it was mainly a response to the grievances of the professions rather than to public concern about the quality of services. But by the end of the 1970s reform could not be avoided any longer. Three main problems were increasingly evident: professional rivalries; poor management and co-ordination; and, in some areas, poor-quality services.

The Primary Health Care Team (PHCT) had been encouraged in the 1960s to improve professional co-operation (Ministry of Health, 1963). This involved the attachment of nurses, health visitors, midwives (and sometimes other professionals, such as social workers) to GP practices. While the PHCT was regarded as a step forward, such arrangements sometimes failed (DHSS, 1981a). GPs tended to dominate, much to the annoyance of the other professions, thus undermining co-operation. In addition, PHCTs were rarely based on explicit agreements about each participant's role and this led to poor co-ordination and a failure to recognise mutual responsibilities.

Primary care also suffered from a fragmented management system. An opportunity was missed in 1974 when Family Practitioner Committees (FPCs) replaced the old Executive Councils in England and Wales. The FPCs' main task, like their predecessors, was to administer the contracts of GPs, dentists, pharmacists and opticians. But they lacked a clear management role. To complicate matters further, other primary care professions, such as district nurses, were from 1974 onwards managed by District Management Teams (DMTs). Collaboration between DMTs and FPCs was poor, with neither willing to accept overall management responsibility (see Ottewill and Wall, 1990). To make matters worse, primary health care services were poorly co-ordinated with community care provided by local government. Attempts to improve co-ordination of health and social services through joint planning had a limited impact, as will be shown in Chapters 10 and 11.

Finally, there was an increasing concern about the quality and effectiveness of primary care services. The Royal College of General Practitioners, in its evidence to the Royal Commission on the NHS (see below), mentioned unacceptably low standards in a minority of practices. There was particular criticism of primary care in inner cities, where needs were often complex and services limited. Initially, worries about effectiveness and quality of services were confined to specific areas or practices. However, the increasing demands being placed on the primary care sector began to generate more fundamental concerns about its ability to deliver high-quality services. There is a further discussion of the development of these services in Chapter 10.

Industrial Action, Professional Power and the Consumer

The 1970s saw a marked deterioration in industrial relations in the health service, reflecting general trends in British society. The government became embroiled in pay disputes with all classes of NHS staff: nurses, doctors and ancillary workers. In addition, the government faced the threat of industrial action from hospital doctors (and some of the unions representing ancillary workers) over the issue of pay beds in the NHS.

Industrial action in the NHS was not new. In 1965 GPs had threatened to resign from the NHS in a dispute over pay and conditions (Rivett, 1998). The differences between the 1970s and previous disputes were in terms of scale, regularity and intensity (Webster, 1996, p. 63). The 1970s not only saw more days lost (298,000 working days were lost to the NHS through industrial action in 1973 compared with only 500 in 1966), but the ferocity of the disputes was of a different order. It was, as Edwards (1993, p. 22) observed, that 'the emotional barriers against strike action in the NHS had been breached'.

Industrial action, based mainly on the protection of the interests of workers and professionals, disrupted services for patients. Yet, surprisingly, this, along with other problems such as the length of waiting lists and the occasional scandals of malpractice or ill-treatment, never seriously damaged the public's support for the NHS and it remained a popular institution, though, as Edwards,

(1993, p. 29) notes, public confidence in the NHS and its management was dented. There was, however, no room for complacency. The growth of the private sector in the late 1970s illustrated that some people were beginning to vote with their feet. There was also a feeling that once support for the NHS began to subside, the whole edifice might cave in.

Certainly, there were signs that patients were not quite as passive as they had once been. Wider concerns about the quality of health services and their responsiveness to consumer pressures grew in the 1960s and 1970s. Notably there were several high-profile scandals in long-stay hospitals, which led to the introduction of the Hospital Advisory Service to report on conditions (Klein, 1983, p. 80). Subsequently, the 1974 reorganisation introduced Community Health Councils to represent patients' views. In 1973 Parliament created the Health Service Commissioner to investigate maladministration in the NHS. There were also moves to improve complaints procedures, though these efforts did not come to fruition for some time (see Chapter 12).

The Royal Commission on the NHS

The accumulation of these various problems by the mid-1970s contributed to a growing sense of crisis in the NHS. The Labour government responded in May 1976 by establishing a Royal Commission to consider 'the best use and management of financial and manpower resources of the NHS' (Cmnd 7615, 1979, p. 1). The Royal Commission was not intended as a tool of radical change; indeed, its membership was carefully selected to avoid such an outcome. Yet it was, as Edwards (1993, p. 37) has noted, 'probably one of the most comprehensive reviews of a health service undertaken anywhere in the world'.

The Royal Commission noted the absence of clear objectives in the NHS and sought to remedy this by setting out seven key objectives. These were: to encourage and assist individuals to remain healthy; to provide equality of entitlement to health services; to provide a broad range of services to a high standard; to provide equality of access to these services; to provide a service free at the time of use; to satisfy the reasonable expectations of its users; and to remain a national service responsive to local needs. The commission's assessment of the situation facing the NHS was less gloomy than most. It identified social and geographical inequalities as being a particular problem, but added that this could not be tackled by the NHS alone. It also urged greater efforts to prevent ill health (through an extension of screening programmes and the compulsory wearing of seat belts by motorists and front-seat passengers). Nevertheless, the commission believed that the performance of the NHS could be improved in many areas, and that much of this improvement could be achieved through greater efficiency.

Many of the commission's 117 recommendations fell on stony ground. For example, it unsuccessfully urged direct accountability of the regional health authorities to Parliament and the abolition of charges. The commission's argument for the abolition of a tier of management below the regional level, however, was enthusiastically pursued, as was the recommendation for a limited list of prescribed medicines. The passage of time also saw the commission's recommendations for medical audit, the extension of screening programmes and the merger of health authorities and family practitioner authorities taken up by government. The acceptance of some of the Royal Commission's conclusions and recommendations by the incoming Conservative Government (see Chapter 5) exemplifies certain continuities in health policy-making. Nevertheless, change was the theme of the 1980s and 1990s in health care, as in many other areas of public policy. These changes arose from the general approach of the Thatcher government, explored in the next chapter.

Conclusion

This chapter has shown that many of today's health and health care issues (problems of funding and finance, access to services, inequalities, problems of accountability and workforce relations, poor co-ordination between agencies, and problems relating to the quality of care) have their origins in the past. Moreover, it has indicated that attempts by Government to deal with these problems have important precedents. Indeed, as will become clear, contemporary reforms often re-open old policy debates and reawaken interest in policy proposals previously disregarded.

_____ *Further Reading*_____

Allsop, J. (1995) *Health Policy and the NHS – Towards 2000*, 2nd edn (Harlow, Longman).

Hodgkinson, R. (1967) *The Origins of the NHS: The Medical Services of the New Poor Law* (London, Wellcome Foundation).

Klein, R. (1983) *The Politics of the National Health Service* (London, Longman).

Klein, R. (1995) *The New Politics of the NHS*, 3rd edn (London, Longman).

Klein, R. (2000) *The New Politics of the NHS*, 4th edn (London, Prentice-Hall).

Mohan, J. (2002) *Planning, Markets and Hospitals* (London, Routledge).

Rivett, G. (1998) *From Cradle to Grave: Fifty Years of the NHS* (London, King's Fund).

Timmins, N. (1995) *The Five Giants: A Biography of the Welfare State* (London, Harper Collins).

Webster, C. (1988) *Health Services Since the War, Volume I: Problems of Health Care. The National Health Service before 1957* (London, HMSO).

Webster, C. (1996) *Government and Health Care, Volume II: The National Health Service 1958–79* (London, HMSO).

Webster, C. (2002) *The National Health Service: A Political History*, 2nd edn (Oxford, Oxford University Press).

Health Policy from Thatcher to Blair

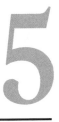

In this chapter the development of health policy under the Conservative Governments of Margaret Thatcher and John Major is examined, along with the implementation of their reforms and their impact on the NHS. This is followed by a discussion of the Blair Government's reform agenda and its approach to the continuing problems of the health care system.

Thatcherism and Health Policy

Margaret Thatcher's victory for the Conservative Party at the 1979 general election is regarded as an important watershed for the welfare state and public services (Timmins, 1995). Her style, approach and policies represented a considerable break with the past (Jenkins, 1987; Riddell, 1991; Young, 1991). Strongly influenced by the New Right perspective (see Chapter 3), the Thatcher Governments attempted to transform many aspects of the postwar settlement, favouring private sector solutions to those offered by the public sector, privatisation to nationalisation, lower taxes above public spending, deregulation to state control. They also promoted self-help and voluntary solutions to social problems and were disposed against interventionist policies to reduce poverty. The Thatcher Governments also pursued a managerialist approach to public services. This led to an increased emphasis upon private sector management principles and techniques, a stronger focus on efficiency, cost control, and performance measurement, and ultimately processes that were intended to mimic market mechanisms.

The NHS, as a key public service and cornerstone of the welfare state, employing over a million people and accounting for around a tenth of public spending, could not escape this political trend. The Thatcher Governments were *conviction* governments, undaunted by powerful vested interests such as the medical profession and the health service trade unions which had held sway over previous governments. Moreover, they benefited from a favourable political environment – long periods in office, large parliamentary majorities, a supportive media, a passive public and a feeble political opposition. However, 'Thatcherism', despite its ideological roots, remained a pragmatic philosophy, lacking coherence and purpose (Gamble, 1994; Young, 1991). There was often a gap between radical intention and outcome (Marsh and Rhodes, 1992), and the NHS was, initially at least, to some extent protected from the Thatcher Governments' reforming zeal by its public popularity and the lobbying activities of producer groups such as the BMA. Other sectors, such as housing, underwent a much more radical change in the 1980s (see Timmins, 1995). Nonetheless, the impact of the Thatcher Governments on health policy and the NHS should not be underestimated. Indeed, the broad approach of these policies survived long after Thatcher herself had left office.

Reorganisation and Management Reform

In retrospect, the Thatcher Governments appear quite conservative in their handling of the NHS during the first two terms of office (1979–83; 1983–7). Initially, continuity rather than change was the order of the day, as the government responded to the recommendations of the Royal Commission established by its Labour predecessor (see Chapter 4). This led to a reorganisation that abolished Area Health Authorities (AHAs) and established a large number of District Health Authorities (DHAs) at local level (see Figure 5.1). Meanwhile, planning and professional advisory systems were simplified (Hambleton, 1983) and detailed central guidelines to the NHS were replaced by a general statement of priorities from the central government department then responsible for health policy, the Department of Health and Social Security (DHSS, 1981b). The approach was decentralist rather than directive, with the government distancing itself from the problems of the service at local level. However, priorities were much the same as under the Labour government, save for an added emphasis on private sector involvement, evident in a reversal of the previous government's policy on NHS pay beds. Health Ministers also established a review of alternative ways of financing health service, though the report was never published (Timmins, 1995, pp. 388–90).

Undoubtedly there were controversies. In 1982, with a general election looming, Thatcher herself famously declared that the NHS was 'safe with us' and that 'adequate health care should be available to all, regardless of ability to pay' (Thatcher, 1982). This followed the leak of a Central Policy Review Staff (CPRS) report on the welfare state that had proposed a raft of controversial measures, such as increased and extended charges for health services (including visits to the family doctor) and an expansion of private health insurance. Although Thatcher allegedly wanted to pursue these ideas (Young, 1991, p. 301), her colleagues persuaded her to reject them. Nonetheless, the media and public hostility towards these proposals did not abate. Although the Conservatives won the 1983 general election by a comfortable margin, they realised they had to tread carefully in future. However, to do nothing was not an option, and

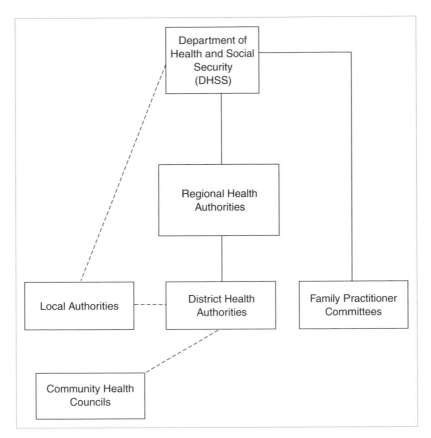

Figure 5.1 The NHS in England, 1982

their resolve to act was strengthened by a series of major strikes among health workers in 1982.

An inquiry was therefore conducted into NHS management, prompted to some extent by industrial action, and partly by the dilemmas posed by decentralisation. As noted earlier, the DHSS had adopted a less interventionist approach. Although this had political advantages – it was believed that local health authorities would be blamed for the shortcomings of the service – it raised issues of accountability. One of the problems with the NHS since its creation was that it was a national service funded mainly out of general taxation, which created pressures to hold the DHSS (and formerly the Ministry of Health) and the NHS to account (see Klein, 1995). These pressures intensified as central government, and in particular the Treasury, sought to restrain public spending and introduce a more managerialist approach to public services. Indeed, prior to the NHS management inquiry the DHSS had already established a system of review, setting clearer central objectives and monitoring health authority performance.

The management inquiry was undertaken by a small team of people with business experience chaired by Sir Roy Griffiths (the deputy chairman and managing director of Sainsbury's). Although its original remit covered England, its recommendations were subsequently applied to other parts of the UK. The Griffiths Inquiry report (DHSS, 1983), which was succinct, focused on the absence of a clear line of management responsibility in the NHS, summed up in the observation that 'if Florence Nightingale were carrying her lamp through the corridors of the NHS today, she would almost certainly be searching for the people in charge' (p. 12). Much of the blame was laid at the door of 'consensus management', the existing method of decision-making introduced in 1974. Under this system, management teams were drawn from a variety of backgrounds including administration, finance, nursing and medicine. In principle, no member of the management team had superior status and each had the power to veto decisions. Although this form of decision-making had advantages, in particular that the management team had to consider different perspectives before arriving at a decision, it was held responsible for delays in decision-making, avoidance of tough decisions, and blurred responsibility.

The inquiry also identified a confusion of responsibilities between the DHSS and the NHS. Echoing an earlier investigation (DHSS, 1976b), it found that the DHSS actually intervened too much in the detailed affairs of health authorities, contrary to the declared policy of decentralisation and delegation, and that this was undertaken in a haphazard and inconsistent way. Furthermore, the inquiry was highly critical of failure to address the needs of consumers and to achieve national policy objectives. It identified an absence of clear objectives for the NHS, and insufficient performance monitoring, while acknowledging the department's recent efforts to introduce performance review.

The Griffiths Inquiry Recommendations

The Griffiths Inquiry recommended the creation of two new boards within the DHSS: a Health Services Supervisory Board (HSSB), chaired by the Secretary of State and responsible for NHS strategy, reviewing performance and allocating overall resources, and an NHS Management Board, accountable to the HSSB for the management of the NHS. The aim was to separate policy (and, by implication, politics) from management. This arrangement got off to a very bad start, with the resignation of the chairman of the NHS Management Board amid allegations of political interference. Secondly, Griffiths recommended that existing arrangements be replaced by general management, defined as 'the responsibility drawn together in one person, at different levels of the organisation, for planning, implementation and control of performance'. It was intended that general managers would take overall responsibility for service performance and management at regional, district and unit level. The rationale for general management was that it would improve leadership, clarify responsibility, promote greater accountability and achieve cost-efficiency. Thirdly, the inquiry argued that accountability would be further strengthened by including units, such as hospitals, within the annual review process currently used to monitor the performance of health authorities, thus creating a line of accountability from service providers up to the Management Board. Fourthly, a key role was identified for health authority chairpersons at regional and district level in the implementation of general management, by taking a lead role in appointments and performance monitoring. Chairpersons would be expected to take on an important leadership role in the organisation of health authority business, as well as having a specific brief to promote efficiency.

The Griffiths report made other recommendations, such as the introduction of cost-improvement programmes to improve efficiency. It recommended the development of management budgeting systems to relate clinical workload directly to resources, and urged that doctors become more closely involved in processes of management and budgeting (see Chapter 9). The report recommended better information about the effectiveness and efficiency of services. It urged managers to evaluate performance, particularly from the patient's perspective, and wanted this to be incorporated in the planning and management of services.

Implementing Griffiths

The Government was keen that general managers be recruited from outside the NHS, in particular from business. But the attractions of NHS management were limited, remuneration packages relatively poor and contracts short-term. Hence, the majority of general managers – around two-thirds – were former NHS administrators. Only a fifth of regional and district general managers, and less than one in ten unit general managers, came from outside the NHS. The remainder were drawn from a nursing or medical background.

The Griffiths report laid the foundations of future management reform. As Edwards (1993, pp. 122–3) reflected, 'there is little doubt that without the development of general management it would have been difficult, if not impossible, to deliver the later reforms' (see also Harrison et al., 1992). Following the implementation of its recommendations, other changes were introduced in an effort to encourage a more entrepreneurial management culture, including new financial incentives for managers, such as performance-related pay and more generous remuneration packages. NHS management structures were reformed so that they more closely resembled structures of decision-making found in the business sector (see Chapter 7). Furthermore, an array of management techniques used widely in commercial organisations were imported into the health service. Finally, the advent of the NHS internal market represented an attempt to create a decision-making environment that imitated a commercial environment, with contracts and prices, buyers and sellers.

Management Structures

Griffiths argued for a more streamlined and efficient NHS management system. Central to this philosophy was that once objectives were set, managers should be given the freedom to achieve them. Following Griffiths, general managers re-fashioned their management structures, and because these changes often reflected local personalities and conditions, senior management structures began to diversify. Management structures below board level also began to change, with the introduction of clinical directorates – discussed in Chapter 9. Diversity was further encouraged by the creation of NHS trusts, which were given a certain amount of freedom in determining their internal management arrangements. Nonetheless, there were important continuities. Consensus management, although formally abandoned, persisted to some extent informally (Strong and Robinson, 1990, pp. 143–4). Some health authorities attempted to retain its advantages by emphasising teamwork at board level. Others believed that a 'macho' management style would backfire and that more could be achieved by working constructively with the professions and other staff. Elsewhere, however, new management styles and structures created conflict between managers and staff.

Another important aspect of the new management arrangements was the key role played by health authority (and, later, trust) chairpersons. Evidence concerning the role of health authority members following the implementation of Griffiths indicated that the balance of power within health authorities tended to reside with the chairperson and the general manager (Strong and Robinson, 1990; Ferlie, Ashburner and Fitzgerald, 1993). The chairperson had a key role, not only in the organisation of health authority business but in the appointment of the general manager and in the assessment of his or her performance.

Privatisation

Another important policy of the 1980s was to encourage the private sector. There was a drive to encourage people to take out private health insurance. Private health insurance coverage did increase, from 4 per cent to almost 12 per cent of the adult population between 1978 and 1990, but this was nowhere near the level which some of the Thatcherites wanted. Even the introduction of extended tax relief (to the over-60s) in 1989 failed to have the desired impact. Efforts to extend competitive tendering in the NHS, whereby the private sector would compete with current 'in-house' provision of services such as cleaning, catering and laundry, also faced problems. This policy, introduced in 1983 in England and Wales, was strongly resisted by the trade unions and by some health authorities. However, private contractors were accused of poor standards of service. In addition 'in-house' bids were often successful. Eventually the rules were changed to benefit external contractors, though 'in-house' bids continued to win the majority of contracts. However, the policy did increase the use of casual workers and reduce unionisation in these services. It also tended to reduce costs further in the short term, as the 'in-house' bids had to make cost savings in order to secure the contract in the face of competition. The policy may also have contributed to poor standards of hygiene and cleanliness, and thereby to hospital-acquired infections (see Chapter 9).

Radical Reform?: The NHS Internal Market

Following Thatcher's third general election victory in 1987, a period of policy change for the NHS was heralded in the form of the internal market. This policy emerged from a review of the NHS, prompted by a financial crisis (Timmins, 1988). The financial problems of the service had been blamed for ward closures and the cancellation of operations. Professionals, trade unions and patients complained vociferously about the state of the NHS, and their cause was taken up in the media and in Parliament. When the offer of additional funding failed to stop this criticism, the Prime Minister announced a full-scale review of the NHS, which bore all the hallmarks of the Thatcher Government's policy style: speedy, secretive and leader-driven (Butler, 1992; Griggs, 1991). Thatcher chaired the review committee, which consisted of her health advisor, Sir Roy Griffiths, health ministers and Treasury ministers. There were no formal consultations with organised interests, though medical and management opinion was 'sounded out'. In addition, individuals and organisations submitted their ideas for reform.

The review focused on two main areas. Alternative systems of finance – such as insurance-based systems (see Chapter 6) – were ruled out largely because the tax-funded system was viewed as having several advantages, notably low revenue-collection costs. There was, however, some support (notably from Thatcher herself) for encouraging private insurance through extending tax relief. This was opposed by the Treasury, and a compromise was reached in the form of the extension of tax relief on private health insurance for the elderly, referred to earlier. The review concentrated mainly upon the allocation of resources within the NHS. There was some support within the review team for greater competition within the NHS and for a decentralisation of management responsibility. Competition had been championed by a number of economists, politicians and think tanks (Brown et al., 1988; Butler and Pirie, 1988; Owen, 1988; Redwood, 1988; Whitney, 1988). They drew on ideas from overseas, particularly from the US, where increasing competition, in the form of Health Maintenance Organisations (HMO) had been credited with promoting greater cost-effectiveness. Particular interest was shown in the arguments of Alain Enthoven (1985), an American academic who, a few years earlier, had suggested competition as a remedy for the problems of the NHS. Interestingly, Enthoven's ideas had been considered before by the NHS Management Board and rejected, though experiments based on his ideas were initiated (see Butler, 1992, pp. 23–4; Owen, 1988, pp. 102–6).

Exhibit 5.1 Health Maintenance Organisations and Managed Care

The number and coverage of Health Maintenance Organisations (HMOs) grew in the USA during the 1980s and, by the end of the decade, one in five of the population was enrolled in such schemes. Although there was considerable variation between different schemes, the principle was much the same. HMOs agree to cover the cost of the care of enrolled members when they need it, while exercising control over how these services are funded and provided. The development of HMOs and other forms of managed care arose out of concern among those who funded health care, principally large employers and the state, about the rising cost of health care. They believed that HMOs would increase competition and lower costs, while at the same time seeking to improve the quality of service. Others were less sanguine, pointing out that HMOs underprovided services for the poor and chronically ill (Petchey, 1987). Some HMOs succumbed to financial pressures or scandals, and there was a move towards mergers, thereby reducing competition. Later studies indicated that HMOs could lead to a reduction in the quality and availability of services while not achieving the efficiency gains predicted (Salmon, 1995; Himmelstein et al., 1999). Particular criticism was levelled at for-profit HMOs, which grew rapidly in the 1990s. Ironically profitability began to fall, leading many HMOs to cut back on benefits and increase co-payments. In the US, however, there has been some backlash against HMOs. Patients now have stronger rights, following the passage of new legislation, and greater discretion is being introduced into the system, alongside appeal mechanisms, in order to head off legal action.

HMOs – and other forms of US managed care – emerged as a means of dealing with the high and rising cost of care, and, to some extent, the fragmentation of the US system of health care. But, despite their shortcomings, and with due regard to the problems of international comparison, some of the techniques they deployed – such as utilisation management and review (for example, authorisation of hospital admissions), physician profiling (comparing doctor's performance), disease management (organising care through guidelines and protocols), and financial incentives – have been linked to improved cost-effectiveness (see Robinson and Steiner, 1998; West, 1998; Grembowski et al., 2002). It has even been argued that US managed-care systems compare favourably with state health care systems such as the NHS. One study argued that a non-profit HMO achieved better outcomes than the NHS at similar cost owing to better integration of services, competition and superior IT systems (see page 151). Useful lessons may be learned from such systems (Fairfield et al., 1997), and the NHS has already introduced some of the techniques found in the US, such as clinical guidelines for example. However, caution should be exercised when importing approaches from other health care systems – particularly those such as the USA that have performed poorly on measures of cost and equity. Moreover, the NHS is itself a managed care system, and one that has had a relatively good track record in providing cost-effective, comprehensive care. Indeed, if the US experience is anything to go by, managed care could be seen as a vehicle for changes that increase bureaucracy, undermine professional autonomy, restrict access to services, and create further opportunities for the private sector.

Enthoven in fact warned against importing the HMO model into the NHS. Subsequently, the more radical schemes, involving the private sector and private funding to a greater extent (see, for example, Goldsmith and Willetts, 1988) were rejected by the Government review. There was, however, more support for schemes that encouraged a quasi-market within the NHS, especially 'fund-holder' schemes that gave GPs a key role in purchasing care from other providers (Bevan et al., 1988; Bosanquet, 1986; Culyer, Brazier and O'Donnell, 1988). These ideas apparently had a strong influence on the review, evident when the government's planned reforms were announced in the White Paper, *Working for Patients*, published in 1989 (Cm 555, 1989).

Working for Patients

The White Paper covered a wide range of proposals, some new and others modified from previous initiatives. The policy/management division proposed by Griffiths was resurrected with the creation of an NHS Policy Board, responsible for policy and strategy in the NHS, and a Management Board, to advise on policy and responsible for the day-to-day management of the service. The Policy Board comprised ministers and senior civil servants, specialist advisors, people with experience in managing large business and public sector organisations among others. The Management Board, headed by the Chief Executive of the NHS consisted of senior managers (finance, human resources, and so on). The NHS was subsequently renamed the NHS Management Executive (and then later, the NHS Executive). It became the headquarters of the NHS and in 1992 was relocated in Leeds, away from the London-based Department of Health (though it remained part of the department).

Other proposals in the White Paper included a change in the structure and management of health authorities. New bodies, called Family Health Service Authorities were given the task of managing family practitioner services. Both they and the District Health Authorities were expected to become more managerial in outlook and were reconstituted in ways discussed later in this chapter. The White Paper also proposed the extension of the Resource Management Initiative which aimed to relate clinical workload to resources (see Chapter 9).

The centrepiece of the reforms was the establishment of a division between purchasers and providers (see Figure 5.2). In future, services for NHS patients would be purchased on their behalf by GP fundholders and District Health Authorities (DHAs). GP practices that opted to join the fundholder scheme would be given a budget to purchase care for individual patients up to a financial limit. For more expensive services and for patients whose GP was not a fundholder, the DHA would pay for treatment. On the supply side, NHS hospitals and other provider units would supply services and earn revenue on the basis of service contracts. They could apply for trust status, and were encouraged

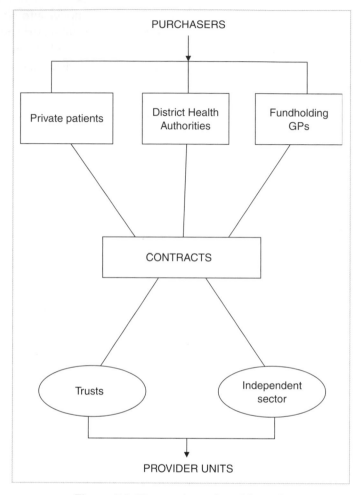

Figure 5.2 The purchaser/provider split

to do so by the promise of greater freedom to manage services. Those that did not remained under the direct management of health authorities. Notably the 'internal' market acknowledged private patients and private hospitals. There was a recognition that the boundaries between the NHS and the private sector markets would become increasingly blurred, as NHS hospitals contracted with private 'purchasers' of care and NHS purchasers contracted with private providers.

The reforms were enacted by the NHS and Community Care Act, 1990 (the community care element of the reforms is discussed in more detail in Chapter 11). Despite the controversy surrounding the legislation, and the opposition from professional groups and trade unions, it passed through Parliament with relative ease, thanks to the government's large majority. Once the legislation was in place, however, the government began to adopt a more cautious approach. The next general election was looming, and the government recognised that their policy was unpopular. The commercial language used by ministers to describe the reforms began to change. There was less talk of 'markets' and 'purchasing' and more emphasis on 'commissioning' services (Ham, 2000, p. 29). The pace of reform slowed (Butler, 1992). Thatcher, concerned about the impact of the reforms in the pre-election period, asked her advisors to investigate and was told that in the absence of systems of financial and management information, the internal market would not work (Ham, 2000, p. 11; Timmins, 1995, p. 471; see also Audit Commission, 1991; NAO, 1989, 1995). The Secretary of State for Health, Kenneth Clarke, argued that the reforms should be implemented, and the Prime Minister eventually agreed (although the community care sections of the Act were not implemented until after the 1992 election).

Although the reforms had the green light, implementation was gradual. Rather than introducing trust status and fundholding all at once, applications were invited from GP practices and hospitals to join the schemes. As a result, the reforms were phased in, beginning with the first wave of 57 provider units and 306 GP practices in 1991. Further 'waves' followed until by the mid-1990s almost all NHS providers in England were trusts and about half of patients in England and Wales were covered by GP fundholders. The implementation of the reforms in other parts of the UK proceeded more slowly (see Exhibit 5.2).

Exhibit 5.2 NHS Reform in Other Parts of the UK

The Conservatives' internal market reforms were implemented at different speeds in different parts of the UK. In Scotland, fundholding and trust status was slower to develop. By 1996 the majority of people north of the border were still covered by non-fundholding GPs, while the health care providers on the Scottish isles remained directly managed by health boards. As is often the case, in Northern Ireland the health reforms were implemented later than in the rest of the UK. But, by the same token, the features of the internal market as originally implemented survived longer there than elsewhere.

The Labour government's health reforms coincided with a fresh attempt to introduce devolution in the UK (Pollock, 1999). As a result, the Scottish Parliament acquired the power to make primary legislation in areas such as health, and to vary income-tax rates. In Wales, the powers and responsibilities of the Secretary of State for Wales were transferred to the Welsh Assembly, including those relating to health, such as health promotion, the allocation of resources, the organisation of the NHS and the holding of NHS bodies to account. These changes, along with attempts to devolve power to a Northern Ireland Assembly, increased the scope for diversity between the different health care systems (see Jervis and Hazell, 1998).

In Wales, for example, a separate White Paper on the NHS was published in 1998 (Welsh Office, 1998a). In contrast to England, the Welsh decided not to proceed with Primary Care Trusts. The task of advising health authorities on commissioning was undertaken by Local Health Groups (LHGs), similar to the Primary Care Groups in England, though these tended to be slower in developing their commissioning role than their English counterparts (Audit Commission, 2000a). The LHGs, unlike the English PCGs, were established so as to be consistent with local authority boundaries. They placed a high value on building

$\longrightarrow$

Exhibit 5.2 continued

→

collaborative links with local government and the voluntary sector. Subsequently, the Welsh NHS Plan also differed considerably from its English counterpart (National Assembly for Wales, 2001a). For example, it was more strongly oriented towards public heath. New structures were set up to implement the plan in the form of an All Wales Health and Wellbeing Council. Health authorities were abolished, and local health groups replaced by Local Health Boards (LHBs) responsible for commissioning and providing services. However, most health services other than primary care remained with NHS trusts. Also LHBs were required to operate a much more explicit partnership approach with local government and the voluntary sector. The Welsh Plan also included commitments not found in the NHS Plan for England, such as the freezing of prescription charges, the extension of free prescriptions to under-25s, free dental checks for under-25s and over-60s, and a new free eye-care service. Moreover, unlike England, there were no plans to abolish Community Health Councils. The Welsh NHS also differs from England in its planning and performance management system (see Exhibit 7.1).

Scotland also began to develop a distinctive approach (see Nottingham, 2000). In its White Paper on the NHS, the Scottish Executive did not create primary care groups (PCGs), but established PCTs at the outset (Secretary of State for Scotland, 1997). These were given responsibilities for community health services, mental health, continuing care for elderly people, services for disabled persons and primary care. GPs were encouraged, but not compelled, to join local health care cooperatives (LHCCs) under the auspices of the PCTs. The LHCCs were expected to lead service improvement and promote co-operation between practices (see Hopton and Heaney, 1999; Woods, 2001). Both primary care and hospital trusts were brought under new unified health boards, in effect bridging the division between commissioning and providing care. It was subsequently proposed that trusts be completely abolished (Scottish Executive, 2003a). New bodies – community health partnerships – were also proposed as a means of integrating services within the Health Board areas (see Exhibit 7.1 and Chapter 10). These would replace the LHCCs. Scotland also has a different system for setting and monitoring clinical standards and for managing the performance of NHS organisations (see Exhibit 7.1). Like Wales, Scotland embarked on an ambitious public health strategy, and this was reflected in the priority given to health promotion and prevention of disease in the Scottish NHS Plan (Scottish Executive, 2000a).

As Deffenbaugh (2002) has noted, the Scottish NHS has been less interested in partnerships with the private sector and has placed more emphasis on working with the voluntary sector and local authorities. The NHS in Scotland has adopted a unified health board structure that includes strong local authority representation. Another important difference may arise from the Scottish Executive's decision to fund both personal and nursing care in residential and nursing homes (in England and Wales the government decided that only the latter would be provided free by the state). The Scots may also receive free eye and dental checks if current proposals succeed (see Chapters 10 and 11).

With regard to Northern Ireland, the suspension of the Assembly and Executive coupled with the delayed implementation of earlier reforms, produced a complicated situation. A number of ideas were put forward, including the abolition of GP fundholding. The overall task of planning and commissioning services was given to the Four Health and Social Care Boards in the province. These commission care from 19 trusts responsible for providing health and social care. In addition, local health and social care groups have been established to develop primary care within each of the Health and Social Care Board areas. It is expected that these groups will be given greater responsibility for commissioning services in the future.

The Government adopted a 'steady state' approach, ensuring that contracts reflected existing patterns of activity. Initially, the vast majority were 'block contracts' where providers received a fixed price for services. More flexible contracts, such as cost and volume contracts (where providers received a fixed sum for a basic level of treatment and additional payments beyond this level of activity) and cost-per-case contracts (where providers receive a set price for each case) became more common. Plans to charge providers for the use of capital (buildings, equipment, and so on) were postponed. The introduction of weighted capitation – basing purchasers' budgets on the size of their resident populations adjusted in order to indicate health care needs – was delayed for practical reasons. However, political calculations were also relevant here; not only was there a lack of accurate measures of need at the local level, but the implementation of changes based on needs would have led to a shift in resources away from London and the south-east and placed even greater financial pressures on the London hospitals. In the event, the government established an inquiry to examine reform of hospital services in the capital and gave additional funding to London health authorities to ease their financial problems (Tomlinson, 1992).

Attempts to dilute and slow down the reforms preceded the ousting of Thatcher as Conservative Party leader and Prime Minister in 1990 (Ham, 2000, p. 51; see Lee-Potter, 1997). What would have happened if Thatcher had continued is uncertain. Thatcher denied that she ever wanted fundamentally to change the NHS, and stated that although she wanted a flourishing private sector, the NHS and its principles were a 'fixed point' in her policies (Thatcher, 1993, p. 606). Others, including some of her own Cabinet colleagues, doubt that she was a great believer in the NHS and suggest that she preferred policies that encouraged 'better-off' people taking out private insurance (Ham, 2000, p. 9).

Implementation: The Major Years

Thatcher's successor, John Major, was believed to be a supporter of the NHS. He reiterated his commitment to the service in his first conference speech after becoming leader, where he ruled out charges for hospital treatment, visits to the doctor, and privatisation of health care (Major, 2000, pp. 391–2). Nonetheless, his government decided to continue the task of implementing the NHS internal market. Other important policy developments occurred in this period, including a further NHS reorganisation, the launch of the *Patient's Charter*, and the introduction of the *Health of the Nation* strategy.

The post-1992 election period saw some relaxation of the cautious 'pre-election' approach described earlier. GP fundholding was extended to smaller practices and covered a greater range of services. The number of trusts increased and now included community health services as well as hospitals.

There was greater use of more flexible types of contract, though the shift was perhaps not as dramatic as envisaged, while competition was reduced as a result of mergers between trusts. The DHAs also began to merge with each other, their number halving in England between 1991 and 1995. There was also considerable regulation of the market by the NHS Executive and the regional bodies, strengthened by organisational changes (Allen, 2002).

A 'Quiet' Reorganisation

The DHAs began to work more closely with Family Health Service Authorities (FHSAs) which had taken over the responsibilities of the Family Practitioner Committees in 1991. The FHSAs had been introduced with the aim of bringing a managerial approach to the family practitioner services. Compared with the old FPCs, FHSAs were smaller bodies, had fewer professional representatives and included executive directors as well as non-executive directors on their board. DHA boards were also reconstituted in 1991 along similar lines with executive directors (including the general manager, finance director and director of public health).

In 1995 the Government decided to legislate to integrate DHAs and FHSAs in England and Wales. The new bodies were to be known simply as Health Authorities. Meanwhile, the regional tier of health authorities in England was abolished and replaced by regional offices of the NHS Executive. The regional offices were expected to be less independent than the bodies they replaced. Their role was advise the NHS Executive on resource allocation, to implement central policies and directives, and to manage the performance of health authorities and trusts. They also had important roles with regard to other activities including the oversight of medical education, research and development, and public health.

Further Changes

Gradually, relations between groups opposing the internal market reforms and Government began to improve (see Ham, 2000; Lee-Potter, 1997), though not quite returning to their initial position (see Baggott and McGregor-Riley, 1999). The Government made overtures to the professions in order to secure their co-operation in specific areas of health policy, such as primary care. In the mid-1990s, modifications were made to the rules of the internal market (DoH, 1994a), and guidelines were introduced in an attempt to improve co-operation, planning and accountability at the local level (DoH, 1995e). A national cancer plan was introduced (DoH, 1995a), an admission that market forces alone could not secure major changes in services. In response to the criticism that the internal market had increased bureaucracy, the Government introduced measures to reduce management costs. More generally, the internal market became a much more centralised process than Thatcher originally envisaged. The powers of central government increased, through reorganisation and the abolition of regional health authorities, the introduction of performance indicators, league tables, and tighter systems of target-setting and performance review. Despite the rhetoric of decentralised commissioning, the system was more like a command economy than a marketplace.

Finally, the Major Government introduced several important health reforms during the 1990s. First was the *Patient's Charter* of 1992, discussed further in Chapter 12, which set out service standards, expectations and rights. Although not legally binding, it established explicit minimum standards for a range of services, which were increasingly specified in performance-review processes, targets and service contracts. Other targets for improvement were introduced by the *Health of the Nation* strategy, launched in 1992 (and discussed in more detail in Chapter 13). This set out targets for the reduction of illnesses, such as cancer and heart disease, as well as key risk factors, such as smoking and obesity. This was an important break with Thatcherism, whose adherents had been openly hostile to the idea of a health strategy.

Interestingly, both the *Health of the Nation* strategy and the *Patient's Charter* drew on ideas advanced by the opposition parties. However, the identification of health priorities and a more consumerist approach to standards was actually compatible with a more managerialist approach to health care which the Thatcher Government had engendered. Both facilitated the setting of targets and standards and the development of performance-management systems. The Major Government also continued to promote other policy ideas generated by Thatcher's policy. It extended competitive tendering to more NHS support services including clinical support services, it extended the Private Finance Initiative (PFI) to health care, and it imposed strict efficiency targets on the NHS (see Chapter 6).

Evaluating the Conservatives' NHS Internal Market

It is possible to reach broad conclusions about the internal market (for general reviews see Mays, Mulligan and Goodwin, 2000; Le Grand, Mays and Mulligan, 1998). Nonetheless, there are enormous difficulties in attempting to assess its impact (see Baggott, 1997; Powell, 1997). First, the Thatcher Governments, and subsequently the Major Governments, ruled out independent evaluation of the reforms. However, researchers rushed to fill the vacuum and produced a considerable body of evidence. Secondly, the reforms were constantly modified for both political and technical reasons while being implemented. Thirdly, the introduction of new initiatives, such as the *Patient's Charter*, for example, coincided with the internal market reforms, making it difficult to disentangle their relative impact. Fourthly, there was an underlying and longer-term impact of previous reforms; for example, it is widely acknowledged that the implementation of the Griffiths management report laid the foundations for the internal market (Harrison et al., 1992). Finally, the reforms evolved over time and those involved learned from their experience and modified their behaviour. Bearing in mind these caveats, we shall now explore the impact of the internal market on efficiency, accountability, service co-ordination, quality, choice and equity.

Efficiency

According to Maniadakis, Hollingsworth and Thanassoulis (1999), hospital productivity rose, by around 7 per cent in the period 1991–6. Soderlund et al. (1997) also revealed productivity improvements associated with trust status between 1991 and 1994. Meanwhile, Mulligan (1998) found that cost-efficiency (measured by changes in NHS activity relative to resources) improved by 1.95 per cent per annum following the introduction of the internal market up until 1995/6, compared with 1.54 per cent in the period 1980/1 to 1991/2. Improved cost-efficiency was also suggested by falling average costs in services such as maternity, geriatrics and acute services.

However, it has been argued that these efficiency measures were inappropriate – in particular because they failed to capture improvements in services. Critics noted that measures emphasised outputs rather than outcomes, and placed importance on the acute sector at the expense of primary and community services (Clarke, McKee and Appleby, 1993). Measures of activity – which from 1988/9 were based on Finished Consultant Episodes (FCEs) rather than on Individual Patient Episodes – were believed to have exaggerated changes in productivity and efficiency (Hamblin, 1998, pp. 104–5). Another criticism was that the statistics were inaccurate, owing to poor data collection or deliberate efforts to distort performance outcome. Indeed, a possible explanation for the hospital productivity improvements by trusts was that hospitals intentionally understated productivity before achieving trust status so that they could demonstrate a marked improvement afterwards (Soderlund et al., 1997). It also appears that other factors not directly associated with reform affected productivity, such as technical change.

Others questioned improvements in allocative efficiency, arising from the transfer of funds between different providers (see Mays, Mulligan and Goodwin, 2000). Indeed, it is possible that the efficiency of the health care system as a whole may have been impaired by the internal market reforms. By creating pressures to reduce the length of hospital stays and the number of beds, incentives were created to shift costs on to others such as primary and community care providers, as well as individual patients and carers. This also meant that the capacity of the NHS to deal with sudden upturns in demand was undermined (Capewell, 1996).

Claims that the internal market improved efficiency were further challenged on the basis of the additional administrative and transaction costs it generated, including new contracting, costing and payment systems. Although there was a lack of reliable information about administrative and transaction costs, there was anecdotal evidence about the administrative cost of extra-contractual referrals, which in some cases exceeded the cost of treatment (Butler, 1995), and regarding higher management costs for fundholders (Dixon and Glennerster, 1995; Audit Commission, 1996a). The numbers of management and administrative staff increased following the introduction of the market, though the beginning of this trend predated the reforms. The expansion of staff post-1991 may have been due to other reforms – such as the *Patient's Charter* standards, the extension of resource management and clinical audit – as well as job reclassification. Indeed, some studies found little evidence that overall management costs increased following the introduction of the internal market (see Soderlund, 1999).

It appears that the reforms had a differential effect on efficiency. For example, some GP fundholders secured quicker treatment for their patients and obtained reductions in prices of treatments (Glennerster, Matsaganis and Owens, 1994, p. 72; Propper, Wilson and Soderlund, 1998), and were able to make cost savings in areas such as prescribing (see Howie, Heaney and Maxwell, 1995; Wilson, Buchan and Whalley, 1995). Yet even these gains were disputed (see Stewart Brown et al., 1995, in relation to prescribing). Moreover, fundholding involved high administration and transaction costs, not met by efficiency savings (Audit Commission, 1996a). On the other hand, the internal market appeared to have adverse effects on the efficiency of others, such as the providers of specialist services (Mullen, 1995; Langham and Black, 1995). It was claimed that purchasers were reluctant to refer patients on grounds of cost and that there was a lack of a fair pricing system which in effect penalised efficient providers. However, these problems were not entirely new, nor were they confined to specialist services (see Adams, 1995; Paton, 1995). Community health services were also believed to have suffered adversely from the introduction of markets and contracting. Not only was it more difficult to specify meaningful contracts in this field compared with, say, acute care (Flynn, Williams and Pickard, 1996), but the internal market seemed to have an adverse effect on the quality of service, and in particular constrained the work of community nurses (Tinsley and Luck, 1998).

Quality and Choice

There was little direct evidence to show that the overall quality of care improved or deteriorated following the introduction of the internal market (see Le Grand,

Mays and Mulligan, 1998). Most evidence cited in favour of the reforms was indirect, relating to the specification of standards in contracts rather than actual achievements (Carruthers et al., 1995; Coulter, 1995). Other indirect evidence included a survey of public health doctors (Marks, 1995) who believed that on balance the reforms had a positive impact on quality of services. Other studies gave examples of how fundholders secured a better quality service, such as a quicker response rate to their referrals (Glennerster, Matsaganis and Owens, 1994), though non-fundholders also claimed success here (see Graffy and Williams, 1994; Black, Birchall and Trimble, 1994).

It is difficult to substantiate an argument that the reforms produced a marked improvement in quality. The Audit Commission (1996a) found that only a third of GP fundholders claimed evidence-based medicine influenced purchasing, and few had access to clinical audit information that might inform such decisions. Furthermore, evidence suggested that contractual specifications of quality were ignored in practice (Baeza and Calnan, 1997). Other studies suggested a decline in quality. Maniadakis, Hollingsworth and Thanassoulis (1999) argued that increases in volume of services may have compromised service quality, and scaled down their previously reported increase in productivity as a result (to 2 per cent). Propper, Burgess and Abraham (2002) found that in the 1990s hospitals in more competitive areas had higher acute myocardial infarction (AMI) death-rates. They argued that this provided some evidence that the internal market had an adverse effect on quality. Meanwhile, Paton (1998, p. 105) suggested that quality improvements focused upon marginal aspects rather than upon clinical services. It is possible that improvements may also have been variable across different areas of care. In their study of GP fundholding, Howie, Heaney and Maxwell (1995) found that although for most conditions the quality of care had been maintained after the introduction of the scheme, in some areas the quality of service had declined.

Turning to choice and flexibility of services, again it is difficult to establish whether this improved or deteriorated. In terms of the individual patient choice the internal market appeared to have hardly any impact. This was because patients had no direct choice over treatment options. Instead, choice was exercised through other agents, GPs and health authorities, who varied in their commitment to gauge the views of individual patients and the public and act on these findings (see Chapter 12). It was argued that GP fundholders were more willing to take into account patients' preferences compared with non-fundholders, had more leverage over providers and considered a wider range of providers when making referrals (see Glennerster, Matsaganis and Owens, 1994; Howie, Heaney and Maxwell, 1995; Audit Commission, 1996a). However, some studies revealed a reduction in choice following the reforms (see Fotaki, 1998), supporting criticisms that contracts constrained flexibility when referring patients to secondary providers.

Finally, one of the arguments in favour of the internal market and fundholding in particular was that it would release an entrepreneurial spirit which would produce innovation and service improvement. Research has indicated that the entrepreneurialism of GPs varied. Ennew et al. (1998) concluded that some fundholders, particularly those who were early entrants to the scheme, were more entrepreneurial in outlook – more willing to secure a better deal and introduce innovative services – than others. Moreover, less than half of fundholders demonstrated genuine innovations and some non-fundholding GPs had also demonstrated such improvements (Whynes, 1997). In addition, while new services – such as outreach clinics (where specialists hold clinics in GP surgeries) – were introduced, there were doubts about their cost-effectiveness (Roland and Shapiro, 1998; Leese, 1996).

Accountability, Planning and Co-ordination

The reforms appeared to strengthen financial accountability, though this was more to do with the introduction of external auditing and resource management systems. Certainly, the internal market placed great emphasis on budgets, contracts and financial control. However, financial controls were unable to prevent inefficiency and fraud (see Chapter 6) and did not assuage concern about the financial accountability of fundholders. The impact of the reforms on other aspects of accountability is even harder to judge, largely because of the many factors involved. Take clinical accountability, for example, which was shaped by developments in clinical audit, professional regulation and user involvement. Meanwhile, political and managerial accountability was influenced by the introduction of systems of performance review, and wider public perceptions about responsibility for services.

With regard to planning and co-ordination, the internal market appeared to have an adverse effect. The reforms were blamed for producing poor communication and distrust between the different participants, making it difficult to plan future service provision (Ferlie, 1994; Audit Commission, 1993a, 1993b). The Major Government sought to address this planning guidance. However, the failure of NHS bodies to work with each other, and with other agencies such as social services, was not new (see Chapter 4). Nonetheless, there was much anecdotal evidence that the internal market impeded collaboration (Hadley and Goldman, 1995; Rea, 1995). In particular, the creation of two different systems of purchasing – health authorities and GP fundholders – was seen as a barrier to coherent planning and co-ordination of local services.

Equity

One of the most controversial criticisms of the internal market was that it created a two-tier system. It was argued that patients of fundholders received a superior service and could be 'fast-tracked' into secondary services as well as receiving better primary care. There was evidence that fundholders' patients received quicker hospital treatment (Kammerling and Kinnear, 1996) and experienced shorter waiting times (Dowling, 1997). Yet inequities may have been exaggerated or short-term (Glennerster, Matsaganis and Owens, 1994). It should be noted that there were inequities between fundholding practices, as their funding was related not to patients' needs but to historical factors. Moreover, there was evidence that some 'high cost' patients fared less well under fundholding (Howie, Heaney and Maxwell, 1995).

'Cream-skimming' had also been identified as a potential problem of the internal market (see Glennerster, Matsaganis and Owens, 1994). This is where purchasers of care seek to deter or offload patients who carry a high financial risk. Fundholders had some incentive to do this, though their financial liabilities were capped for each patient and excluded 'high cost' care and treatment. Doctors agreed that there was an incentive to remove patients, though these related more to drug budgets and to payments for prevention and health promotion rather than fundholding (Pickin et al., 2001). Though anecdotal examples were found, only one study provided systematic evidence of fundholders being more likely than non-fundholders to remove patients from their list, and even here the difference was small (O'Reilly et al., 1998).

Other Effects

A number of other consequences were highlighted by researchers. It was generally agreed that fundholding shifted the balance between primary and secondary care, though the extent of this shift was disputed (Chapter 10). Another possible impact was upon relationships between managers and doctors, some arguing that the internal market gave more leverage to managers than the Griffiths management reforms (Harrison et al., 1992). However, it has since been shown that managers depended on professionals to make the contracting system work and that, combined with the continued social and cultural authority of consultants, managers' ability to control professionals was limited (Griffiths and Hughes, 2000).

The Evolution of Commissioning and Contracting

The internal market evolved over time. As the 1990s unfolded, the commissioning and contracting process began to change. Despite the conceptual simplicity of the purchaser–provider split, many different models emerged (see Chappel et al., 1999). Alongside standard GP fundholding came a more limited scheme for smaller practices called 'community fundholding', and also multifund schemes, where practices joined together under a single management structure. As the standard scheme expanded beyond the original list of services to include virtually all elective and community health services, total fundholding schemes – covering potentially all hospital and community health services – were introduced on an experimental basis. Meanwhile, health authorities began to create commissioning groups, increasingly on a locality basis, to discuss service priorities and commissioning. In some areas these were primarily aimed at engaging non-fundholding GPs, in others there was closer working between fundholding and non-fundholding practices. These various arrangements are discussed further in Chapter 10.

Although the purchaser–provider divide was modelled on a classical form of contracting, relying on formal rules and contract specifications, a form of relational contracting – where informal relations and norms play a crucial part in determining outcomes – emerged. The market was not a competitive one and the process appears to have been focused on securing change through negotiation rather than by switching contracts (see North, 1998; Flynn Williams and Pickard, 1996; Bennett and Ferlie, 1996; Paton, 1998; Le Grand, Mays and Mulligan, 1998; Dopson and Locock, 2002). This occurred because the scope for competition was small; there was a lack of alternative providers in most areas, reduced further by trust mergers. Although adversarial approaches to contracting were deployed, purchasers and providers acknowledged the benefits of co-operation and used the contracting process as a means of negotiating change. Moreover, central government increasingly emphasised planning within the market, which further reduced the scope for competition. Furthermore, the high administrative and transaction costs deterred the development of highly specific contracts. Despite a shift towards cost and volume and cost-per-case contracts, block contracts continued to dominate, though they did become more detailed.

Those adopting a strict New Right perspective will have been disappointed. Green (1990, p. 3), viewed the reforms as 'a great missed opportunity'. As Mohan (1995, p. 221) correctly perceived, the changes were not a systematic imposition of a coherent blueprint, but part of a pragmatic and tactical approach. Hence the internal market was introduced cautiously and gradually, and was hedged with controls and regulations. As a result, according to Le Grand, Mays and Dixon (1998, p. 30), 'the incentives were too weak and the constraints were too strong'. But there is wide agreement that the internal market did make a difference in a number of respects, notably in promoting managerial, cultural and organisational change. The reforms also enhanced the status of general practice within the British health care system. By giving GPs a key role in the commissioning process, it paved the way for a further series of reforms under the next Government.

New Labour and the NHS

The Blair Government stated that it wanted to pursue a Third Way in health (see Chapter 3), steering a passage between the 'Old Labour' 'command and control' approach and the Conservative's internal market philosophy. This led to a configuration of hierarchies, networks and markets (Exworthy and Powell, 1999), which combined centralised performance management with a highly regulated contracting process. Although new Labour promised greater localism, with the promise of change through consensual partnerships at local level, in practice it proved to be a centralising force (see Dixon, 2001, p. 25; Powell, 1998; Harrison, 2001; Klein, 1999).

Public spending on health was constrained by a commitment to adhere to the Conservative Government's spending plans, though additional funds were allocated from contingency funds. According to Toynbee and Walker (2001, p. 120), the Conservatives had no intention of maintaining these plans had they been re-elected. The Blair Government continued the policy of using private finance to build and run hospitals – the Private Finance Initiative (see Exhibit 6.1). But while this reflected an acknowledgement that the private sector would play a greater role in the NHS in future, other moves, such as the decision to abolish tax relief for the elderly on health insurance premiums showed the new Government in a different light.

This ambiguity was evident in the decision to retain the purchaser–provider split in England and Wales, while pledging to end the Conservatives' internal market. Longer-term service agreements would replace contracts and there was a commitment to reduce management costs substantially. The emphasis was on planning and collaboration rather than competition, though, as already noted, the trend was already in this direction. GP fundholding was to end and be replaced by local commissioning bodies. These bodies, known as Primary Care Groups (PCGs) in England, would operate initially under health authorities. These resembled the more inclusive forms of commissioning schemes that had begun to emerge as the internal market developed. It was envisaged that the PCGs would have the option of becoming Primary Care Trusts, free-standing bodies accountable to health authorities for the commissioning of care and for the provision of community health services. This later became compulsory. Notably, arrangements differed considerably across the different parts of the UK. In Scotland, for example, the purchaser–provider split was abandoned (see Exhibit 5.2).

Like its Conservative predecessor, the Blair Government emphasised the importance of primary care. It experimented with new forms of primary care provision, using the Conservatives' 1997 Primary Care Act as a basis for these innovations (see Chapter 10). It also introduced new services such as NHS Direct, where people could get advice over the telephone about health problems and conditions, and Walk-in Centres. However, the acute sector remained a high priority. Indeed the key health target in New Labour's five 'pledges' to the electorate in 1997 was to reduce hospital waiting lists by treating 100,000 additional patients.

New Labour placed greater emphasis on collaboration in promoting improvements in the quality of health care and in population health. A statutory duty of co-operation was placed on health authorities and trusts and they (along with local authorities) were required to contribute to Health Improvement Programmes drawn up by health authorities (see Chapter 7). Health bodies and local authorities were required to work together effectively on issues such as social care, drawing up joint investment plans, for example. Legislation was also introduced to make it easier for health and local authorities to pool service budgets. Meanwhile, new bodies, Health Action Zones, were introduced to improve health standards where needs were greatest by improving joint working between health service bodies, local government agencies and the voluntary and private sector (see Exhibit 10.2).

As well as improving co-ordination and planning, the Blair Government was keen to set standards of care and to ensure that access to high-quality services was fair (see Chapter 8). Bodies at national level were established to issue guidelines on the cost-effectiveness of treatments and to monitor the quality of health care, in the form of the National Institute for Clinical Excellence (NICE) and the Commission for Health Improvement (CHI) respectively. A new regulatory body was also established to regulate social care and private health care in the form of the National Care Standards Commission. A duty was placed on trusts to safeguard the quality of care and they were required to implement a new system of clinical governance; professional bodies were told to strengthen systems of self-regulation. In a further move, a new performance assessment framework was introduced into the NHS in England. This focused on six areas (health improvement, fair access, effective delivery of appropriate services, efficiency, patient/carer experience, and health outcomes). This evolved with further performance measures, including clinical indicators to assess the outcomes of health care. The Government embarked on a programme of National Service frameworks (NSFs) setting out principles and standards of service provision in a range of condition areas and for population groups (such as coronary heart disease, mental health, older people). These frameworks were based on clinical advice, evidence and inputs from others such as service users (see Exhibit 7.4).

Finally, the Blair Government placed a higher priority on public health and health inequalities compared with its predecessor. An enquiry was established to examine health inequalities, an issue which the Conservatives had largely ignored. New public health policies focused on tackling the social, economic and environmental factors in ill health. This was seen as task for both Government and the individual, and was heralded as a move away from the victim-blaming approach of previous Governments, while raising hopes of a more co-ordinated strategy across Government than hitherto. A Green Paper on the subject was published in 1998, with a White Paper the following year. These policies and the record of the Blair Government in this field are discussed further in Chapter 13.

The NHS in Crisis – Again

The Government's policy on health care was set out in a White Paper of 1997, *The New NHS, Modern, Dependable* (Cm 3807, 1997). There followed a honeymoon period, where Government's policies attracted little public criticism. Even where serious problems did come to light – as in the Bristol case (see Chapter 9) – it was the professional organisations and local NHS bodies which came under attack. Indeed, this and other cases – such as the Shipman case – strengthened the Government's call for improvements in professional regulation and stronger quality control.

But as the self-imposed public spending constraints began to bite, Government faced growing accusations about underfunding and lack of service capacity. This was reflected in waiting lists, which remained high. Cases where operations had been cancelled or postponed rose, with fatal consequences for some. Media attention intensified in a similar way as it had done during the late 1980s. One of the most prominent cases covered concerned Mavis Skeet, whose throat cancer operation was cancelled several times, until it was found to be inoperable. The breaking point came in 2000 when Lord Winston, a Labour peer, pioneering fertility doctor and TV personality, stated that health care provision was 'deeply unsatisfactory' for many people and that the reforms had done little to address this. Although he later retracted some of his comments, the pressure did not abate. Tony Blair himself committed the Government to raising health spending as a proportion of national expenditure to the level of the European average, though there was disagreement about what exactly this meant (see Chapter 7). Nonetheless, a large increase in spending (over 6 per cent per annum after adjustment for inflation) was announced in the 2000 Budget.

The NHS Plan

This new-found generosity had a price: the Government established a fresh review of the NHS. To facilitate the review the Government undertook a hurried consultation of staff and the public. This was seen by some as a rather token exercise, though over 210,000 people responded. The Government also established

Modernisation Action Teams (MATs) in six areas of the NHS:

- *Partnership*: making sure the different parts of the health care system worked together effectively.

- *Performance*: improving clinical performance and health service productivity.

- *Professions*: increasing the flexibility of training and working practices in the context of an expansion in the NHS workforce.

- *Prevention*: tackling health inequalities and focusing the health system on preventing avoidable illness.

- *Patient care*: ensuring fast and convenient access to services.

- *Patient empowerment and information*: giving patients a bigger role in their own care.

The MATs consisted of doctors, nurses and managers, as well as civil servants and ministers. People from user, carer and other voluntary organisations were also involved in this process. The MAT reports were considered by the Government and led to the NHS Plan, published in the summer of 2000 (Cm 4818, 2000). Separate plans were subsequently published for Wales and Scotland (see Exhibit 5.2). Key aspects of the NHS Plan will be examined in more detail in the following chapters. However, the main commitments are given in Exhibit 5.3.

Exhibit 5.3 The NHS Plan

The NHS Plan, published in July 2000, outlined a range of targets and initiatives. Some were new, others echoed earlier commitments. Separate plans were subsequently issued for other parts of the UK and these are referred to in Exhibit 5.2. The Plan ruled out changes in the way in which the NHS was funded. It upheld the main principles of the NHS and reiterated the importance of free care at point of delivery. It established that nursing care (but not personal care) would be free to all in residential and nursing homes (see Chapter 11)

The Government's targets, identified in the Plan, took the form of inputs – 7,000 extra beds and 100 new hospital schemes by 2010, 7,500 more consultants, 2,000 new GPs and 20,000 more nurses in addition to a further 6,500 other health professionals. In relation to outputs, the Government reiterated the commitment to reduce the major causes of mortality and morbidity in line with its earlier White Paper, *Saving Lives*, and added further targets relating to the reduction of health inequalities (see Chapter 13). With regard to services, the main targets covered patient access to primary care, cancelled operations, and out-patient, in-patient and Accident and Emergency waiting times.

Important changes included an expansion of intermediate care facilities (such as community hospitals, nursing homes and intensive rehabilitation services, as well as non-residential care places and integrated care teams to provide care at home), diagnostic and treatment centres to increase day surgery and 'short stay' treatment. The Plan stated that two-thirds of all out-patient appointments and in-patient elective treatment would be prebooked by ⟶

Exhibit 5.3 continued

→

2003/4 (and all by 2005). All Primary Care Groups were expected to become Primary Care Trusts – free-standing bodies responsible for commissioning secondary care services as well as providing primary care and community health services. The Plan also identified ways of improving joint working between the NHS and other care providers. It proposed new care trusts to combine health and social services. A greater role for the private sector was highlighted. Private sector management teams would be able to take on the management of failing hospitals and run new diagnostic and treatment centres. Also, a concordat between the NHS and the private sector was promised to clarify their respective roles.

A new performance-management system was announced in the Plan. Trusts that were judged to have performed well could earn autonomy and have more freedom to spend funds for service improvement. Those that performed less well would be more tightly regulated. A Modernisation Board was proposed, to oversee the planned improvements. Meanwhile, local authorities were promised powers of scrutiny over NHS services, including major service reorganisations, which could be referred to a new Independent Panel on Reconfiguration.

Changes for the professions included new contracts for consultants and GPs, including a proposal to limit private practice for new consultants. The Plan reiterated a commitment to give nurses new roles and responsibilities. It identified a new post of 'modern matron' who would have a clear brief for clinical standards and the quality of the patient experience. In line with current initiatives, improvements in professional regulation were promised, and a commitment to improve collaboration and teamwork between different professions was outlined.

The Plan claimed to place patients at the centre of the NHS. Some of the long-standing complaints of patients about the quality of the caring environment – in particular, hospital food and hygiene – were explicitly addressed, including plans to improve catering services and clearer responsibilities for food quality and hygiene. An entire chapter was devoted to patient and public involvement, proposing radical changes to the system including greater patient and public representation on key national committees and boards, the establishment of patients' forums and new advice and advocacy services within trusts, counterbalanced by the planned abolition of Community Health Councils.

Finally, a number of commitments were made in the public health field, including a free fruit and vegetable scheme for children, new health inequalities targets at national level, and closer working relationships between agencies responsible for public health (see Chapter 13).

Source: Cm 4818 (2000) *The NHS Plan: A Plan for Investment. A Plan for Reform*

The reception given to the NHS Plan was generally positive. There were obvious controversies, including the proposed abolition of the Community Health Councils and a proposal to limit private practice for new consultants. The new structure appeared to be highly centralised, with a plethora of bodies at national level regulating or overseeing health care. This was balanced by a promise that trusts could 'earn' autonomy from the centre. Some of the targets – on waiting times, for example – were regarded as very ambitious, even considering the additional expenditure. Another criticism was that public health was in effect being downgraded by the renewed emphasis on health service reform (see Chapter 13).

Unlike the previous White Paper of 1997, the NHS Plan explicitly acknowledged the role of the private sector in health care. Subsequently, a concordat was drawn up between the NHS and the private sector, its implications explored more fully in Chapter 6. But the Government ruled out any major change to the way in which the NHS was funded, a position supported by a Treasury Review, published in 2002 (Wanless, 2002). Nonetheless, there were marginal changes: the 2002 Budget provided additional spending on the NHS, funded by a new 1 per cent rise in National Insurance contributions.

The Blair Government had clearly shifted position. It now explicitly backed a greater role for the private sector. A move towards a more pluralistic and competitive health care market was clearly being sanctioned. In a related move, following a European Court judgement, NHS patients were allowed to have their treatment overseas paid for by the British tax-payer, opening up the prospect of greater cross-border competition for patients (see Chapter 12).

The NHS Plan precipitated a further reorganisation in England, implemented in 2002 (for organisational changes in Scotland, Wales and Northern Ireland see Exhibit 5.2). The NHS regions were reduced, both in number and in their role, and were later abolished, health authorities were reconstituted as Strategic Health Authorities and primary care groups were corralled into primary care trusts. Subsequently, the Government proposed new foundation trusts, remaining part of the NHS, but promised greater freedom from central government. The significance of these changes is explored in later chapters.

Conclusion

As noted in the previous chapter, many problems faced by Government in the health field are not new, and policy debates have often reawakened interest in earlier attempts to solve these problems. Moreover, despite Governments having different ideological stances and political styles, there has actually been a high degree of continuity. This is largely because they have faced the same constraints when embarking upon reform. First, the high profile of the NHS and the broad political support for its principles has made it difficult to introduce changes that appear to challenge these principles. Secondly, Governments have faced technical difficulties, particularly with regard to information about costs and the quality of care, which have limited the implementation of new policies. Thirdly, Government has remained highly dependent on professional expertise, notably that of the medical profession but increasingly that of management expertise too, to deliver its policies. A fourth factor, which has inhibited attempts genuinely to decentralise the NHS, has been the demands of political accountability. The fact that the NHS remains largely funded out of national taxation and is regarded as a key responsibility of central government, has made it extremely difficult for Government to shift responsibility for the service on to managers and professionals at local level.

So far the policies adopted by the Blair Government appear to have strengthened these factors. As Klein (1999) has noted, this Government's approach was likely to fuel public expectations. Initially, at least, it adopted a more centralised approach and identified itself clearly with the future success or failure of the service. Also, by refusing to consider other forms of funding, it reiterated that national government should be the central focus of political accountability. Subsequent chapters discuss in detail how these policies have developed in a range of key policy areas.

Further Reading

Butler, J. (1992) *Patients, Policies and Politics: Before and After 'Working for Patients'* (Buckingham, Open University Press).

Edwards, B. (1993) *The National Health Service: A Managers Tale 1946–92* (London, Nuffield Provincial Hospitals Trust).

Glennerster, H., Matsaganis, M. and Owens, P. (1994) *Implementing GP Fundholding: Wild Card or Winning Hand?* (Buckingham, Open University Press).

Ham, C. (2000) *The Politics of NHS Reform 1988–97 – Metaphor or Reality?* (London, King's Fund).

Klein, R. (2000) *The New Politics of the NHS*, 4th edn (London, Prentice-Hall).

Le Grand, J., Mays, N. and Mulligan, J. (1998) *Learning from the NHS Internal Market: A Review of Evidence* (London, King's Fund).

Lee-Potter, J. (1997) *A Damn Bad Business: The NHS Deformed* (London, Indigo).

Timmins, N. (1995) *The Five Giants: A Biography of the Welfare State* (London, Harper Collins).

Webster, C. (2002) *The National Health Service: A Political History*, 2nd edn (Oxford, Oxford University Press).

Health Care Funding and Independent Sector Provision

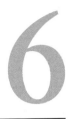

This chapter examines the way in which health care in Britain is funded. It explores health care financing mechanisms, recent policies on public and private expenditure on health care, and the contribution of independent providers to the British health care system.

Funding Health Care

Between 1948 and 1997 health care expenditures rose from 3 per cent of World Gross Domestic product (GDP) to almost 8 per cent (WHO, 2000, p. 95). Despite this, health care systems continued to face substantial financial pressures from rising public expectations, increasing demand, and financial pressures associated with new technologies. In the UK context, it has been argued that these pressures will widen the gap between the demand and supply (see Healthcare 2000, 1995), the implication being that state-funded systems such as the NHS would become unsustainable. This gloomy scenario has been challenged, critics arguing that the NHS could meet future demands for health care (Wordsworth, Donaldson and Scott, 1996; Frankel, Ebrahim and Davey Smith, 2000). Nonetheless, this debate stimulated interest in alternative forms of funding health care (see Maxwell, 1988; Mossialos et al., 2002; Freeman, 2000; BMA, 1997, 2001; Scott, 2001; Wanless, 2001; Gladstone, 1997; Green and Irvine, 2001).

General Taxation

The main source of funding for the NHS is general taxation, which has several advantages. It is a relatively efficient method of raising revenue. Funds are accrued through the existing tax system, so no additional costs are incurred. Funding through general taxation provides strong financial discipline and helps control health costs. This is because Government becomes, in effect, the 'single payer' for health care. Those providing health care cannot easily increase their income by raising prices or premiums, as in private insurance and social insurance systems (though the state does endeavour to influence prices in such systems). Also, in a general-tax-funded system, the financing of services is divorced from provision, and this is an important factor in promoting equitable access to services. Because access is not tied to the individual's financial contribution, the provision of care is more likely to be based on principles of clinical need, than on an entitlement through their financial contribution.

Health care systems funded from general taxation redistribute resources in a number of ways: from the healthy to the sick, from the wealthy to the poor, and from those who are of working age to the elderly and children. As long as the tax system is progressive – richer people paying proportionally more tax on their incomes than poorer citizens – a health care system funded from general taxation will redistribute towards those on lower incomes (Wagstaff et al., 1999). However, for each individual, contributions and benefits will tend to balance out over a lifetime. People use the service more when they are children and when they become old, while contributing more to the costs of the service in their healthier years.

The main disadvantage of general taxation is that it ties health services closely to the state of the economy and to the taxation policies of central government. Economic recession reduces tax revenues and can adversely affect the health budget. Even in prosperous times, health budgets may suffer if Government gives priority to low taxation over public services. A further problem is that if the financial discipline imposed by a tax-funded system is too strong relative to health care demand, it could produce a reduction in the quality and availability of services. Indeed, critics of general-tax-funded systems argue that they promote excessive rationing and poor-quality services (Redwood, 2000). However, again much depends on the priority given to health spending relative to other priorities. A reliance on general taxation will not automatically lead to a shortage of resources, though it does give Governments more power to constrain health budgets if they are committed to do so. Tax funding has also been blamed for making the health care system less responsive to patients' needs and choices (Redwood, 2000). Because resources for health care are separated from provision, the patients cannot use 'purchasing power' to effect change. However, this is less an intrinsic problem of tax funding,more a failure to devise mechanisms of service planning and provision that articulate user perspectives (see Chapter 12).

Hypothecated Taxes

Hypothecated taxes have been advanced as a means of explicitly identifying taxes for funding health care and 'ring-fencing' them for this purpose (Jones and Duncan, 1995; Bailey and Bruce, 1994). The main argument in favour is that by making the cost of health services more explicit, people will tolerate tax increases to pay for better health care. Supporters of hypothecation argue that the system of funding public services, including health, should be much more transparent so that people can judge for themselves the costs and benefits of taxation (Le Grand, 2000). Although there is evidence that people are happier to see tax rises to pay for health rather than other services (Fabian Society, 2000, p. 8; Hedges and Bromley, 2000), it is uncertain whether persistent increases in a specific health tax would receive continued public support.

Indeed, a hypothecated health tax may encourage citizens to think in narrow terms about what each is getting for his or her money (Bennett, 2000). In contrast, the pooling of resources through general taxation allows the state to maintain services that benefit all, taxpayers and non-taxpayers alike, and to protect services that may be less popular but nonetheless vital to a comprehensive welfare state. Hypothecated taxes may also impede a comprehensive approach in other ways. By focusing on the funding of the health care system, the role of other services which have important implications for health services, such as social care, housing and education, could be ignored. In an era of pooled budgets and inter-agency initiatives to improve health and social care, hypothecation looks somewhat out of place.

Hypothecated taxes have been criticised for their inflexibility, particularly with regard to new, unexpected increases in demand. They can also narrow the tax base, reducing the proportion of people contributing revenue. Much, however, depends on how such a tax is implemented. Most proposals involve a tax on earned income. This exempts those not working, which is good from a redistributive point of view because this excludes unemployed, ill and elderly people. However, it also exempts those with large investment incomes, reducing their contribution to the cost of health services, and this is likely to be regressive, placing a greater burden on the poor.

Local Taxes

This discussion has assumed so far that health taxes will be collected wholly by national government. However, health services may be funded to some extent from local taxes, as in Sweden for example. Local taxation implies greater accountability of health services to the local community, and may overcome the criticism that centralised tax-funded systems are unresponsive to local needs. But there is a downside. Local taxation places more emphasis on local economic and political factors. This increases the likelihood of disparities between local areas, often related to their prosperity, compounding local variations in socio-economic, geographical and demographic factors. Moreover, studies of equity in the financing of health care have found that systems that depend to some extent on local taxes tend to be less progressive than others (Wagstaff et al., 1999).

General, hypothecated and local taxation are the main options for a tax-funded health care system. However, other supplementary sources have been suggested. For example, specific 'earmarked' taxes on goods and services, particularly those linked with ill health such as alcohol, tobacco and junk food.

Social Insurance

A common method of raising revenue for health care is through social insurance, whereby individuals are compelled to contribute a share of their income to a state or licensed sickness fund. When the individual needs health care, the fund pays the provider. People who cannot afford contributions because of unemployment, infirmity or low income are usually exempt. Social insurance schemes are therefore rated highly on equity grounds, though it is possible that some people (refugees, travellers, homeless people, for example) may not be entitled to care, compared with a tax-based system where no evidence of contributions is usually required.

The NHS is still partly financed by social insurance, in the form of National Insurance contributions from employers and employees. Approximately an eighth of the NHS budget comes from this source. This is a legacy of Lloyd George's scheme, introduced in the early years of the twentieth century (see Chapter 4). The contributory principle was extended in 2003 with the imposition of a rise in National Insurance contributions to support increased health spending. However, National Insurance payments do not carry an entitlement to health care and are not transmitted directly from individuals to the NHS but through a transfer from the National Insurance Fund. In reality this is a kind of hypothecated tax (see above). It bears little resemblance to the social insurance systems, such as those in Europe for example, where a range of sickness funds are financed by contributions from employers, employees and citizens. Such systems, compared with tax-funded systems, are associated with additional choice to patients. Indeed, some countries, notably Holland and Germany, have encouraged greater competition between funds in recent years (Dixon and Mossialos, 2001; Mossialos et al., 2002).

One of the main disadvantages of social insurance is that, while providing universal coverage, it is usually funded by a smaller proportion of the population than is the case under a general-tax-based system – the burden falling mainly on employers and employees. Social insurance systems can also be more regressive than general tax-funded systems (see Wagstaff et al., 1999), but much depends on who is covered by the system and, in particular, whether higher earners are excluded (their absence makes the system more regressive). Another disadvantage of such systems is their high administrative costs, particularly where there are a large number of insurance funds. There are also fewer incentives to control costs in such systems, although most countries with social insurance have sought to introduce regulations and incentives to impose greater financial discipline.

Private Insurance

In most health care systems, private insurance supplements other methods of funding. Private insurance may be taken out to pay for services not covered by the state scheme (as in France), or by individuals who want a quicker or more responsive service (as in the UK) or by people 'opting out' of state systems to make their own arrangements for funding health care (as in Holland and Germany for example). Few systems depend on private insurance for the majority of their citizens' health care needs. Even in the USA, where over half of the population is covered by private insurance schemes, this only accounts for around a third of health care expenditure.

While private insurance tends to deliver a responsive service to those who can afford it, there is no guarantee that it will provide appropriate or good-quality care. Indeed, private insurance systems have incentives to overprovide care. Even though patients are now better informed and more willing to challenge professionals, they remain at a disadvantage in terms of knowledge and information, and are still vulnerable to exploitation. This creates problems for those wishing to contain health costs. It is no coincidence that those countries which are most heavily dependent on private insurance funding are those which also face the greatest difficulties in controlling costs (Scott, 2001). Private insurance systems also have high administrative costs, largely because of the large number of transactions and the multiplicity of agencies involved in purchasing care, providing care, billing, and regulating services. In the USA it has been estimated that around a quarter of the cost of health care is absorbed by administration (Woolhandler, Himmelstein and Lewontin, 1993).

Systems that depend heavily on private insurance rate poorly on equity considerations because they link the availability of treatment closely to the ability to pay. Yet those who need health care the most tend to be the least likely to be able to pay for it. They struggle to afford the premiums and tend to settle for a less comprehensive package of care. Some people on low incomes, unemployed workers, older people and the chronically sick, are unable to afford any coverage at all. Hence there is a need for state-funded schemes, such as the Medicare scheme in the USA for the elderly, and the Medicaid scheme for the poor. However, not all those without private insurance are covered: approximately forty million Americans fall into this category.

The impact of private insurance on equity is more ambiguous when it is used to supplement tax- and insurance-based systems. Wagstaff et al. (1999) demonstrated that in such systems private insurance is in fact progressive, placing a higher financial burden on those with higher incomes (see also Propper and Green, 2001). This is because private insurance is an expensive commodity for which wealthier people pay a premium. However, if the privately insured receive a superior service this could contribute to unacceptable inequities of outcome, even though the richer are paying more for health care as a proportion of their income.

Charges and Co-Payments

Direct user charges make up a small proportion of health service spending, largely because of the high cost and uncertain demand for health care (Robinson, 2002b, p. 161). No comprehensive health care system could be based on up-front charges for services because most potential users would be unable to fund their treatment. However, charges are seen as a useful way of raising additional revenues for health care systems providing they do not distort clinical priorities. It has been suggested that patients in the future will demand better-quality non-clinical services (such as access to computer and entertainment facilities when in hospital), and for these they must pay extra. But where does one draw the line? Charges for improvements in food or accommodation services may seem optional extras, but it can be argued that edible, nutritious food and pleasant accommodation are essential components of good-quality care.

Charges for clinical services are more controversial. However, in tax-funded systems such as the NHS, charges have been levied almost since the beginning of the service (on prescriptions, optical and dental services and certain appliances, for example). Other countries impose a charge for visiting the doctor (Sweden and Portugal, for example) or for hospital stays (Austria, Germany and Belgium, for example). The amount of money that could be raised by charges is substantial, though much depends on exemptions. The BMA (1997, 2001) calculated that £1.25 billion could be raised by a £40 fee for food and accommodation in hospital, while a £10 fee to see a GP could raise £3.3 billion (or £2 billion with exemptions for the elderly and children).

The problem with charges, however, is that they compound problems of access to services and discriminate against those on low incomes and those who genuinely need services (Dixon and Mossialos, 2001; Elofsson, Unden and Krakau, 1998; Newhouse and the Insurance Experiment Group, 1993; Robinson and Chalkley, 1998; National Association of Citizens' Advice Bureaux, 2001). As Wagstaff et al. (1999) remarked, charges or 'out-of-pocket payments' are a highly regressive means of raising revenue, though again much depends on the exemptions given to groups such as the chronically ill, elderly and children. Obviously, if exemptions are generous then the system will be less regressive, but will also raise less revenue.

A further problem is collection costs. There is often a reluctance to pay at point of delivery, and it is often seen as inconvenient or inappropriate to collect the charge at this time. This means that a system of accounts administration and revenue collection is needed. But, given that most charges tend to be small, collection costs can easily exceed revenues. Indeed, because of this, it may actually be more cost-effective to provide a free service than levy small fees.

Other Sources of Funding and Resources

Of all the other alternatives, perhaps the most important is funding from charitable sources. As noted in Chapter 4, voluntary and charitable organisations have a long history of funding (and providing) health services in the UK. Even today there is much reliance on charitable resources to supplement state funding (see Mohan and Gorsky, 2001). This takes many forms, such as fund-raising for research and for the provision of health services, the use of charitable funds for equipment, and National Lottery funding. The amount of money involved is considerable, and indeed there has been criticism that charitable funding, rather than providing an additional or enhanced health services, is actually replacing state funding. There has been particular criticism of the use of National Lottery funds for vital equipment, such as that used in the diagnosis and treatment of cancer. More generally, studies have found that in the NHS core services have been funded by charities (Fitzherbert and Giles, 1990; Fitzherbert, 1992). The amounts raised by charities on behalf of the NHS is substantial. According to the National Audit Office (NAO, 2000a), charitable funds associated with the NHS held assets of £1.8 billion and spent £322 million in 1998–9. A report from the Charities Aid Foundation (2001) found that, in London, money spent by charities in support of the NHS amounted to almost a tenth of income from government.

Another potential source of funding is from the sale of assets and trading income. Since the late 1980s NHS organisations have been encouraged by government to generate resources. This has led among other things to an expansion of private health care provided by the NHS, and an expansion in sales of land and buildings. Although the amounts of money raised in this way are still relatively small, they make an important contribution. Moreover, it should be noted that health service funds can also be generated from third parties who are paying for specific services or who are in some way liable for costs. In the NHS, for example, organisations requiring specific services (such as the use of its facilities or equipment) are charged for this. Another aspect is the treatment of road accident victims, the cost of which can be recovered from insurance companies.

Public Expenditure and the NHS

Having reviewed the various sources of funding for health care, this section explores public expenditure on health care in the UK. The proportion of public spending devoted to the NHS, which remained around 10 per cent in the 1950s and 1960s, increased during the 1980s and 1990s, rising to 16 per cent by 2000. Meanwhile, NHS expenditure grew as a percentage of GDP from 3 per cent to 5.5 per cent between 1949/50 and 1996/7, while in volume terms (after adjusting for inflation) expenditure increased by 235 per cent over this period (Appleby, 1999a). As Table 6.1 shows, the NHS received above-average inflation increases in its budget during the eighties and nineties.

Underfunding

The Conservative governments of Thatcher and Major were nonetheless criticised for allocating insufficient resources. The actual growth rate for health spending under the Conservatives was smaller than official figures suggest (see Table 6.1).

In the 1980s and 1990s, the increase in NHS funding was lower than the Department of Health's estimate that at least 2 per cent per annum was needed to meet the costs of changing disease patterns, new forms of service delivery, demographic changes and developments in medical technology (Social Services Committee, 1986, p. 26). On this basis the NHS was seriously underfunded; the cumulative shortfall for the 1980s alone was estimated at £4.4 billion (NAHAT, 1990). Evidence of underfunding was also supported by international comparisons (Pritchard, 1992). By the end of the 1990s the UK still spent less on health care than comparable countries (see Figure 6.1).

Table 6.1 Growth rate for health spending, 1983–2001

Government	Period	Annual percentage	
		Increase in spending on NHS (after adjustment for general inflation)	Increase in spending on NHS (after adjustment for health service inflation)
Thatcher	1983–7	2.1	0.9
Thatcher/Major	1987–92	4.1	2.0
Major	1992–7	2.6	1.4
Blair	1997–2001	4.7	4.1

Source: J. Appleby and A. Coote (2002) *Five Year Health Check: A Review of Government Health Policy 1997–2002*, pp. 11–12

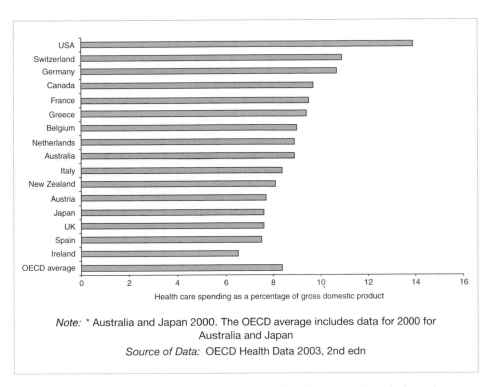

Health care spending as a percentage of gross domestic product

Note: * Australia and Japan 2000. The OECD average includes data for 2000 for Australia and Japan

Source of Data: OECD Health Data 2003, 2nd edn

Figure 6.1 Cross-national comparisons of health expenditure (selected OECD countries), 2001*

However, the underfunding thesis has been criticised on several grounds. Much depends on value judgements about the need for increased spending (Dixon, Harrison and New, 1997). Critics have argued that there is no commonly agreed indicator of need, and estimates are based largely on guesswork (Social Services Committee, 1986). They have also pointed out that sums spent on health care are not necessarily good indicators of quality and cost-effectiveness (Haywood, 1990). There are also doubts about the validity of international comparisons of health expenditure (discussed further below) which can exaggerate differences in funding levels between countries.

It should be noted that the level of UK *public* spending on health care is close to the average for industrialised countries. So the main difference between the UK and most other comparable countries lies in private expenditure. Private health spending in the UK, despite its recent growth, remains a relatively small proportion of the total. For this reason, some have argued that private payments should be increased rather than further public expenditure (Whitney, 1988).

The Impact of New Labour

In the Blair Government's first term, the annual average increase in NHS spending was 4.7 per cent after adjusting for the general rate of inflation (see Appleby, 1999a; Appleby and Coote, 2002, ch. 2). Further increases – amounting to 6.3 per cent per annum for 2000/1 to 2003/4 – accompanied the NHS Plan. In 2000, as noted in Chapter 5, Tony Blair declared that spending would rise to match the European Union average (Richards and Brown, 2001). At the time the total amount of public and private health care expenditure as a propor-tion of GDP (the standard measure of national income and expenditure) was 6.8 per cent in the UK compared with 8 per cent across the European Union (excluding the UK). However, this figure was based on an 'unweighted' average and did not reflect the different population sizes of EU countries.

The EU 'weighted' average (excluding the UK) was in fact 8.9 per cent (Emmerson et al., 2002; see also Towse and Sussex, 2000). One study estimated that it would require almost £10 billion to make up the difference between the UK level of spending and that of the EU (Emmerson et al., 2002). Moreover, the figure would be even greater if, as was likely, other EU countries invested a higher proportion of their GDP in their health care systems in future years. The weighted EU average, excluding the UK, was estimated to reach 10.7 per cent of GDP by 2005/6 (Appleby and Boyle, 2001), which would require an increase in spending of approximately £30 billion (Appleby and Coote, 2002, p. 15).

Estimates were, however, hampered by problems of inter-country comparisons of expenditure (see Schieber and Poullier, 1992; Dixon and Mossialos, 2001). What counts as health spending varies between countries. For example, nursing home care is included in measures of health spending in some countries but not others (BMA, 2001; Towse and Sussex, 2000). Moreover, as suggested earlier, levels of spending do not guarantee high-quality health care, good access to services or efficiency. Indeed, the NHS is acknowledged as relatively good at controlling costs, and it may well be that it does not require the same level of funding as continental systems which have the added burden of higher transaction costs (Jones, 2001). Furthermore, the costs of treatment tend to be lower in the NHS compared with other countries – one study found that of 89 procedures, 46 cost less in the NHS than in five other European health care systems (Hospital HealthcareCom, 2002).

Finally, it should be noted that the Blair Government's original 8 per cent target related not simply to NHS spending but to health care spending as a whole. Its achievement was not dependent wholly on NHS spending and at least some of the growth would have to come from private health care spending (Towse and Sussex, 2000; Appleby and Boyle, 2000). Failing this, even more resources would have to be invested by the public sector.

The Wanless review

The new spending commitment was followed by a Treasury review of health spending headed by Derek Wanless, former Chief Executive of NatWest Bank. The review examined the 'technological, demographic, and medical trends over the next two decades' affecting the UK health service and attempted 'to identify the key factors which will determine the financial and other resources required to ensure that the NHS can provide a publicly funded, comprehensive, high quality service available on the basis of clinical need and not ability to pay' (Wanless, 2001, p. 1). An interim report was published which noted that health outcomes (life expectancy for women at both birth and age 65, and for men at age 65, and infant mortality for both sexes) were generally worse for the UK relative to seven comparable European and Commonwealth countries. It found no justification on grounds of equity or efficiency for changing the current system of financing through general taxation.

Wanless's second report (2002) provided a detailed analysis of trends and scenarios that might affect the demand for health care and the resources available to meet this. The main influences on resources included: government commitments to improve the quality of the health service; increasing public and patient expectations regarding the quality of care and greater choice; advances in medical technologies, including drug therapies; changing health needs of the population (though his report noted that the changing age structure of the population would have less impact than many assumed); the rising costs of health care resources, including skilled staff; potential improvements in productivity, especially from Information and Communication Technology (ICT), as well as changes in the skill mix of staff and improvements in management, and a more coherent approach to service planning and provision, notably with regard to health and social services.

Recognising that many variables could shape the demand for health care, Wanless identified three future scenarios:

- ■ *Solid progress:* where people became more willing to adopt healthy lifestyles and make appropriate use of primary care services. Health status is improved overall and socio-economic health inequalities are reduced. Meanwhile the health service becomes more responsive to people's needs, with high take-up rates of new technologies and ICT as well as greater efficiency in the use of resources.

- ■ *Slow uptake:* where health status does not improve significantly and health inequalities are unchanged. There is little change in lifestyles and the frequency of consultation with doctors remains at the same level for the same level of need, though there is a increase in chronic ill health experienced by the over-65s. The service is slow to respond to investment and the speed of improvement is limited, with slow uptake of new technologies. Other potential improvements, such as those arising from better use of the workforce and ICT are not fully realised.

■ *Fully engaged*: People live longer and in better health compared with the other two scenarios. There is a dramatic improvement in health status and public engagement. People have changed their lifestyles to improve health and this reduces their demands on health services, though their expectations are high and they demand high-quality care. Health inequalities are also reduced. Meanwhile the health service responds effectively, with improvement in ICT, changes in skill mix and the rapid uptake of new technologies.

The review set out detailed financial projections for each scenario. In the early years there was little difference in the estimates, largely because the impact of most changes, particularly technology and changes in lifestyles, would be in the longer term. At the end of the twenty-year period, however, significant differences were evident between the scenarios (see Table 6.2). For example, the most pessimistic 'slow uptake' option required health service spending to reach 12.5 per cent of GDP by 2022 compared with 10.6 per cent if the most optimistic, 'fully engaged' scenario was to come to pass.

Table 6.2 UK health spending summary

		Projections			
	2002–3[1]	2007–8	2012–13	2017–18	2022–3
Total health spending (per cent of money GDP)[2]					
Solid progress	7.7	9.4	10.5	10.9	11.1
Slow uptake	7.7	9.5	11.0	11.9	12.5
Fully engaged	7.7	9.4	10.3	10.6	10.6
Total NHS spending (£ billion, 2002–3 prices)					
Solid progress	68	96	121	141	161
Slow uptake	68	97	127	155	184
Fully engaged	68	96	119	137	154
Average annual real growth in NHS spending (per cent)[3]					
Solid progress	6.8	7.1	4.7	3.1	2.7
Slow uptake	6.8	7.3	5.6	4.0	3.5
Fully engaged	6.8	7.1	4.4	2.8	2.4

Notes
[1] Estimates
[2] All figures include 1.2 per cent for private sector health spending
[3] Growth figures are annual average for the five years up to date shown. (Four years for the period to 2002–3)
Source: D. Wanless (2002) *Securing our future health: taking a long-term view – Final report* (HM Treasury).

The second report by Wanless (2002) made several other key points;

■ There are significant pressures on *social care* caused by demographic change and in particular the growing elderly population.

■ The impact of increases in spending in the short term will depend heavily on the full delivery of workforce expansion plans, otherwise the result will be higher costs due to staff shortages. Early action is needed to avoid capacity constraints in the medium term by increasing staff numbers and changing the skill mix.

■ High-quality health care will not be guaranteed by simply spending more money. Radical reform is also needed.

■ The National Institute for Clinical Excellence (NICE) – see Chapter 8 – should examine older technologies and practices to assess their cost-effectiveness.

■ National Service Frameworks (see Chapter 7) should be rolled out across the health service and in future should include estimates of resources necessary for their delivery.

■ A major programme is needed to establish an effective ICT infrastructure in the NHS.

■ Evidence-based principles are needed for public health expenditure decisions in order to get maximum benefit from investment in health promotion and disease prevention.

■ Rigorous and regular independent monitoring of health spending is needed to ensure efficiency in the use of resources. However, the audit process needs to be 'in the round' rather than tied to a small number of targets.

■ The balance of health and social care is still skewed too much to the use of hospital beds, and more diagnosis and treatment should take place in primary care.

■ Greater public engagement is needed, and the governance of local health care delivery could include community representation, including patients and the business community.

■ Greater local freedom can improve the overall health service significantly, allowing innovation and experimentation in resource management.

The final report reiterated the interim findings that the current method of funding the NHS through taxation was relatively efficient and equitable. Wanless himself argued that, while it would be inappropriate to fund clinical services through an extension of 'out-of-pocket' payments, there might be some scope to extend these to non-clinical services. However, his report did not rule out broader changes, stating that 'the way in which the resources are raised to fund health and social care will continue to be an issue for consideration in the light of the UK's overall economic performance'.

The Blair Government, while welcoming this endorsement of the tax-funded system, was ready to consider alternative sources of funding. It announced a large increase in the health budget in 2002, of 7.5 per cent per annum over a five-year period. This totalled over £40 billion, a 43 per cent rise after adjusting for general inflation. The Government estimated that this would bring UK health expenditure to 9.4 per cent of GDP by 2007–8 (Brown, 2002). Boxed in by an earlier pledge not to raise basic or higher rates of income tax, the Chancellor funded this by raising national income contributions by 1 per cent on all employers and employees (and the self-employed) from April 2003, while excluding those on very low earnings. This increase applied above the current earnings limit for National Insurance contributions and was, all but in name, a rise in income tax. But by placing greater reliance on a social insurance funding stream based on earned income, these additional resources would in future be raised from a narrower funding base.

Other changes to the funding system have occurred at the margins. These included extending the National Lottery's role in raising funds for NHS services and increased charges for treating road accident casualties. At the time of writing it has been announced that hospitals will get greater powers to recoup the costs of treating other accident victims, such as those injured in falls as a result of negligence. This move will raise premiums and, despite the avowed intentions of Government, shift the emphasis on to private insurance. The Blair Government also experimented with earmarked taxes on specific goods. In 2000, the tax on tobacco was increased and the additional revenue earmarked for use in the NHS.

Increasing Private Expenditure?

One way of increasing health care resources is to encourage private expenditure (Redwood, 2000). The UK still has relatively low levels of private health care expenditure (see Figure 6.2). In 1998 just over 16 per cent of UK health spending came from private sources. Nonetheless, this is still a substantial contribution, and represents almost a doubling of the level of the late 1970s. In some areas of care, the contribution of private expenditure is even greater (see Table 6.3): elective surgery, for example, with around a fifth of certain procedures including abdominal hernia repair, varicose vein procedures and hip replacement, being funded privately in England and Wales (Williams et al., 2000). This increase is part of an international trend among industrialised countries, and there has been an average increase of 0.6 per cent across OECD countries between 1980 and 1990 in private health expenditure (Propper and Green, 2001).

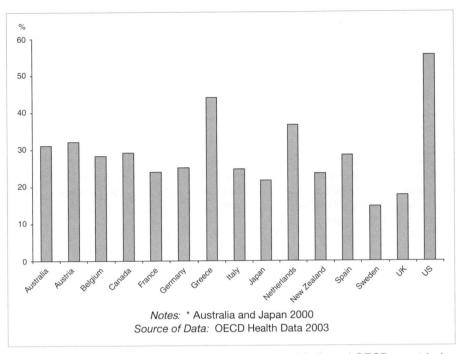

Notes: * Australia and Japan 2000
Source of Data: OECD Health Data 2003

Figure 6.2 Proportion of health care privately funded (selected OECD countries), 2001* (private expenditure as a percentage of total health care spending)

Private insurance

In 2000, 11.5 per cent of the UK population had private health insurance (Laing and Buisson, 2001). The majority of private health insurance schemes (around two-thirds) are organised by employers. A further 1 per cent are covered by company medical schemes which pay for health care treatment directly rather than on an insurance basis. The majority of private health insurance schemes (around two-thirds) are organised by employers. In the 1980s, Government actively encouraged private health insurance and extended tax relief for certain people, notably the elderly (see Chapter 5). Other factors (see Besley, Hall and Preston, 1996; Calnan, Cant and Gabe, 1993) contributed to this trend, such as industrial action in the 1980s, the popularity of health insurance as an employment benefit, dissatisfaction with NHS waiting lists, and perceived shortcomings in NHS services. In addition, direct payments for health care increased as people self-funded treatment using sources such as savings and loans. Over a fifth of private spending is self-funded (Laing and Buisson, 2001). The level of private health insurance, which peaked in the early 1990s, has over the last decade remained fairly stable. The Blair Government signalled its initial disdain for this form of funding by abolishing tax relief for health insurance for

Table 6.3 Public/private mix: Summary of selected markets

Market	Year to which relates	Basis of partition	Public finance public supply (%)	Public finance private supply (%)	Private finance public supply (%)	Private finance private supply (%)
Elective surgery – UK residents[1]	1997/8	cases	85.7	0.8	1.2	12.2
Acute psychiatric treatment[2]	2000/1	beds	87	8	small	5
Long-term nursing/residential home care of elderly people[3]	2000/1	occupied beds	17	56	2	25
Long-term nursing/residential home care of mentally ill people[2]	2000	occupied beds	26	73	small	small
Long-term nursing/residential home care of learning disabled people[2]	2000	occupied beds	21	79	small	small
Maternity – UK residents[4]	1999	birth	99.5	small	small	0.5
Abortions – UK residents[5]	2000	cases	46	28.5	small	25.5
General practice[6]	1998	consultations	97	0	0	3
Dentistry[7]	1998/99	cash	43	0	19	38

Notes
[1] See Laing's Healthcare Market Review 2001/2002, Laing & Buisson, ch. 2
[2] See Laing's Healthcare Market Review 2001/2002, Laing & Buisson, ch. 5
[3] See Laing's Healthcare Market Review 2001/2002, Laing & Buisson, ch. 6
[4] Office for National Statistics, Birth Statistics
[5] See Laing's Healthcare Market Review 2001/2002, Laing & Buisson, ch. 2
[6] See Laing's Healthcare Market Review 2001/2002, Laing & Buisson, ch. 4
[7] UK Dental Care 1999, Laing & Buisson
Source: Laing & Buisson, 2001.

the elderly soon after taking office, and continued to resist this as an option for generating additional funding for health care.

Charges

Charges rose as a proportion of total spending during the 1980s, largely as a result of new eye and dental test fees, and increased charges, for prescriptions and dental care. They raised 4.5 per cent of NHS revenue in 1990–1, but only 2.1 per cent by the end of the decade. The Blair Government indicated that it had no plans to extend charges for health care. However, the Prime Minister did speculate about the possibility of introducing additional copayments in the public sector (Smith, 2003). There is considerable scope for further charges, which may be exploited in the future, including charges levied on services that contribute to patient comfort, but which are not part of personal health care. Broader service charges may also encourage the scope for charging. It should also be noted that when services are moved out of the hospital setting into social care settings (see Chapter 11), opportunities for imposing charges occur.

Impact of increased private funding

Propper and Green (2001) found that reforms aimed at increasing the role of the private sector in financing health care would be likely to increase health care expenditure, though administration costs would probably rise. Greater inequity was likely, but might be moderated if the richer members of society were prevented from opting out of the NHS. Similarly, greater regulation might be needed to maintain access and equity in systems using what is in effect 'parallel private insurance' (Stewart, 1999), which could lead to an increase in health care costs.

Although the Blair Government rejected moves to encourage private health expenditure, it did begin to promote independent sector involvement in the provision of NHS services, discussed later in this chapter. In addition, it was enthusiastic about using the private sector to raise funds for capital developments in the NHS in the form of the Private Finance Initiative (see Exhibit 6.1).

Exhibit 6.1 The Private Finance Initiative (PFI)

Under the Private Finance Initiative (PFI), a public sector organisation contracts with a consortium involving private sector firms to design, build, finance and operate a facility. In the context of the NHS this is usually a hospital, though schemes are being extended into other services. Contracts are long term, the typical PFI contract in the NHS being 30 years, though some are longer. In the early 1990s the NHS was urged to explore private finance options. But the process proved highly complex, and private sector was deterred both by the high cost of bidding for contracts and the risk involved in such ventures. To deal with these problems, changes to bidding procedures and clarification of legal liabilities were introduced.

Following the Labour's Party's victory at the 1997 general election, the PFI policy was pursued even more vigorously. Despite earlier opposition, the Labour leadership backed PFI, believing it could secure additional capital investment without adding significantly to public expenditure in the short term. A new procedure for prioritising and evaluating capital NHS projects was introduced. Between 1997 and 2001 major PFI schemes (those costing over £25 m) worth £300 m were completed, and a further £7 billion worth of projects was approved. Meanwhile, public funding for major projects shrank to little over 2 per cent of the total, though it remained a substantial source for smaller projects. PFI was described as 'the only game in town' for major capital development (see Ruane, 2000).

The NHS Plan proposed an expansion in the capital programme, funded by PFI. It also envisaged a broader role for PFI in the redesign of local health services (so that PFI hospital schemes could, where appropriate, include the redevelopment of NHS primary care and intermediate care). Meanwhile, other schemes were proposed, including the NHS Local Improvement Finance Trust (NHS LIFT), which combines public and private finance in the development of primary care facilities (Pollock, Player and Godden, 2001; Glendenning and Bailey, 2000; Appleby et al., 2001). The Blair Government sought to moderate criticism of PFI. Clinical support services such as pathology and radiology were excluded from future schemes. Trade unions were promised a role in scrutinising the employment 'track record' of shortlisted bidders.

$\longrightarrow$

Exhibit 6.1 continued

→

The Government also proposed that more information be made available to staff and public about planned PFI schemes. It also pledged that in all new PFI deals, workers would remain NHS employees.

Nonetheless, the debate over PFI remains highly controversial (see Ball, Heafey and King, 2000; Ruane, 2000; Dawson, 2001; Monbiot, 2001; IPPR, 2001; Health Committee, 2002a; NAO, 2002a, 2003a). The main advantages claimed are that it secures additional capital funds for the NHS, given public spending constraints, and that these funds become available more quickly than under a publicly financed scheme (Smith, 1999). Furthermore, it is argued that PFI contributes to the effectiveness of capital projects by drawing on the skills and expertise of the private sector in several areas, including the management of risk, efficiency in the use of resources, and innovation in design and organisation of facilities (see Office of Government Commerce and Commission for Architecture and the Built Environment, 2000).

Have these gains materialised? Certainly, there has been a major expansion of capital projects in recent years. There is evidence of value for money, but this is based mainly on attitude surveys of those involved in the contracting process (NAO, 2001b). Indeed, there is little to suggest that PFI schemes are necessarily better value for money than publicly funded capital projects (NAO, 2002a), though most appear to offer initial benefits in terms of price certainty and delivering on time. Notably, the IPPR (2001) did not find that PFI had yielded significant gains in the NHS, though it urged improvement and experimentation in public–private partnership arrangements rather than their abandonment.

Could capital developments have been funded to a greater extent by public money? It might have been cheaper in the long term to have done so. Governments can borrow at low rates of interest and it is difficult to see how PFI could be less costly than public funding. A former Treasury advisor has conceded that conventionally funded schemes are more cost-effective than PFI and that the pursuit of the latter has been the result of political imperatives rather than based on evidence (Sussex, 2001; see also Dawson, 2001). Moreover, the PFI option has often been more expensive than predicted. There has been criticism of the high costs of negotiating and implementing PFI contracts, with large fees paid to advisors. Critics point out that payment for PFI schemes absorbs a large proportion of trust expenditure. In one study of new hospital schemes, the cost of capital had risen from an average of 8 per cent to 27 per cent of annual revenue expenditure (Pollock et al., 2002).

Some believe that PFI schemes represent poor value for money. Research has shown that planned bed numbers for PFI schemes are lower than current levels of provision, with reductions ranging from 5 to 40 per cent (Pollock et al., 1997). Although there may be a case for reducing acute beds (to fund places in other community-based facilities, for example), the overall picture is at odds with the findings of the Government's own inquiry (DoH, 2000c) and the NHS Plan which promised an expansion in bed numbers.

The argument that PFI schemes are more innovative in design or organisation has been challenged (IPPR, 2001). Indeed some PFI schemes have had significant design problems, and have been criticised for paying insufficient attention to factors affecting the patient's well-being (Mathiason, 2000). Another common criticism is that PFI makes large profits for the private sector firms involved. These profits can be increased further by 'refinancing', where the consortium borrows against future revenue once the facility has been built. This can be done relatively cheaply because future earnings are now relatively secure, enabling repayment of debts, reduction of costs and increased profits (McKendrick and McCabe, 1997; Dawson, 2001). This angered critics, because the transfer of risk is supposed to be one of the key reasons for choosing PFI (Pollock, 2002). Government responded by

→

Exhibit 6.1 continued

⟶

seeking a proportion of any refinancing gains (NAO, 2002a) although supporters of PFI argue that the main risk lies in the building rather than the servicing aspects of the contract.

Furthermore, PFI contracts may prevent the NHS from responding to new challenges in the future (Public Accounts Committee,1996a).Technological developments could render current facilities inappropriate, as more patients are treated at home or in community settings. The closure of a PFI facility represents a large liability for providers and may prove unpalatable. As Dawson (2001, p. 484) has observed, this maximises the cost to the NHS of adjusting to change.

On the other hand, PFI may have been unfairly blamed for some of the problems of procuring and implementing such large-scale projects (Dawson, 2001). The history of hospital building before PFI was not a happy one, with many cases of design problems, cost-overruns and inefficiency. Similar arguments could be made about other perceived consequences of PFI, such as hospital reconfiguration and closures, which have attracted local protest. Another reason why PFI has attracted much blame has been a lack of transparency in decision-making (Dawson, 2001). Because PFI is in effect a commercial transaction it is bounded by confidentiality requirements (Pollock et al., 1997), which makes it impossible for outsiders to evaluate. Hence the issue remains highly controversial, dominated by ideology and political imperative rather than reason and evidence.

Efficiency and Value for Money

The Blair Government, like the previous Conservative Governments of Major and Thatcher, sought to make existing public sector resources go further. This involved the promotion of evidence-based practice, a framework for improving the quality of services and a system for assessing the cost-effectiveness of interventions. These are discussed in later chapters. It also introduced measures aimed at improving efficiency.

Improving efficiency

From the mid-1980s the NHS introduced Cost Improvement Programmes (CIPs) to release resources for patient care. According to the Audit Commission (1999a, p. 51), a majority of trusts had undertaken CIPs in areas such as reducing management costs, grade and skills-mix reviews, contracting out, estate rationalisation, drug controls, surgical and medical supplies, and purchasing. Of these, most success was reported in purchasing, estate rationalisation and reducing management costs. Although the search for efficiency was laudable, a number of problems were associated with the CIPs. They tended to focus on short-term savings and could raise costs in the longer term (NAO, 1989). They imposed costs on other agencies or individuals, potentially increasing the overall costs of health care. Furthermore, plans to secure efficiency gains were not always achievable or fully implemented. One study found that only a fifth of potential savings were actually realised (Audit Commission, 1994a).

In 1992 efficiency targets were introduced for health authorities, initially 2 per cent, rising to 3 per cent in later years. This, coupled with financial requirements placed on trusts (to break even year on year and to achieve a rate of return of 6 per cent on capital), placed tight financial constraints that led to a perpetual search for savings. However, these targets proved to be a blunt instrument and did not necessarily improve the use of resources. Indeed, the measure of efficiency adopted by the Conservative Government – the Purchaser Efficiency Index – was heavily criticised for not taking into account the effectiveness and quality of services provided. It was blamed for encouraging 'gaming', where managers sought advantage by meeting targets rather than seeking genuine improvements (see Goddard, Mannion and Smith, 2000).

Despite criticising the previous Government's approach, the Blair Government imposed similar constraints in the form of a 3 per cent efficiency target, later reduced to a 2 per cent minimum 'productivity' target. However, this was part of a new Performance Assessment Framework, which covered a wider range of factors. In addition, changes to trusts' financial regime were made, supposedly to enable them to take a longer term view of efficiency gains.

The Blair Government, like its predecessor, sought to reduce administration costs. It introduced a cap on management costs (Cm 3807, 1997, p. 19) and abolished the previous Government's internal market with a view to saving £1 billion in its first term. Some observers cast doubt on this approach, however, noting the high management costs associated with Labour's reorganisation (Croxson, 1999). It emerged that the Government adopted a highly selective approach to the measurement of management costs. The number of senior managers in the NHS rose by 17 per cent (and their salaries bill by over a fifth) in the period, 1997–2000 (Appleby, 2001). Interestingly, costs associated with the Blair Government's modernisation programme were excluded from the management cost figures while there was some double counting of cost savings from the changes to the internal market.

Costing

A national schedule of reference costs was introduced to provide information on the unit costs of treatments and procedures across different hospitals (and, later, community health services). In addition, a reference cost index was produced, which compared the costs of providing the range of services by an NHS organisation with the national average. The aim was to place pressure on 'high cost' trusts (and PCTs) to explore ways of reducing their unit costs.

Although in theory this approach would enable a more accurate base for comparison, there were practical problems (see Grout, Jenkins and Propper, 2000; Dawson and Street, 2000). These stemmed largely from the difficulties in measuring costs consistently. A range of factors affect cost variations, such as the size of a hospital or its location, the range of services available, and the ways in which costs are apportioned. Following criticisms that the original measures were too crude, changes were made in the calculation of reference costs (see Dawson and Street, 2000). The Department of Health also clarified the costing methodology used by NHS bodies in an effort to improve consistency. The initial schedule of reference costs covered only a fifth of trust expenditure. More areas of expenditure have since been incorporated and additional data used to compile the figures. The 2001 schedule covered over four-fifths of hospital and community health services expenditure and 100 per cent coverage is planned for 2004 (DoH, 2002b).

Yet the new reference cost system is regarded by many as irrelevant (see Dawson and Jacobs, 2003). One of its shortcomings has been a failure to combine cost and outcome data. Costs tend to rise, at least in the short term, as a result of initiatives that improve the quality of service and transfer patients to more appropriate settings. By focusing on costs rather than quality, these measures create perverse incentives, discouraging the kind of changes that might improve the efficiency and responsiveness of the service in the longer term. Some argue that this creates an imperative towards mediocrity as hospitals strive to move towards the standard cost index score (Llewellyn and Northcott, 2002). The Performance Assessment Framework introduced by the Blair Government declared an intention to take a broader view, balancing cost and quality considerations. However, there is still a strong imperative to make productivity gains, largely through short-term measures that can damage long-term efficiency, such as freezing job vacancies and reducing beds.

It remains to be seen whether the emphasis on reference costs will produce greater efficiency. The lesson seems to be that the availability of information alone will not improve efficiency (York Health Economics Consortium and MSA Health and Social Research Consultancy, 1999) and the scope for 'gaming' remains considerable. Moreover, there are doubts about the scope for further efficiency gains, particularly as in the period 1994/5 to 1999/2000 no reduction occurred in acute trust unit costs or in the variance of unit costs over time (Dawson and Jacobs, 2003). Even so, the Department of Health has claimed that the variation in costs has since narrowed (see DoH, 2002c).

Another suggestion for improving efficiency is to create an element of competition between providers of health care. This was the rationale behind the Conservative Government's internal market. Although the Blair Government claimed to have abolished this system, the purchaser–provider split remained intact. Moreover, it subsequently shifted ground by encouraging a plurality of supply or, in other words, competition. It began to endorse greater choice, and proposed a system where resources would follow the patient based on a proposed single tariff for each treatment (see Chapter 7). Similarly with regard to support services, although the Government abandoned its predecessors' policy of requiring health authorities to subject these services to competitive tendering, the drive to cut costs and prove that the maximum value was being derived meant that the momentum to 'market test' services was actually maintained.

Efficiency watchdogs

Other institutions are involved in identifying ways of improving value for money. The Audit Commission, which was established initially to promote value for money in local government services, extended its brief to the NHS in 1990. As well as commenting on aspects of efficiency in a range of areas including, for example, the work of hospital doctors, day surgery, mental health, and accident and emergency services, the Commission has assessed the broader impact of health reforms on services. However, from 2004 the Audit Commission's value-for-money studies will be absorbed by a new body, the Commission for Healthcare Audit and Inspection (CHAI). It will, however, retain its auditing role, which involves appointing auditors for NHS bodies.

The House of Commons' Public Accounts Committee also has a role in examining NHS spending and investigating inefficiencies and financial mismanagement. For example, it has issued critical reports on issues such as hospital building programmes, the education and training of health professionals, clinical audit and preventive medicine. Another body, the National Audit Office, prepares the way for PAC inquiries and highlights waste, financial mismanagement and inefficiency. In recent years it has produced reports on outpatient services, the management of surplus property, NHS Direct, the Private Finance Initiative and charitable funding in the NHS. Meanwhile the Parliamentary Health Select Committee monitors Government spending plans for health and the impact of health programmes and policies. It has issued reports in recent years on public health, mental health and consultants' contracts. Finally, new bodies have been established to counter fraud in the NHS, which has been estimated at over £100 million a year (Audit Commission, 2001a). A Directorate of Counter-Fraud was set up in 1998, followed by a Counter-Fraud Operational Service, comprising specialist teams.

The Independent Sector

In all health care systems there is a balance between public and private sectors (Scott, 2001). Indeed, the British health care system has never been totally dependent on state-financed and state-run services. As Salter (1995) pointed out, the majority of the NHS budget is spent on services provided by the private sector (such as drugs, equipment, construction) and on services provided by independent contractors. For example, most GPs are not salaried employees but independent contractors who receive payment on the basis of a negotiated service contract. Private and voluntary organisations (which together comprise the independent health sector) also provide services on behalf of the NHS. The picture is complicated further by the fact that the NHS supplies some services in a private capacity. For example, patients may pay privately for treatment in an NHS hospital. Indeed, the NHS is the largest single supplier of private treatment and acute health care in the UK, with a market share of around 14 per cent (Laing and Buisson, 2001). NHS consultants, though salaried public sector employees, are permitted to undertake some private work, either in the NHS or in private clinics. Also, as noted earlier, the voluntary sector plays a significant role in both the financing and the provision of health care.

The Size and Growth of the Independent Sector

It is difficult to estimate the size of the independent sector, largely because it is so diverse. It consists of private (for profit) organisations, and voluntary (not for profit) organisations as well as individual practitioners working partly or wholly in a private capacity. It includes a considerable range of health care services, from acute hospitals and nursing homes through to dentistry and alternative medicine. In short, estimates of the size of the sector depend crucially on how 'independent health care' is defined.

A more fruitful approach is to examine the contribution of the independent sector to different areas of health care (Laing and Buisson, 2001; Table 6.3 earlier). The sector provided 19 per cent of hospital and nursing home services by value in the UK in 2000. Within this, the contribution of the independent sector varied considerably: under 1 per cent of maternity care, 13 per cent for elective surgery, over 50 per cent of abortions, and over 80 per cent of long-term nursing and residential care for elderly people. The independent sector also makes a significant contribution to primary care. Although its share of general practitioner services is small, at around 3 per cent, it makes a major contribution to the supply of dental services (38 per cent).

It is similarly difficult to estimate trends accurately in independent provision. However, it is clear that the share of hospital and nursing home care has increased since the early 1980s. According to Laing and Buisson (2001, p. 46), this share doubled between 1986 and 1992 (largely due to the expansion of long-term care in the independent sector in this period) and has since levelled off. Another area of growth has been private dentistry, discussed further in Chapter 10.

These general trends mask important developments within the independent sector. First, there has been a growth in 'for-profit' health care provision. In the independent acute sector, the majority of beds are now in 'for-profit' hospitals, a reversal of the position in 1979 (Laing and Buisson, 2001). Furthermore, because voluntary providers now operate in a much more 'commercial' environment – they now have to compete to win business and contracts – the differences between for-profit and not-for-profit providers have been eroded considerably.

Implications of a Greater Role for the Independent Health Sector

There are two main arguments in favour of an expanded role for the independent sector. First, it is argued that it contributes to the overall resources of the health care system. According to this view, one patient treated in the independent sector (whether privately- or NHS-funded) is one less on the waiting list for treatment. Secondly, it is suggested that the NHS has much to learn from the independent sector, in particular from its management systems and its approach to costing and service organisation.

Taking the first point, critics argue that the independent sector does not necessarily make a positive contribution to health care resources. Indeed, it can be argued that the UK independent sector draws resources away from the NHS. Two-thirds of NHS consultants engage in some private practice. It is argued that this creates incentives to build up private case-loads, resulting in a poorer service for NHS patients (who consequently may boost a consultant's private workload even further by deciding to pay for timely treatment). Yates (1995) found that over half of orthopaedic surgeons and ophthalmology consultants undertook two or more private clinics a week. But this does not mean that their NHS patients were adversely affected. The proportion of NHS consultants doing private work and neglecting NHS duties is regarded as fairly small (around 1 per cent in Donaldsons' 1994 study). Moreover, some consultants exceed their NHS contracts *and* do private work (Monopolies and Mergers Commission, 1993). However, the Audit Commission (1995c) found that a quarter of consultants with the heaviest private workloads carried out less NHS work than their colleagues. Furthermore, Yates (2002a) reported that the amount of private work undertaken by orthopaedic consultants was inversely related to NHS waiting times and argued that private work had a detrimental effect on NHS productivity.

Although no conclusive evidence about the relationship between consultants' NHS and private work exists, a more transparent approach is required, involving a clearer separation of public and private practice, along with the removal of incentives to build up NHS waiting lists (Keen, Light and Mays, 2001). Some have gone further, including the Health Committee (2000a) which urged the Government to adopt a long-term aim that consultants should not undertake private practice. Subsequently, in the NHS Plan, the Government proposed a seven-year ban on private practice for new consultants. This was later replaced by a Code of Conduct on private practice and changes to consultants' terms and conditions aimed at preventing their private practice from undermining NHS care.

The other main criticism is that the independent sector makes an insufficient contribution to activities such as research and development, or staff training. Yet it benefits considerably from these 'public goods' when it employs doctors, nurses and other health care workers. The independent sector also benefits from having the NHS as an essential 'back-up' service. Patients needing emergency care can be transferred to the NHS, with the costs falling on the tax-payer. Although, the independent sector has improved facilities in this area, it is still regarded as being at a disadvantage in this respect (Keen, Light and Mays, 2001). The independent sector plays a small role in training staff but it is expected to make a greater contribution in the future.

Comparing the independent sector and the NHS

There is very little evidence on the comparative performance of the independent sector and the NHS. However, in 2002, a controversial study of the relative efficiency of the NHS and a California-based health care organisation Kaiser Permanente (hereafter Kaiser) was published in the British Medical Journal. Kaiser is a non-profit Health Maintenance Organisation (HMO – see Exhibit 5.1) with over 6 million members in California (three-quarters of the total membership, the remainder based in other states). Members receive services through Kaiser-owned hospitals and independent physician groups. The article concluded that there was a similar per capita cost between the two systems (after adjusting for factors such as differences in benefits, population characteristics and 'the cost environment'). However, it found that Kaiser members experienced more comprehensive, convenient and timely services and had lower rates of acute hospital usage.

The study was criticised on several grounds, most concerning problems of comparison (see Appleby, 2002). Kaiser did not provide a comprehensive service (it excluded long-term psychiatric and dental care), nor did it provide services to the very poor, who are among the largest users of health care. The authors' attempts to adjust for these factors were regarded by some commentators as inadequate. Other adjustments (such as that which raised NHS costs substantially to reflect the higher input costs faced by Kaiser) were also contentious. Finally, it was also noted that the objectives of the two systems are very different and this makes it difficult to compare them.

There is some data on the comparison of independent sector and NHS management. A large-scale study of public and private managers found that NHS managers were rated more highly than private sector managers by their subordinates in terms of interpersonal skills, intellectual ability, change management and entrepreneurialism (Alimo-Metcalfe and Alban-Metcalfe, 2002). Moreover, it should be noted that provider organisations in the independent sector tend to be smaller than in the NHS and differ in many important ways, notably in relation to their objectives, the scope of activities, their accountability framework and their environment. The management task is perhaps not as challenging as that faced by NHS managers. In particular, managers in private hospitals do not operate in the highly political context faced by their NHS counterparts.

Although there is no comparative research on the quality of service, it should be noted that the independent sector has not escaped criticism of its standards of care (Health Committee, 1999b; Keen, Light and Mays, 2001). Indeed, a number of high-profile cases have revealed unsatisfactory standards of practice in independent hospitals, in particular a lack of peer review and poor back-up facilities. These exposed the weaknesses of the current regulatory framework in the independent sector, while the increasing use of the independent sector by NHS patients (see later) highlighted the need for common standards with the NHS (see Health Service Commissioner for England, 2002). Indeed, some of the worst examples of poor and unsafe practice in recent years have involved doctors who undertook private practice as well as NHS work (see Chapter 9).

The NHS as a Supplier of Private Health Care

As mentioned above, the NHS is a key player in the private health market. Financial pressures in the late 1980s, combined with additional freedoms to generate income from private patients, led many trusts to invest in facilities for private patients. By the mid-1990s there were 72 dedicated private units in English NHS hospitals, providing 1370 beds (National Economic Research Associates, 1995). As a result, the NHS share of private treatment and acute health care rose. However, this market share had been even larger before. In 1972 the NHS had almost half of the private health care market (Laing and Buisson, 2001, p. 71). Restrictions on pay beds, industrial action affecting private wards and the expansion of independent hospitals all combined to reduce this.

A study of private treatment in NHS hospitals suggested that, despite the expansion of NHS private work, private patients remained a small part of the business of the NHS (less than 1 per cent of finished consultant episodes 1989–95, according to Williams, 1997). It concluded that although private patients were admitted sooner for potentially serious conditions and much sooner for less urgent conditions, private patients did not prejudice the treatment of NHS patients. However, a subsequent analysis (Williams and Pearson, 1999) found that official data underestimated private patient activity, implying that the impact of private patients on NHS care had been underestimated.

Collaboration Between the NHS and the Independent Sector

The NHS has worked with the independent sector in a number of ways. One of the main areas of collaboration has been the use of the latter's excess capacity to meet NHS performance targets on waiting lists and times. NHS spending on health care in the independent sector remains small, around 5 per cent of the total NHS budget. Even so, this has grown from a small base and is likely to rise further in view of the government's support for public–private partnerships in health.

Public–private partnerships require a closer working relationship with the independent sector in the planning of services. As Doyle and Bull (2000) have argued, the private sector and the NHS have tended to operate in isolation and need to actively engage with each other to ensure that all health care resources are deployed to achieve national aims. In particular, they noted the potential benefits of improved co-operation for training and development, technology and costing, and research and development, among others. The Blair Government sought to improve collaboration by agreeing a concordat with the independent sector in 2000 (Independent Healthcare Association and Department of Health, 2000) which stated (p. 2) that 'there should be no organisational or ideological barriers to the delivery of high quality health care free at the point of delivery to those who need it, when they need it'. The concordat was intended as an enabling framework and signalled a commitment to include the independent sector in service planning. This would mean: closer involvement of the independent sector in planning, with local agreements on its role; commissioning or subcontracting services from it, and ensuring that services met NHS quality standards. Three areas of care were identified as potential areas for closer working between the NHS and the independent sector: elective care, critical care and intermediate care. In addition, closer co-operation was urged in local workforce planning, to ensure an adequate supply of trained and qualified staff. The document also urged both NHS and independent sector employers to provide information on adverse clinical effects, clinical performance and the treatment of NHS patients.

Subsequently, further emphasis was placed on the partnership role of the independent sector, particularly with regard to expanding the capacity of the health care system (DoH, 2002d). The Government proposed that new 'fast track' Diagnostic and Treatment Centres (DTCs) would be developed in partnership with the independent sector. These specialise in routine diagnosis and elective surgery operations. By 2003, 15 had been established by the NHS in

England, and one by an independent provider, BUPA. In addition, a range of Independent Sector Treatment Centres (ISTCs) were also introduced. The Government had previously announced that overseas medical teams could be brought in by the NHS to provide treatment. This was effectively superseded by the ISTCs, which involve overseas staff. It appears that NHS staff will also be seconded to these new centres, fuelling criticism that they will draw resources away from the NHS (Carlisle, 2003a). Also, it was made clear that a new system of franchising, whereby poorly performing trusts could be taken over by new management teams, would be open to private firms as well as NHS organisations. In 2003, the Good Hope hospital in Sutton Coldfield was the first to be franchised out to a private company. Furthermore, following landmark court cases, patients were allowed to travel to other countries for treatment, paid for by the NHS. Later, the Government offered NHS patients waiting more than six months for treatment a choice of where to be treated, including abroad or in the independent sector.

The policy of closer co-operation with the independent sector has been interpreted in radically different ways. For some, the greater use of the independent sector could pose a threat to the NHS (see Health Committee, 2002a). The NHS may be open to commercial exploitation, providing a low-risk market for the underutilised facilities of the independent sector. Furthermore, as a result of the geographical imbalance in the independent sector (a third of acute private hospitals are located in the south-east – The Fitzhugh Directory, 2002) opportunities for using independent providers will vary between different areas of the country. This could disadvantage NHS patients in areas with few independent providers. Further problems may arise if independent hospitals are allowed to choose the cases they treat (the suggestion being that when a fixed price is paid, the more costly patients may not be accepted for treatment and therefore lose out). There is also a 'thin end of the wedge' argument that once the role of the independent sector in treating NHS patients reaches a significant size, it will begin to exert leverage over local NHS priorities, processes and plans, to the disadvantage of patients.

Others take a different view (see Higgins, 2001a), arguing that in reality the concordat and other initiatives strengthens state regulation of the independent sector. For example, the independent sector is increasingly required to contribute to health service planning, and is expected to contribute to other activities such as training. From 2004 it will be regulated by the same body responsible for quality in the NHS, the Commission for Healthcare Audit and Inspection. Another argument is that the independent sector will actually be weakened by the new partnerships. Indeed, reduced waiting times may undermine the market for private health insurance, making the sector more dependent on the NHS as a customer and more sensitive to its needs. It is also possible that the NHS may take over private facilities, as occurred in 2001 when the private Heart Hospital in London was acquired by University College London NHS Hospitals Trust (NAO, 2002b).

An alternative perspective is that these new developments will make very little difference. Indeed, a survey of acute trusts in 2001 found that although NHS expenditure on services provided by the independent sector had increased sharply, there was little sign of private and voluntary providers being involved in long-term planning (Sussex and Goddard, 2002; see also Moore, 2003a).

Conclusion

The British health care system is still predominantly a public service model. However, important changes have occurred over the last two decades, reflecting global and ideological factors (Scott, 2001). As a result, there has been a shift towards a greater dependence on private funding and independent provision. However, this process has been far from straightforward and its implications unclear. The independent sector (and the wider commercial sector) has become more closely involved in the provision of NHS health care and facilities. Indeed, the current policy is to encourage a plurality of supply for NHS services, including NHS organisations (which are themselves diverse), public–private partnerships, and private, voluntary, and even overseas providers.

But what does this mean? It may result in a more efficient service with taxpayers getting better value for money. This may be combined with better standards overall, as non-NHS providers submit to greater state regulation and contribute ideas and resources to the health care system as a whole. Others, however, take a less sanguine approach (see, for example, Mohan, 2002, ch. 10), arguing that an important transformation of the British health care system is taking place that reflects wider changes in the welfare state. According to this view, the new regime provides greater opportunities for private profit, the reduction of entitlements to free care, and the prospect of greater inequity and selectivity. From this perspective, moves to extend the involvement of the independent sector therefore involve a reconceptualisation of the NHS, mark an important change in its culture and ethos, and undermine its collectivist principles.

_____ *Further Reading*_____

Fitzhugh Directory, The (2002) *Independent Healthcare and Long Term Care* (London, Health Care Information Service).

IPPR (2001) *Building Better Partnerships: The Final Report from the Commission on Public Private Partnerships* (London, IPPR).

Keen, J., Light, D. and Mays, N. (2001) *Public–Private Relations in Healthcare* (London, King's Fund).

Laing and Buisson (2001) *Laing's Healthcare Market Review 2001/2002* (London, Laing and Buisson Publications).

Mossialos, E., Dixon, A., Figueras, J. and Kutzin, R. (eds) (2002) *Funding Health Care: Options for Europe* (Buckingham, Open University Press).

Scott, C. (2001) *Public and Private Roles in Health Care Systems. Reform Expenses in Seven OECD Countries* (Buckingham, Open University Press).

Wagstaff, A., van Doorslaer, A., van der Burg, H., Calonge, S., Christiansen, T. et al. (1999) 'Equity in the Finance of Health Care: Some Further Comparisons', *Journal of Health Economics*, 18, 263–90.

Wanless, D. (2002) *Securing Our Future Health: Taking a Long Term View Final Report* (London, HM Treasury).

Health Care Policy, Planning and Management

Introduction

This chapter explores the organisational structures, networks and processes that underpin policy development and planning in the NHS, including the mechanisms that allocate resources within the service. It begins with an overview of the structure of the NHS. This is followed by an analysis of the relationships between central government and local NHS organisations and how these have developed under the Blair Governments. Finally, key problems are identified along with further suggestions for reform.

NHS Structure and Organisation

The current structure of the NHS in England is shown in Figure 7.1 (for a discussion of variations in different parts of the UK, see Exhibit 5.2 and Exhibit 7.1). The precise relationships between these various bodies are described in the following sections.

Central Government

Health policy making is a cross-government activity involving a wide range of departments and agencies (see Ham, 1999a). Government has acknowledged that the factors that determine good health can be shaped by the activities of a range of government bodies, and that policy making and implementation needs to be 'joined-up' more effectively (Cm 4386, 1999). Aside from the Department of Health, other departments and agencies have an interest in health issues. The Department for Education and Skills (DfES), for example, has responsibilities for health promotion in schools and for programmes of higher education, including medicine and nursing. The Department of Work and Pensions (DWP) is responsible for state financial support to elderly, chronically ill and disabled people, and low-income families, groups that include the largest users of health and social care. The Department of the Environment, Food

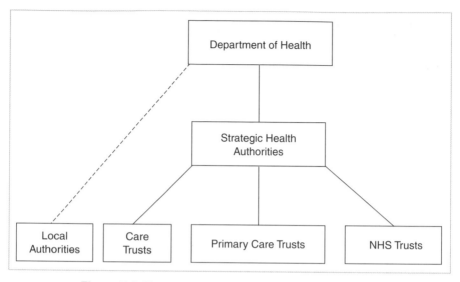

Figure 7.1 The current structure of the NHS in England

and Rural Affairs (DEFRA) has responsibility for a range of issues that impinge upon public health, such as food production and environmental protection.

The direction and co-ordination of health policy across central government is undertaken by several institutions. Ultimately the Cabinet determines Government policy, though full discussion only usually occurs when there is a major disagreement between departments, when a programme of major reform is being formulated, or in the event of an immediate NHS crisis or threat to the nation's health. Most discussion takes place in Cabinet Committees, which are essentially subcommittees of Cabinet. The Cabinet Committees most likely to discuss health policy issues are Domestic Affairs, Science Policy, Public Services and Public Expenditure, Welfare Reform, Social Exclusion and Regeneration, Older People, Drugs Policy and Children and Young People's Services. Interdepartmental committees of civil servants also discuss health policy issues affecting more than one department.

The Treasury plays a key role in health policy. It monitors the Department of Health's performance and expenditure against objectives set out in its 'Public Service Agreement'. Meanwhile, the Cabinet Office, which has a brief for modernising public services, seeks to promote improved performance and greater responsiveness to consumers across public services, including health. This is discharged by the Prime Minister's Office for Public Service Reform, which has a brief to improve public services. Also located in the Cabinet Office are the Prime Minister's Strategy Unit and the Prime Minister's Delivery Unit. The former seeks to develop policy on long-term and cross-cutting issues, including health-related matters. The Delivery Unit seeks to monitor the progress of Government initiatives in key public services such as health, to ensure that departmental targets are met and service improvement policies implemented.

Recent Prime Ministers have taken a close interest in health policy. This was true of Margaret Thatcher (who initiated a major review of the NHS in the late 1980s), John Major (who prompted the development of the *Health of the Nation* Strategy and the *Patient's Charter*) and, more recently, Tony Blair (who initiated the process that produced the *NHS Plan*). The Prime Minister's Office monitors developments in health policy and can influence the detail of initiatives – such as National Service Frameworks (see Exhibit 7.4), for example.

The Office of the Deputy Prime Minister (ODPM) also has an important co-ordinating function with regard to health. It oversees issues relating to regeneration, and regional and local government. The Government Offices of the Regions, which now have a public health function – regional Directors of Public Health are now based there – operate under the aegis of this department. Furthermore, the ODPM is host to two units which seek to bring together government initiatives that have an important bearing on health and wellbeing: the Neighbourhood Renewal Unit and the Social Exclusion Unit.

Several other agencies have a specific brief to improve and/or protect health. These include non-departmental executive health bodies such as the Commission for Healthcare Audit and Inspection (see Exhibit 9.2) and the Human Fertilisation and Embryology Authority. Others, such as the Food Standards Agency, the Health and Safety Commission and Sport England, are engaged in activities that have important health implications. In addition there are a host of advisory bodies, such as the Committee on the Safety of Medicines, the Scientific Committee on Smoking and Health and the Standing Medical Advisory Committee. Although these various bodies are outside the direct control of Government departments, they are accountable to Parliament through ministers. Ministers can influence them through appointments, performance review, and financial mechanisms. Furthermore, the statutory functions of these organisations can be altered by ministers, though substantial changes usually require parliamentary approval.

The Department of Health

The Department of Health is the lead organisation for health matters in England (and on UK-wide issues). Health and health care in Scotland, Wales and Northern Ireland is the responsibility of the Scottish Executive (Health Department), the National Assembly for Wales, and the Department of Health, Social Services and Public Safety in Northern Ireland, respectively.

The Department of Health (DoH) is headed by the Secretary of State for Health who has a statutory responsibility to promote and protect the health of the nation, to provide a National Health Service, and for social care, including the oversight of personal social services provided by local authorities. Given this broad remit, the department is at the centre of key policy development and planning processes in health and social policy, some of which extend into other spheres within central government and others which extend 'downwards' into the NHS. The DoH is responsible for the overall performance and management of the health care system, for standard-setting, for ensuring effective regulation and inspection of health services, and has powers to intervene when serious problems arise in the operation of services. The structure of the department is shown in Figure 7.2. Five ministers assist the Secretary of State for Health, who is ultimately accountable for policy and the overall management of the department. The ministers are drawn from the House of Commons, and one from the House of Lords who acts as the spokesperson for the department in this chamber. Each minister below Secretary of State level has responsibility for specific policies and services (for example, public health). Ministers' roles include the direction of policy, participating in interdepartmental activities (such as Cabinet committees), being accountable to Parliament, and acting as the department's spokesperson in Parliament and in the media.

In 2003, the DoH employed over 3000 civil servants. This number is expected to fall to over 2000 by 2004 following a restructuring of the department. Civil servants' roles include advising, briefing and supporting ministers (though ministers also have their own special advisors, who play an important role in maintaining political lines of communication; see Ham, 2000, pp. 46–7), managing and co-ordinating policy development, and the implementation of policy. They are organised into various groups, as shown in Figure 7.2. The department is managed by a board consisting of the Chief Executive of the NHS along with heads of the three main groups and other key personnel, including the Chief Medical Officer and the Chief Nursing Officer. The Chief Executive of the NHS, who also serves as the Permanent Secretary (the chief civil servant) in the DoH is responsible for the day-to-day management of the department. Between 1989 and 2000 the two posts were separated in an attempt to distinguish policy from management.

Civil servants in the DoH come from a range of professional, scientific and administrative backgrounds, including medicine, nursing and management. There have been efforts to increase the number of civil servants with an NHS management background in recent years. As part of a wider initiative across government, the DoH has also attempted to recruit people from business and the voluntary sector, often on a short-term or seconded basis. These developments have implications for the culture of the department, with the civil service's traditional approach being modified by this infusion of 'new blood', which some claim has a more positive attitude towards risk-taking and an emphasis on practical outcomes of policy (see Day and Klein, 1997 for further discussion).

Other key organisations include the Modernisation Board, which monitors the implementation of the NHS Plan. The board is chaired by the Secretary of State for Health and consists of members drawn from national health organisations (such as Royal Colleges and the BMA), managers and professionals working in

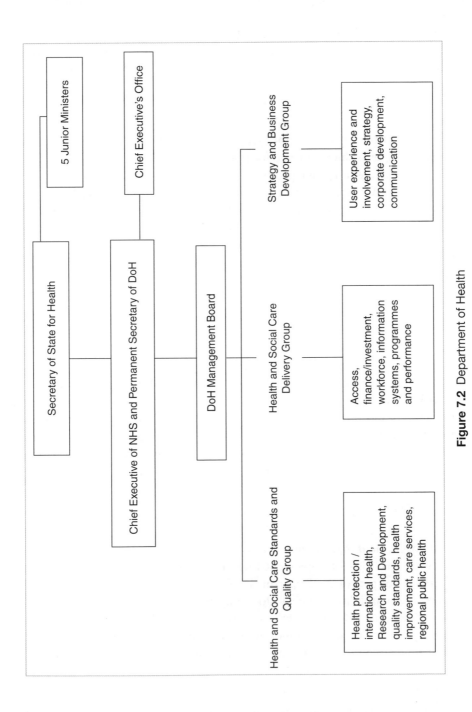

Figure 7.2 Department of Health

the NHS and a number of patient and citizen representatives (who comprise a third of its membership).

The Department of Health also has six executive agencies which are responsible for specific services and which operate at 'arm's length' from the Department, though they are accountable to ministers for their activities. They are the Health Protection Agency, the Medicines and Health Products Regulatory Agency, NHS Estates, the NHS Pensions Agency and the NHS Purchasing and Supply Agency. In addition, there are a number of Special Health Authorities including the Health Development Agency (which is responsible for providing evidence for policy and practice in improving public health and reducing health inequalities), the Prescription Pricing Authority, the National Blood Authority and the National Institute for Clinical Excellence (see Exhibit 8.2). The department is also festooned with advisory committees, working parties and task forces. These include people from outside government, including those working in the NHS and the voluntary and private sectors. Examples include the external advisory groups that supported the development of the National Service Frameworks (see Exhibit 7.4).

Formal contacts between the department, the NHS and outside organisations and experts are complemented by a range of informal contacts, including meetings, delegations and briefings. Civil servants and ministers are regularly in contact with senior figures in the health professions and in NHS management, and, increasingly, representatives of voluntary organisations and patient groups (see Allsop, Jones and Baggott, 2002) on matters of policy. Commercial interests, such as contractors, the private health care industry, medical equipment manufacturers and the pharmaceutical industry also seek to influence ministers and civil servants on policy issues. These organisations, along with individual experts in clinical, scientific and management fields, constitute a network within which health policies are formulated.

Policy and Planning at the Local Level

Central government may develop national priorities and standards, but if agencies at local level do not implement them they will be rendered meaningless. The NHS is not part of the Department of Health, and the latter, though having overall responsibility for policy, does not directly operate services. However, the department has a range of methods to persuade, cajole and coerce the NHS. Before we examine these, it is important to describe the current structure of the NHS in England and the functions of the principal organisations.

Strategic Health Authorities

The 28 Strategic Health Authorities (StHAs) in England are accountable to the Secretary of State for Health for the strategic management of the NHS in their area. The performance of each StHA is monitored by the DoH. Serving populations of around 1.5 million, StHA functions include developing local health strategies and ensuring their coherence, holding to account local health service commissioners and providers – NHS trusts and PCTs – ensuring high-quality services, and building capacity and support for improved performance locally, notably in areas such as clinical governance and the development of clinical networks. More specifically, they are expected to develop strategies for capital investment, information management and workforce development. StHAs are the main conduit for implementing central initiatives such as National Service Frameworks and are expected to ensure that such plans are integrated at the local level. StHAs are also charged with ensuring strong and coherent professional leadership and involvement of all professional groups, especially medicine and nursing. Their brief includes supporting improvements in patient and public involvement. StHAs are also expected to broker solutions to conflicts between different organisations in the local health care system.

Primary care trusts

Primary care trusts, of which there are currently over three hundred in England, are responsible for determining local population needs, planning, and ensuring that appropriate services are in place. They are responsible for drawing up local delivery plans which set out the aims of the local health care system and how these are to be pursued. PCTs are responsible for securing the provision of primary care, community health, mental health and acute secondary care services, personal medical services, medical, dental, pharmaceutical and optical services and emergency ambulance and patient transport services. They manage the contracts of family health service providers, including GPs. They are charged with primary care development and managing clinical performance within their organisations. They are also responsible for public health and public involvement. PCTs discharge their various roles by commissioning services from providers, such as acute trusts for example. It is envisaged that they will control 75 per cent of the NHS Budget by 2004, and an even larger share in the future. In addition, PCTs provide some services directly themselves (see Chapter 10) and have a brief to promote a more integrated health and social care system. PCTs are expected to engage with other agencies to ensure co-ordination of planning and community engagement, integrate service delivery and contribute to wider programmes that impact on public health and safety. Each PCT is accountable to the Secretary of State for Health through a Strategic Health Authority.

NHS trusts and foundation trusts

NHS trusts provide a range of hospital and specialist health care services. Most of their services are commissioned by PCTs. They are accountable to the Strategic Health Authority for their area. NHS trusts may apply to become Foundation Trusts (DoH, 2002e). Initially, this option is only available to trusts that have been adjudged 'high achievers' according to performance management criteria. Foundation status has been heralded as a means of giving these organisations greater freedom. Foundation trusts have been promised more autonomy over board and governance structures and greater powers over assets and financial resources. However, they will be expected to comply with NHS standards and targets (see Exhibit 7.2).

Care trusts

Care trusts work across health and social care, especially where closer integration is required, such as mental health. The precise functions of a particular Care Trust is determined by local partnerships between the NHS and local authorities (see Exhibit 11.2). They are also accountable to the Strategic Health Authority and to the relevant local authorities.

Local authorities

Local authorities have a range of health and social care functions. They provide and commission social care, and have important responsibilities with regard to environmental health. The Health and Social Care Act 2001 gave unitary, metropolitan and county councils powers to scrutinise health services, establishing overview and scrutiny committees for this purpose. Meanwhile, in terms of broader health issues, local authorities were given powers, in the Local Government Act of 2000, to promote the economic, environmental and social well-being of their area (see Chapter 13).

Private and voluntary organisations

Increasingly the NHS is seen as a plurality of organisations rather than a single monolithic structure. Health and social care may be commissioned by NHS bodies, but may be provided by private and voluntary sector organisations, such as private clinics or charities. These are important stakeholders in the provision of care, and increasingly demand a say in local and national policies. At the same time their increased involvement in care provision may lead to greater regulation of their activities (see Chapter 6).

Exhibit 7.1 Policy, Planning and Management in Scotland and Wales

The Scottish Executive Health Department (SEHD) is responsible for health policy and the NHS in Scotland. It sets priorities and reviews the performance of the 15 unified health boards, which are responsible for planning, health improvement, service provision and financial matters, including managing the performance of primary care and hospital services in their areas. The SEHD is also responsible for a number of special health authorities including

$\longrightarrow$

Exhibit 7.1 continued

the Scottish Ambulance Service, the Common Services Agency and the Health Education Board. The department seeks to promote improvements and changes in the NHS through a Centre for Change and Innovation. It should be noted that, in Scotland, trusts are to be abolished – some health boards have already done this. Community Health Partnerships are to be established in each NHS board area to co-ordinate the planning, development and provision of services. These bodies will plan primary and community-based services and build networks with local authorities, hospitals and specialist services, and the voluntary sector.

Scotland has its own Performance Assessment Framework (PAF), which differs from England in several ways. There are seven areas of assessment: improving health and reducing inequalities; fair access to healthcare services; clinical governance; quality and effectiveness of healthcare; patient experience and service quality; involving public and communities; and staff governance and organisational and financial performance and efficiency. There is more discretion in Scotland for local health boards to develop their own indicators and measures to reflect local circumstances. The Scottish PAF embodies a different approach, setting explicit success criteria for each area of assessment, and allows qualitative evidence to be used as well as quantitative indicators. It is geared more to identifying good practice, with the performance review focusing on examples of strong performance as well as weaknesses. The Scottish system does not involve a composite indicator or star rating, as is currently the case in England.

Scotland has a different system of standard-setting and quality assurance. A number of organisations emerged in the 1980s and 1990s, including the Clinical Resource and Audit Group (CRAG), which promoted clinical audit and evidence-based health care. CRAG funded the Scottish Intercollegiate Guidelines Network (SIGN) established by the Royal Colleges and other professional bodies in Scotland to produce multidisciplinary clinical guidelines in areas such as cancer and coronary heart disease. Another body, the Health Technology Board for Scotland (HTBS), was established to assess the cost-effectiveness of new technologies. Meanwhile, a Clinical Standards Board for Scotland (CSBS) defined and implemented national standards for health services. These standards were of two types: those generic to all clinical services and those specific to particular conditions.

The number of bodies involved, and their various functions, was confusing (see Scottish Executive Health Department, 2000a) – SIGN and HTBS, for example, undertook functions that were combined in one body in England and Wales, the National Institute for Clinical Excellence (see Exhibit 8.2). This confusion led to some rationalisation of these activities. In January 2003, a new body, NHS Quality Improvement Scotland, was created by the amalgamation of the CSBS, HTBS, CRAG and two other bodies: the Scottish Health Advisory Service (which inspected services for vulnerable people) and the Nursing and Midwifery Practice Development Unit. The new body is responsible for improving clinical effectiveness and ensuring that the NHS in Scotland provides service to nationally agreed standards. It will have greater powers of inspection and means of enforcing improvement, and will be able to conduct investigations into service failures.

The Welsh Assembly Government sets the key objectives, priorities and targets for the NHS in Wales. It monitors the performance of local health boards (LHBs) and trusts through three regional offices. Local health boards have a statutory duty to work in partnership with local authorities and in conjunction with other local stakeholders in order to formulate health, social care and well-being (HSCWB) strategies based on national and local priorities. Each local health board must also produce an annual service and commissioning plan which

---

Exhibit 7.1 continued

⟶

details how the objectives of the HSCWB strategy is to be pursued in practice. The commissioning of secondary care is co-ordinated by Secondary Care Groups that include local
authorities, local health boards and trusts. These also monitor provider performance for
secondary care and consider service development proposals from providers. In addition,
trusts must develop annual operational plans which detail objectives, and delivery plans which
reflect the plans of service commissioners. There are no foundation trusts or care trusts in
Wales. Service targets cover broadly similar areas as in England, such as health improvement
and access to services. However, there are differences – notably a greater emphasis on public
health following the commitments made in the Welsh version of the NHS plan – and variations
arising from the fact that the Welsh have their own version of NSFs. There is an NHS
Performance Assessment Framework in Wales, but there is less reliance on composite indicators than in England, and no star rating system. A framework for continuous improvement
was proposed in 2002, which seeks to assess all-round performance in the context of local
resources and problems, and is currently being implemented. This is focused more upon producing future improvement than punishing poor performance. The Welsh NHS does draw on
guidance from other expert bodies when implementing clinical governance and establishing
priorities. The Commission for Healthcare Audit and Inspection (see Exhibit 9.2) has overall
responsibility for encouraging improvement in health and health care in Wales. Also it should
be noted that NICE guidance applies to Wales.

Central–Local Relations

The relationships between central government and the local NHS in England
will now be examined. A useful approach is to explore the different ways in
which central government has sought to influence local activity: through organisational reform, priority setting and performance management, resource allocation, appointments and cultural change.

Organisational Reform

As McLachlan (1990) observed, NHS reorganisation became something of
an obsession in the 1970s and 1980s. The aim was to produce formal structures
that produced maximum accountability upwards (to the Department of Health),
while delegating operational responsibility downwards to service providers.
According to Harrison and Wood (1999), more recent reorganisations adopted a
different approach. Rather than simply creating a 'blueprint' of new command
and control structures, reforms such as *Working for Patients* aimed to create an
organisational context that promoted new ways of working by 'incentivising' certain behaviours or activities. Although this did occur, notably with regard to GP
fundholding, these reforms prompted further structural changes, such as the creation of new health authorities and the abolition of regional health authorities.

On taking office, the Blair Government modified the structure of the NHS in a way that arguably reduced local autonomy. GP fundholding was replaced by commissioning through primary care groups (PCGs) covering larger populations. On the other hand, the devolution of health authority commissioning to the PCGs was seen as a decentralist measure. Similar ambiguity surrounded the transfer of functions to PCTs following the NHS Plan. These bodies acquired functions from the health authorities and from the smaller and more localised PCGs. Nonetheless, the Blair Government maintained that this reorganisation would shift the balance of power to the local level and reduce central intervention (Cm 4818, 2000; DoH, 2001d; Cm 5503, 2002). It also claimed that proposals such as earned autonomy and foundation status would increase local flexibility and freedom.

Organisational charts are perhaps less important than the actual powers of central government over local services. Ministers' statutory powers have increased substantially giving a stronger legal basis for intervention. In the Health and Social Care Act of 2001, the Secretary of State acquired powers to intervene in underperforming NHS organisations, including the removal of members and health authority and trust boards. Interestingly, many of these powers can be exercised through statutory instruments, which attract much less parliamentary scrutiny than Acts of Parliament. By the same token, the statutory duties of health authorities and trusts have increased (with new duties of co-operation, health improvement planning and safeguarding the quality of care), thus widening the scope for intervention.

Priority Setting, Planning and Performance Management

The number of NHS targets has increased in recent years, and they have become more specific and detailed. An internal review by the Department of Health in 2001 found in excess of four hundred targets; subsequently the number of key targets was reduced to 62 (Stephenson, 2003). There are now also additional 'milestones', to monitor progress towards targets.

Priorities, targets and milestones arise from various policy commitments and initiatives. Currently, most stem from the key aim of the Department of Health, 'to transform the health and social care system so that it produces faster, fairer services that deliver better health and tackle health inequalities' (Cm 5403, 2002, p. 18) and the three related objectives: to improve service standards; to improve health and social care outcomes for everyone; and to improve value for money.

In line with these objectives, specific targets have been set for health outcomes and service improvement (see Exhibit 7.2), arising from the *NHS Plan* (Cm 4818, 2000), National Service Frameworks (see Exhibit 7.4) and the White Paper, *Saving Lives* (Cm 4386, 1999 – see Chapter 13).

Exhibit 7.2 Key Targets and Standards for the Department of Health and the NHS in England

1 Reduce maximum wait for out-patient appointment to three months and the maximum wait for in-patient treatment to six months by end of 2005 (with the aim of reducing maximum in-patient and day case waiting time to three months by 2008).

2 Reduce to four hours the maximum wait in Accident and Emergency, from arrival to admission, transfer or discharge, by the end of 2004 and reduce the proportion of people waiting one hour.

3 Guarantee access to a primary care professional within 24 hours and a primary care doctor within 48 hours by 2004.

4 Ensure that by the end of 2005 every hospital appointment will be booked for the convenience of the patient, making it easier for patients and GPs to choose the hospital and consultant that best meets their needs.

5 Enhance accountability to patients and the public, and secure sustained national improvements in patient experience as measured by independently validated surveys.

6 Reduce substantially the mortality rates from major killer diseases by 2010 (heart disease by at least 40 per cent in people under 75, cancer by at least 20 per cent in people under 75).

7 Improve life outcomes of adults and children with mental health problems through year-on-year improvements in access to crisis and mental health services and reduce the mortality rate from suicide and undetermined injury by at least 20 per cent by 2010.

8 Improve the quality of life and independence of older people so that they can live at home wherever possible, by increasing from March 2006 the number of those supported intensively to live at home to 30 per cent of the total being supported by social services at home or in residential care.

9 Improve the life chances of children by improving the level of education, training and employment outcomes for care-leavers aged 19, narrowing the gap between proportions of children in care and their peers who are cautioned or convicted, and reducing the under-18 conception rate by 50 per cent by 2010.

10 Increase the participation of problem drug users in drug treatment programmes by 55 per cent by 2004 and 100 per cent by 2008 and increase year on year the proportion of users successfully sustaining or completing treatment programmes.

11 By 2010 reduce inequalities in health outcomes by 10 per cent as measured by infant mortality and life expectancy at birth.

12 Improve value for money in the NHS and personal social services by at least 2 per cent per annum, with annual improvements of 1 per cent in both cost efficiency and service effectiveness.

Source: DoH (2002f) *Improvement, Expansion and Reform: The Next Three Years Priorities and Planning Framework 2003–06*

Priorities are monitored through the planning and performance review process. Most observers agree that this process became more centrally-directed during the 1980s and 1990s (see Paton, 1993; Strong and Robinson, 1990; Harrison et al., 1992; Klein, 1995). The Griffiths management reforms, which involved the appointment of general managers accountable to the health authority or trust, and the strengthening of performance review processes, were instrumental in this. Annual reviews were introduced in the 1980s, and the system extended down to unit, and subsequently trust, level. Performance indicators introduced in this period, coupled with the standards set out in the *Patient's Charter* of 1991, provided explicit benchmarks for monitoring health authorities' and trusts' activities. The replacement of regional health authorities with regional offices in the mid-1990s compounded this process of centralisation (Day and Klein, 1997, p. 14–15). Not only were they staffed by civil servants, but they had a much more proactive role in reviewing the performance of health authorities and in setting objectives and targets for them.

Initially, the Blair Government continued to strengthen the role of the regional offices (Dopson, Locock and Stewart, 1999). They were given the task of leading performance management and developing new forms of measurement. Meanwhile, health authorities were expected to adopt a more strategic role, with commissioning being increasingly devolved to PCGs/PCTs who would in turn be held to account for their performance. Health authorities were given the task of formulating three-year rolling health improvement programmes (HImPs – later renamed Health Improvement and Modernisation Plans). The introduction of HImPs reflected the Government's aim of creating a more strategic and yet inclusive planning process at the local level. Their formulation was expected to include all relevant stakeholders, including primary care groups, trusts as well as local government, the voluntary sector and the public.

Health improvement programmes

A study of the 1999–2000 HImPs found that national priorities were well represented (Abbott and Gillam, 2000), though only seven (out of 36) contained measurable targets. Most programmes included some public consultation, and most (but not all) mentioned consultation with local authorities and trusts. The priorities of PCGs, which produced their own plans, or 'HImP-lets', did not feature strongly in half of the HImPs examined. Directors of Public Health (Geller, 2001) stated that although many aspects of the HImP process went well (including multi-agency working and agreement of key priorities), problems encountered included short timescales, difficulty in obtaining commitment from some stakeholders, and problems linking HImP aspirations with financial and service planning, including obtaining funding for priorities. Further research (Hamer, 2000) revealed significant barriers to progress. In particular, the emphasis on improving health and well-being was apparently undermined by a lack of shared vision in local and national policies, a failure to include all local stakeholders, in particular local communities, and local structures and organisational boundaries which inhibited partnership working. It was clear that HImPs and local authority plans must be co-ordinated more effectively. Tensions between national and local priorities, and between clinical and social/environmental priorities were also evident. Despite the intended focus on health improvement, many HImPs did not emphasise key health determinants and inequalities (see Chapter 13).

Further changes were made to the planning process following the NHS Plan. Local modernisation reviews were introduced at local level to address key aspects of NHS Plan. The aim was to produce three-to-five-year strategic plans setting out changes and investment needed to achieve targets. Although expected to be consistent with the HImP process, the local modernisation reviews were more sharply focused on national priorities, and directed more explicitly at service improvement rather than on improving health.

HImPs were quite lengthy and detailed documents, not particularly user-friendly, and lacked public profile. There is little evidence about their impact on health improvement and services, though it is acknowledged that they provided opportunities for dialogue between different organisations and, for some, a platform for action (Hamer, 2000). But they operated separately from processes of NHS resource and workforce planning on the one hand, and local authority planning on the other, and this was a key weakness. Subsequently, a new framework, which sought to integrate local planning processes, was introduced (see Exhibit 7.3).

Exhibit 7.3 The NHS Planning System

In 2002, the Department of Health announced a new planning system for the NHS for the period 2003–06. This followed the *NHS Plan* and the *Shifting the Balance of Power* programme, which claimed that greater operational discretion would be given to the 'front line'. The new system responded to specific concerns about the number of targets set by the centre, the number and timing of different planning processes, the lack of integration between them, and the limited achievement of plans in practice. Its main features were as follows:

- A three-year planning cycle (to replace annual plans).
- Alignment of planning timetable with local government.
- A reduction in the number of plans, and of planning requirements (reduction of 80 per cent promised by the Department of Health).
- A single local delivery plan, managed by the Strategic Health Authority.
- Longer lead times for planning.
- Plans to be developed from the bottom up, with PCTs and care trusts producing local plans for health and service improvement. Each trust to produce plans showing how resources are to be deployed to deliver national and local priorities and to fit in with PCT plans. Workforce Development Confederations to contribute to these plans, with the workforce plan being part of the local delivery plan.
- Plans integrated across health and local government. Local authorities to lead in one priority area (life chances for children) and possibly in two others to be decided locally (mental health and older people).
- PCTs to hold provider organisations to account for the services commissioned. Strategic Health Authorities to hold all NHS organisations to account for performance, and they in

→

Exhibit 7.3 continued

⟶

turn to be accountable to the Department of Health. Local authorities' performance in the field of social care to be monitored by the Social Services Inspectorate (superseded by the Commission for Social Care Inspection in 2004).

- Fewer targets, and greater flexibility in the achievement of targets.
- Greater emphasis on holding organisations to account on the basis of actual delivery rather than plans.

Superficially much was devolved to the local level. However, the centre will continue to intervene. Indeed, inspection powers of the centre have been strengthened by the new Commission for Social Care Inspection and the Commission for Healthcare Audit and Inspection which will assess the performance of organisations and publish performance ratings. The Department of Health made it clear that there will be a strengthening of review processes to ensure that NHS organisations are monitoring progress (with 'earned autonomy' for the best performers), and that interventions will take place when performance is unsatisfactory.

Source: DoH (2002g) *Planning and Priorities Framework 2003–06*

The Performance Assessment Framework

The Blair Government had proposed a new Performance Assessment Framework in England (DoH, 1998a, 1999c). Although continuing with the previous Government's approach of using performance indicators, it placed greater emphasis on access to care, and the quality of care provided. The new framework identified six key areas: health improvement (including reducing health inequalities), fair access, health outcomes of NHS care, patient and carer experience, effective delivery of appropriate health care, and efficiency (the Performance Assessment Frameworks for Scotland and Wales are different – see Exhibits 7.1 and 7.4). A range of indicators was used to monitor performance in these areas. Some adjustment was made for factors such as the type and size of hospital and the socio-economic characteristics of the area, for example. Performance tables were published, so that the best and worst performers could be identified.

Shifting the balance of power

Further changes were made to the system of performance assessment in England, as part of the *Shifting the Balance of Power* initiative, which aimed to devolve responsibility for implementation to the 'front line' (DoH, 2001d).

The Government claimed that it was moving from a 'top down' approach that emphasised national standards and accountability towards local leadership, decision-making and accountability (DoH, 2002h).

In line with plans to reward trusts that performed well with lighter regulation and more freedom to innovate (see Exhibit 7.3) – the principle of 'earned autonomy' – the Government initially suggested a 'traffic-light system' to indicate overall performance. Trusts would be given a green, amber or red light, based on their performance against various targets, green-light trusts earning greater autonomy, including, less intensive monitoring, more freedom over investment decisions, and greater autonomy in spending their share of a new Performance Fund. Amid concerns about the public reaction to 'traffic-light' indicators, the idea was replaced by a star rating system, with trusts receiving three, two, one or no stars, based on their performance.

The system was initially applied to acute trusts and later extended to specialist trusts and primary care trusts. Three-star trusts – the best performers – would get the most autonomy. Trusts with no stars would be subject to detailed scrutiny, with their chief executives (and potentially their chairs too) facing dismissal if performance did not improve within the required timescale. In addition, management teams (from NHS and from the private sector) were given the opportunity to take over poor performers, through a process of franchising.

The calculation of star ratings depends on the type of organisation being assessed. Essentially, the rating is determined by a combination of performance indicators and clinical governance reviews undertaken by the Commission for Healthcare Audit and Inspection (formerly the Commission for Health Improvement – see Exhibit 9.2). The star ratings for acute and specialist trusts are based on clinical governance reviews and performance indicators that include the achievement of key targets such as waiting times, financial performance, hospital cleanliness, cancelled operations, improving the working lives of staff. In addition, there are three 'focus' areas which form the basis of the rating: clinical focus (including indicators such as clinical negligence, emergency readmission hospital mortality rates); patient focus (indicators such as complaints and measures of patient experience) and capacity and capability focus (indicators such as sickness absence, junior doctors' hours). Star ratings were applied to PCTs from 2003. Their performance is judged in terms of key targets (such as access to a GP and indicators of financial management). In addition, there are indicators in three further areas: access to quality services (such as access to NHS dentistry, mental health care and sexual health), service provision (for example, patients' complaints, sickness-absence rate and generic prescribing) and improving health (for example, deaths from accidents, circulatory diseases and cancer, and breast and cervical cancer screening).

Problems with star ratings, league tables and performance targets

Star ratings are a composite indicator of performance. The problem with such indicators is that they can oversimplify complex situations. Moreover, they may not reflect the quality of care, as perceived by professionals, managers and patients (see Liberal Democrats, 2003; Audit Commission, 2003b). Composite indicators tend to encourage a crude 'league table' mentality. Goldstein and

Spiegelhalter (1996), in a study of league tables in health and education, argued that they had many shortcomings and that potential users should be wary. They noted that many performance measures are influenced by factors outside the control of organisations rather than by those activities which they can influence. This was echoed, specifically in relation to neonatal care, by Parry et al. (1998), who found that performance measures were unreliable comparative indicators. They argued that comparisons should incorporate key factors that had a bearing on performance measures, such as the volume of patients, staffing policy, levels of risk and aspects of clinical practice.

Performance measurement by targets and indicators can have unintended and dysfunctional consequences (see Smith, 1995). If data is published, it might lead to undesirable changes in practice. For example, it has been reported that cardiac surgeons may be reluctant to take on high-risk cases (Schneider and Epstein, 1996). But even if this is not the case, performance measures may distort clinical priorities. In order to reduce waiting times for surgery, it is possible that non-urgent cases may take priority, because they have been waiting longer. For example, cataract cases may take priority over glaucoma patients, despite the latter facing irreversible damage to their sight as a result (Ferguson, 2002). Targets for individual organisations can also undermine a 'whole system approach' to service improvement. It has been suggested, for example, that targets for admission in Accident and Emergency may have led to patients being kept in ambulances for unnecessarily long periods (CHI, 2003a). The 'distortion effect' of performance targets has been found in other sectors of the NHS and the wider public sector (see Audit Commission, 2003a; NAO, 2003b; Public Administration Select Committee, 2003), including primary schools (Tymms and Wiggins, 2000). Another problem has been the deliberate misrepresentation of data to 'massage the figures' (Goddard, Mannion and Smith, 2000). This includes double counting of cases to maximise productivity measures, biased sampling to give unrepresentative results and selective alteration of data (see, for example, CHI, 2003a). For example, there was particular criticism of the measurement of Accident and Emergency waiting times in 2003 and the manipulation of waiting lists in some trusts (see Chapter 8). There is also human error. For example, in 2002 the Royal National Hospital for Rheumatic Diseases in Bath had its star rating upgraded from two to three following the discovery of a data-collection error by an external contractor (Batty, 2002). It was also alleged that ministers directly intervened in star-ratings. Subsequently, the responsibility for producing the star-ratings was given to CHI and its successor the Commission for Healthcare Audit and Inspection.

Little is known about the impact of performance indicators and targets (Nutley and Smith, 1998). A review of the USA, UK and Australia (McLoughlin et al., 2001) suggested that although it is widely believed that targets and indicators may help monitor performance, not much is known about if, how and why they might be effective. There is evidence that targets may have little impact on the quality of care or patient experience. For example, a study of the two-week target waiting time for women with suspected breast cancer found that although GP referral times to the first hospital appointment improved, time from first appointment to treatment increased (Robinson et al., 2003). In another study, the two-week waiting time for cancer was associated with a substantial waiting-time increase for routine referrals for colorectal cancer but did not necessarily improve the identification of treatable cancers (Jones, Rubin and Hungin, 2001). Indeed, targets and indicators fail to capture the quality of care experienced by the patient. This may be due to a lack of public involvement in formulating performance measures, or in attributing appropriate weightings to the various indicators (Appleby and Mulligan, 2000). It may also be the result of the current obsession with quantitative measures that inevitably mask the subtle, subjective and qualitative aspects of services (see Boyle, 2000).

Under the Blair Government, performance indicators have operated against a background of stronger national-level regulation (DoH, 1998b; Greener, 2003), despite the avowedly devolutionary intent of the *NHS Plan* and the *Shifting the Balance of Power* initiative. This, as some commentators have noted, has been a period characterised by the establishment of new central bodies to perform distinctive tasks (Appleby and Coote, 2002, p. 70). A Modernisation Agency was created as a focal point for leadership development and service modernisation, bringing together initiatives such as the National Patients Access Team, the Clinical Governance Support Team, the National Primary Care Development Team, the Changing Workforce Programme, the Leadership Centre and the Learning Network. However, in 2004 it was announced that this body would be disbanded – see Chapter 9. NICE was established in 1999, and its guidance made mandatory from 2002 (see Exhibit 8.2) and the Commission for Health Improvement (CHI) was set up to monitor service standards (see Exhibit 9.2). Furthermore, other regulatory bodies were created to promote higher standards of care and to protect the public, such as the National Care Standards Commission, the National Clinical Assessment Authority and the National Patients Safety Agency, discussed further in Chapter 9. Also, national standards for prevention, treatment and care for specific diseases and client groups were introduced in the form of National Service Frameworks (see Exhibit 7.4).

Exhibit 7.4 National Service Frameworks

National Service Frameworks (NSFs) set out national service standards and key interventions for a particular condition or population group. In England NSFs have been introduced for mental health (DoH, 1999b), coronary heart disease (DoH, 2000d), diabetes (DoH, 2001r) and older people (DoH, 2001e). Others, for children, renal disease and long-term conditions are being completed. In addition, national standards have been set for paediatric intensive care (DoH, 1998c) and for cancer services (DoH, 2000e). Wales also adopted National

$\longrightarrow$

Exhibit 7.4 continued

$\longrightarrow$

Service Frameworks which are broadly similar to those in England, while Scotland has its own system of clinical guidelines and service standards (see Exhibit 7.1).

Each NSF details national standards along with key interventions, targets and implementation plans. NSFs are comprehensive, covering all stages of a particular condition and multiple aspects of care relating to a particular client group. They are based on scientific evidence and on the perspectives of a range of stakeholders, which contribute to their development. Although each NSF has been developed in a slightly different way, there are similarities (see Hogg, 2002). This involves the appointment of an external reference group (ERG), drawn from various stakeholders: user/carer representatives, professionals and the NHS. This body produces a report, usually based on the work of subcommittees, which focuses on a specific topic. The report is approved by health ministers, the Treasury and the Prime Ministers' office, where changes may be made. The NSF is then published and an implementation group (consisting of various stakeholder interests) monitors progress. Health authorities, PCTs and trusts are expected to acknowledge NSFs when undertaking their various functions (i.e. planning, commissioning, drawing up service agreements, reorganising services, seeking to improve the quality of services and so on).

The main strength of NSFs is that they explicitly set standards in relation to a broad range of services. They do not focus wholly on the treatment of disease, but cover prevention, care and quality-of-life issues. Another positive feature is that they are not simply statements of intent, but are part of an ongoing process that includes implementation. Their main negative feature is that they are inflexible and may date quickly in the light of technological developments. It is also possible that they could lead to certain conditions, namely those not subject to an NSF, being neglected (see British Thoracic Society, 2003, with regard to respiratory disease), though the dangers of this should recede as more conditions are covered. A further problem, noted by some critics, is that they are dominated by medical perspectives. This is reflected in the membership of ERGs, though may be moderated by the participation of other stakeholders such as user and carer representatives.

Resource Allocation Within the NHS

Central government can influence local activity in the NHS through its control of financial resources. As noted in Chapter 6, the vast majority of NHS resources are raised out of taxation and National Insurance contributions. But how is this allocated?

There are two types of financial allocation: capital and revenue funding. The level of capital funding, which is defined as spending of more than £5000 on the acquisition or improvement of buildings and equipment (Healthcare Financial Management Association, 2001, p. 31) makes up approximately 5 per cent of the NHS budget. In England, major capital schemes (valued at over £25 million) require approval from the Department of Health, which prioritises schemes (Cm 5403, 2002, p. 40). Once approved, such schemes can be funded out of public capital funds, but are more commonly resourced through the

Private Finance Initiative (see Exhibit 6.1). Strategic Health Authorities receive 'strategic capital funds' and approve projects up to £25 million. They also allocate capital resources to PCTs and trusts for improving access to services. In addition PCTs and trusts receive 'operational' capital allocations directly. Finally, the Department of Health identifies programme budgets for specific capital investment, such as the development of IT.

In the past, revenue funding has been allocated in several ways: general allocations, specific allocations (for central services and initiatives), and payments to GPs under nationally agreed contracts. General allocations were formerly allocated through regional bodies and subsequently direct to health authorities. Now these funds flow directly to PCTs. Allocations, formerly for one year, are now for a three-year period. From 1999/2000 health budgets were unified, covering three elements: the resources for hospital and community health service (HCHS) spending; prescribing costs; and elements of spending on general medical services (GMS) that were not 'cash-limited' (such as the cost of practice staff, premises and IT).

These general allocations are determined by a formula based on variations in the level of need between different areas. Since the 1970s, central government has challenged the historical distribution of health care resources by using various formulae. The most recent version sets a target allocation for each PCT, based on its population, weighted for certain factors that imply greater levels of need, including age structure and deprivation. An element is included to reflect the variation in the costs of providing services in different parts of the country. Since 2001, allocations have been adjusted for health inequalities based on an indicator of 'avoidable mortality', whereby areas with poorer levels of health receive additional money (Shaw and Smith, 2001).

In addition, a substantial amount of funding (over 10 per cent of NHS spending) is 'top sliced' from the NHS budget to pay for national level bodies (such as NICE and other special health authorities and agencies) and specific programmes or initiatives (primary care, IT, clinical priorities, drugs misuse, tackling waiting lists, education and training, research and development). However, this may not necessarily get through to the services as intended. Research by a cancer charity found that half of cancer networks had not received their expected allocation of funds, and 43 per cent of these had experienced shortfalls of 20–25 per cent (CancerBACUP, 2002). Previously, many of these items were resourced out of a Modernisation Fund (of which about half was held centrally – see Appleby, 1999). These funds were subsumed into other budgets including capital allocations and what is known as 'Centrally Funded Initiatives and Services and Special Allocations' (CFISSA), which accounts for over 15 per cent of the NHS budget.

As noted earlier, a new Performance Fund was introduced following the *NHS Plan*. The idea was that the best performing organisations should be given more freedom to spend additional funds. Those that did not earn their autonomy needed the approval of the Modernisation Agency to spend their 'share' of the fund. Further changes followed the announcement of a new system of allocating resources within the NHS (see Exhibit 7.5 below), and the Performance Fund – which, according to the *NHS Plan*, was intended as an important way of incentivising improvements – was abolished.

Exhibit 7.5 A New Internal Market?

The Blair Government rejected the Conservatives' internal market. GP fundholding was abolished and annual contracting replaced by longer-term 'service level agreements'. But, following the NHS Plan, it began to explore new incentives for providers to respond appropriately to patients' needs and choices (Cm 5503, 2002). This led to the introduction of a new financial system (DoH, 2002i) where PCTs would be permitted to commission services from a range of providers, including the independent sector. It was envisaged that service level agreements would become more flexible, reflecting variations in the volume of services, rewarding providers for additional workload, and punishing those that underperformed.

As the policy developed, it began to resemble the internal market, which emphasised cost and volume contracts as a means of securing improvement in services (see Lewis and Gillam, 2003). However, there are important differences. At least initially, service level agreements are to be held and negotiated by PCTs, in theory reducing transaction costs and side-stepping accusations of a two-tier system that plagued fundholding. Secondly, the new system will operate with a national tariff. Instead of setting their own prices, providers will be given a standard price adjusted to reflect the unavoidable variations in the costs of providing services across the country (such as higher wage levels in the south-east, for example).

It is expected that the national tariff will apply from 2003/04 to additional cases in 15 designated HRGs (Healthcare Resource Groups – clinically similar groups of cases requiring similar levels of resourcing for diagnosis, care and treatment), including coronary bypass and cataract removal. It was proposed that for six other specialties – ophthalmology, trauma/orthopaedics, ENT (ear, nose and throat), cardiothoracic surgery, general surgery, and urology – prices will be locally determined, though adjusted for case mix (the mix of types of patients or treatment episodes) based on average costs for each HRG. It is envisaged that eventually almost all medical and surgical specialities will be funded on a cost and volume basis using the national tariff.

Amid fears that the new system would result in large financial losses in trusts that had high costs, it was proposed that the NHS Bank would provide financial support if needed. This would be funded by levies on trusts that made large surpluses. The NHS Bank was established in 2002 to provide reserves for PCTs and overdraft facilities for trusts.

Sources: DoH (2002i) *Reforming NHS Financial Flows*; DoH (2003a) *Payment by Results: Consultation.*

In the past GPs received funding for 'non-cash-limited' general medical services (GMS) or 'non-discretionary' expenditure. GPs received fees and allowances under nationally negotiated contracts and, unlike other items of primary care expenditure (such as premises and practice staff), this was not capped. It was often argued that this element should be controlled more effectively and allocated on the basis of local needs and priorities. Some changes have now taken place. From 2001, health ministers took into account non-discretionary GMS funding when determining allocations. Subsequently, a single composite target for each health authority was devised, which included non-discretionary GMS. Meanwhile, the formula for determining non-discretionary GMS funding was adjusted to take greater account of deprivation factors and the difficulties of attracting GPs to areas of high deprivation. Other relevant developments included the introduction of personal medical service (PMS) contracts for GPs which could be used to reflect local needs and priorities, and a new national contract for GPs with greater emphasis on service quality, needs and outcomes (see Chapter 10). Notably, the new national contract also led to ending of the non-discretionary element of GMS funding. From 2004 PCTs will receive these funds on a cash-limited basis, reflecting practice needs and workload. It is envisaged that in future this stream of funding will be incorporated along with PMS funding in the unified allocations of PCTs.

Ironically, the emphasis on local flexibility has been accompanied by further centralisation in the allocation of resources. This has been reflected in the use of formulae to allocate funds to the local level that reflect national priorities, in the increased earmarking of funds for specific central initiatives, and in the control of capital investment. However, it seems likely that increasingly resources will flow between providers and commissioners on the basis of performance. Although this may imply greater autonomy, the fact that this occurs in a framework of rules set by the centre will strengthen rather than weaken central power in the allocation of resources.

Appointments and Patronage

The Secretary of State for Health has overall responsibility for over 4000 appointments to public bodies. These include national bodies such as Special Health Authorities and other agencies, as well as Strategic Health Authorities, Primary care trusts and NHS trusts. There have been several changes to the system of patronage over the last decade or so. An important change took place when the composition of health authorities was changed in 1990. The old health authorities were run by boards containing part-time members drawn from a range of backgrounds. Some were nominated by local councils, others appointed from the ranks of NHS staff. In contrast, the new health authority boards combined part-time 'non-executive' members and 'executive' members – those with managerial roles. Some argued that these new structures weakened the role of part-time health authority members, though this was already happening according to other observers (see Ham, 1986; Day and Klein, 1987). However, the role of the chair of the board, a part-time appointment, was strengthened. The chair had a key role in the organisation of business, the appointment of the chief executive, and the monitoring of his or her performance. Studies of health authority decision-making indicate that the chairman–chief executive relationship emerged as the key power axis (Wall and Baddeley, 1998; Strong and Robinson, 1990; Ferlie, Ashburner and Fitzgerald, 1993). By contrast, non-executives faced considerable difficulties and were uncertain of their role (Audit Commission, 1995d; Peck, 1995; Stern, Martin and Cray, 1995), though some non-executives were significantly more successful than others in negotiating a more active role (Ferlie et al., 1996).

Changes to the appointment system

Governments have long been accused of using their powers of the appointment of chairs and non-executive board members to further political ends. These criticisms intensified during the 1980s and 1990s when the Conservative Government was accused of appointing sympathisers to health authorities in order to drive through controversial reforms. The Labour Research Department (1994) found that a quarter of NHS trusts had chairmen or non-executives with strong Conservative connections, and that the number of non-executives with such connections outnumbered those with links to other parties sixfold. However, political allegiance as a proportion of all non-executives was relatively low – estimates varied between 10 and 20 per cent; (Ashburner, 1993; NHS Trust Federation, 1995). The new health authorities established in 1990 contained more business and self-employed people, who might be expected to have Conservative sympathies (Pettigrew et al., 1991; Labour Party, 1992). Meanwhile, women and ethnic minorities were under-represented. Less than a third of non-executive members were female, rising to 39 per cent in 1995. Only 2.5 per cent of non-executives were categorised as 'non-white' (Pettigrew et al., 1991), rising to 5 per cent by the mid-1990s (Aanchawan, 1996).

Allegations of bias undermined the legitimacy of health authorities and trusts and, coupled with broader concerns about probity and accountability (Cadbury, 1992; Cm 2850, 1995), resulted in changes in the system of appointment. Non-executive positions (including chairs) were advertised, and vacancies filled by individuals on a regional list, who had to declare their political allegiance and other details. Appointments were scrutinised by panels which had one-third of members independent of the Department of Health. However, when Labour came into power in 1997 the appointments procedure was amended to give local authorities and MPs an opportunity to nominate candidates. This favoured those with political links and allegiances. Labour also continued a practice begun by the Conservatives of allowing MPs to comment on shortlists for health authority and trust chairs. A further requirement under the new regime was that non-executives should live locally and demonstrate a commitment to the NHS.

The need to appoint members of the new primary care group boards, and a decision not to automatically reappoint health authority and trust members and chairs when their current terms of office ended, led to predictions of an influx of Labour sympathisers. Between 1997 and 1999 Labour activists represented between a third and a quarter of 'politically active' appointees, though political activists represented only a quarter of the total number of appointees (see Office of the Commissioner for Public Appointments, 2000). The proportion of board members from ethnic minorities rose (reaching 12 per cent of NHS board members in 2002), as did the proportion of women on boards (almost half in 2002). Complaints about political interference in board appointments continued (see Select Committee on Public Administration, 2000). The Commissioner for Public Appointments, Dame Rennie Fritchie, reported that 'the process has become politicised in a systematic way' (Office of the Commissioner for Public Appointments, 2000, p. 26) and that in some appointments political allegiance had been paramount. Her report also mentioned that there had been cases where people had been short-listed and recommended, but that their appointment had not been made on merit.

Further changes

The Government responded by changing the appointments procedure yet again. Since 1 April 2001 all appointments to the boards of NHS trusts, health authorities and primary care trusts have been undertaken by the NHS Appointments Commission. Although the Secretary of State's direct role in appointments has formally been superseded, it should be noted that the Appointments Commission is a special health authority and therefore subject to ministerial direction. The Secretary of State determines the criteria for appointment and sets out key objectives (for example, equal opportunities and community representativeness). Interestingly, following the introduction of the new system, the proportion of Labour supporters on NHS boards *rose* to 26.5 per cent of all appointments in 2001–02, compared with 17.5 per cent the previous year (see Cole, 2002a, p. 24; Health Committee, 2002b, annex 3).

Ministers still have considerable patronage within the NHS. This has enabled them to appoint sympathisers to key posts, especially the chairs of health authorities and trusts, and now PCTs as well as other key agencies and committees. Although this helps to drive through change, it does not guarantee total obedience for several reasons: first, party activists are not in the majority; secondly, they cannot always be relied on to agree with government; thirdly, most non-executive members lack the knowledge, skills and resources to challenge local management. The crucial appointment is the chair, who, in conjunction with the chief executive, has considerable impact on local strategy. From the point of view of central government, these are the most important individuals in securing national policy objectives at the local level.

Networks

Central–local relations are mediated through networks as well as hierarchies. Indeed, considerable emphasis has been placed on networks as a means of improving services in recent years. The managed clinical network is the most advanced form of this arrangement (see Kunkler, 2000). This was defined in a Scottish context as 'linked groups of health professionals and organisations from primary, secondary and tertiary care, working in a coordinated manner, unconstrained by existing professional and health board boundaries, to ensure equitable provision of high quality, clinically effective services' (NHS Management Executive in Scotland, 1999). Such networks involve lead clinicians developing strategy, setting priorities for funding, relationships across traditional boundaries, involvement of several disciplines, peer review and quality assurance, and involve guidelines and protocols (see Baker and Lorimer, 2000). In England and Wales too, there has been much emphasis on building stronger clinical networks in areas such as cancer and coronary heart disease, for example. These are seen as important in developing good practice and improved services, especially in the context of National Service Frameworks (see Exhibit 7.4). In addition, collaboratives have been introduced to identify current problems in providing services and possible solutions, and to develop ways of sharing good practice and innovations (see Chapter 9).

Problems of Policy and Planning

Too Much Centralisation?

There has been much criticism of the Government's approach to NHS planning and organisation in recent years. Organisations as diverse as the BMA, the King's Fund, and the Institute of Directors, have argued that central government has adopted an overcentralised approach, leading to 'micromanagement' of the NHS. Others have endorsed this view (see Paton, 1998; Mohan, 2002; Klein, 1999; Dixon, 2001; Hughes and Griffiths, 1999). Critics believe that this leads Government to focus on the achievement of central performance targets rather than the experience of patients. As already noted, targets may be well-intentioned, but can impose a simplistic approach on a complex organisation with adverse consequences.

Central government's desire to control the NHS has been manifested in a permanent revolution of its structure and operation, ranging from full-scale reorganisation to wide-ranging changes in planning and management processes. Some have labelled this 'redisorganisation' (Smith, Walshe and Hunter, 2001). The exercise is certainly counterproductive at least in that continual reorganisation causes dislocation and the movement (and loss) of staff with important knowledge and skills. It is also possible that centralisation has undermined the capacity of managers and professionals to deliver service improvements. This may occur in a number of ways. Management and staff are afraid to speak out, for fear of being accused of disloyalty and disciplinary action (see Chapter 9). Another feature of this has been declining levels of trust within the NHS, leading to low morale and increased alienation and cynicism about change. These factors can combine to produce 'dysfunctional behaviour' – where staff engage in activities that inhibit service improvement. This might include massaging data or failing to identify problems that subsequently intensify. However, it is possible that patients may actually benefit where managers and professionals adopt strategies to moderate the impact of ill-thought-out policies (Clatworthy and Mellet, 1997; Hughes and Griffiths, 1999).

Too Much Politics?

According to Ian Bogle (2002), then chairman of the BMA Council, the NHS had become 'the Punch and Judy show of British Politics'. The metaphor of the NHS as a political football is also a common one, which most commentators agree inhibits informed debate about the real problems it faces. Health has been a top priority for recent Governments, and their credibility has often been judged on their stewardship of the NHS. The Blair Government continued this trend by embarking on a high-profile reform programme. As Klein (1999) commented, this was a high-risk strategy because it raised expectations and centralised policy, thereby increasing the political costs of failure. Hence the political stakes are high, adding impetus towards command and control. Moreover, the strength of media and public interest in health issues places Government policy under great scrutiny. Not surprising then that Government is under pressure to control the agenda and identify simple targets that it can claim to have met.

The command and control culture in the NHS is part and parcel of the new managerialism in Britain's public services, which involves the setting of central targets, regular and intrusive monitoring, and the identification of 'failures' and their replacement by others, including the private sector (see Chapter 3). This approach may work in some private enterprises, but not all, and may be highly inappropriate to public services (see Boyne, 2001). Chapman (2002) argues that the current model, where problems are reduced into 'rationally-managed' components, is inappropriate to modern government, largely because it does not account for the complexity of networks and cultures of public service provision. A holistic and systemic approach to policy that takes into account these subtleties is regarded as more appropriate. This involves interventions based on learning about what works, an emphasis on promoting improvements for users, a focus on the processes of improvement, closer engagement with stakeholders in developing innovations and achieving improvements, implementation to foster innovation, and the embodiment of evaluation and reflection. Policy-makers at the centre have a role, but this is limited to setting the direction of change, outlining the boundaries of policy, allocating resources, granting permission for new developments and experiments, and specifying the requirements for evaluation.

Hunter (2000) expressed similar ideas. He argued that command and control culture had been a major source of problems, and noted that the Blair Government in many respects continued and extended the approach of its Conservative predecessor towards managing the NHS. In his view this was mistaken and Governments must adopt a new approach, which focuses on longer-term planning and strengthening trust in the NHS. This must deal with the complexity of the NHS and its various professional subcultures rather than seek to impose uniformity by central direction.

Freedom for the NHS?

Recent policy initiatives have paid lip-service to less authoritarian approaches to improving services. Indeed, the Blair Government proclaimed a desire to shift the balance of power in the NHS to the front line (though some commentators doubt that this will lead to greater autonomy – see Hunter, 2000). Other policy initiatives which have been heralded as part of a more devolved approach include Foundation trusts (see Exhibit 7.6). Nonetheless, there is considerable cynicism about decentralisation in practice, given the high political stakes. Indeed, rhetoric about decentralisation has been accompanied by greater centralisation in practice (Hughes and Griffiths, 1999).

Exhibit 7.6 Foundation Trusts

As part of its stated aim to devolve responsibility for service provision down to local level, the Blair Government proposed foundation trusts (DoH, 2002e). Acute and specialist trusts (but not mental health trusts) in England may apply for foundation trust status, which, the Government argued, will give them greater autonomy from central government. Initially, the scheme will be open only to the highest-performing trusts (that, is those awarded three stars in the performance ratings). However, the Secretary of State for Health envisaged that all acute and specialist hospitals would become foundation trusts within 'four or five years'. It also possible that foundation status could be extended to mental health trusts, independent sector hospitals, primary care trusts and care trusts in the future. The policy draws on two main sources: interest in new forms of public ownership that might strengthen community ownership of organisations; and the experience of devolved hospital management schemes in other countries, notably Spain, Sweden and Denmark.

Despite a wide recognition that greater decentralisation in the NHS was necessary, the reforms proved controversial (see Health Committee, 2003a for discussion of the key

$\longrightarrow$

Exhibit 7.6 continued

arguments). One of the main issues was that additional freedoms promised to foundation trusts would place others at a disadvantage. The promised freedoms included the ability to retain surpluses and to decide how to spend these funds, additional powers to borrow from public and private sectors and to sell assets, and greater flexibility to pay and reward staff. If these were realised, foundation trusts would be able to compete more effectively with non-foundation hospitals, for example, through their greater capacity to improve facilities and attract staff. Coupled with the new system of financial flows, where revenue would be more closely linked to workload, foundation status risked creating wider inequities in services. The Government responded by emphasising that foundation trusts would remain within the NHS, and would be subject to regulation. A new independent regulator was created to authorise the framework for each foundation trust, including conditions with regard to the range of services provided, the level of private practice, a list of protected assets that cannot be sold, and restrictions on borrowing. Although constituted in law as independent public benefit organisations, the Government has stated that foundation hospitals remain part of the NHS, will not be able to extend charges to NHS patients, and will be bound by the duty of co-operation with partner organisations. The standard of care provided will be subject to regulation by the Commission for Healthcare Audit and Inspection (CHAI), while the ability of the foundation trusts to raise capital is restricted by a formula linking borrowing to the ability to repay.

Others were critical not of the freedoms but of the additional regulation this would bring. Recalling the promised freedoms of hospital trusts in the Conservative reforms of the 1990s, they were cynical about the scope for autonomy (see Robinson, 2002c). Moreover, as one observer noted, the scheme would result in a 'cacophony of accountabilities' (Klein, 2003), with foundation trusts at the junction of conflicting pressures to conform to national standards and local priorities. The Government stressed that foundation trusts would be accountable to local communities. Their governance structures were required to grant membership rights to service users and carers, local residents and staff. Although the precise details would be determined by the foundation trust itself, these members would elect the majority of a governing board that would oversee a board of directors responsible for running the organisation. However, there were doubts that most ordinary people would join and that only activists would participate. Indeed, the Government acknowledged this by allowing foundation trusts to introduce schemes whereby people opted out of membership rather than opting in, in an effort to maximise membership. Similarly, the Government backtracked on a proposed membership fee of £1 – stating that this was a token payment, and would be levied at the discretion of each foundation trust – following criticism that people should not be subjected to an additional charge. There was also concern that the governing body was toothless. The Government made it clear that it could not veto strategy, or intervene in day-to-day affairs. The governing body's role in appointing the chair and non-executive members of the board of directors was also diluted by giving extended tenure to current post-holders. Meanwhile, there was strong criticism of the inconsistency of the proposed governance structures of foundation trusts with the new system of patient and public involvement that was being implemented (see Chapter 12). Originally, the Government decided that foundation trusts would not require a Patient and Public Involvement Forum, though this was later conceded.

Another worry was that foundation trusts would undermine interagency relationships and thereby damage the health care system at local level. There was no requirement to include social services, for example, in the governance arrangements of foundation trusts (although there had to be a local government representative). While primary care trusts were expected

→

Exhibit 7.6 continued

⟶

to have representation, this was fairly minimal amounting to a requirement that at least one member of the governing board should be drawn from a local PCT. Although PCTs hold most of the budget for health care, this may not give them much leverage over foundation trusts, particularly as the latter will be able to claim added legitimacy, as mutual organisations. This, it has been argued, could bring about a shift in emphasis away from the principle of a primary-care-led NHS that had become established in the 1990s (Walshe, 2003b). However, it is difficult to predict the impact on relationships between primary and secondary care, and several scenarios are possible (see Lewis, Dixon and Gillam, 2003a).

Despite its large majority in the House of Commons, the Blair Government struggled to get the necessary legislation through. Concessions were given, including a promise that there would be a review of the initial wave of foundation trusts. However, 32 trusts had already been lined up to follow the first wave of 25 foundation trusts. Eventually the Health and Social Care Act (Community and Health Standards) 2003 – which enacted foundation hospitals – was passed. It remains to be seen whether the critics' fears are justified.

Set the NHS free?

Others have argued that the only solution is for central government to divest its powers of micromanagement. Several authoritative reports have recommended that the NHS be given a certain amount of formal independence. The Commission on the NHS (Hutton, 2000), an independent body of experts established by the Association of Community Health Councils for England and Wales (ACHCEW), called for the NHS to be given its own constitution in order to protect its founding principles. It stated that the NHS should become a public corporation at arm's length from Government, with its own board and operational freedoms. It recommended that the NHS become a democratic organisation with elected health authorities at local level and eventually regional assemblies taking on the function. Similarly, a report from the NHS Alliance (2000), a body representing primary care organisations, reported that the NHS Executive (the part of the DoH then responsible for running the NHS) should be separated from Government and restructured as an executive, non-departmental public body.

Further momentum was added by a King's Fund (2002) report which recommended that the NHS be instituted as a corporation, arguing that a clearer separation between Government and the service was needed. Ministers would set policy objectives, set a framework for policy and practice developments, and allocate overall resources. An NHS corporation would then decide how best to meet these objectives, being responsible for standards, regulation, institutional learning and local resource allocation, without direct political interference from central government. A further analysis found potential advantages included greater parliamentary scrutiny, debate and accountability, and possibly greater commitment to and ownership of national health standards and targets (Dewar, 2003).

Caveats

Yet such an approach has dangers and challenges. In the absence of democratic mechanisms, the NHS could in effect be run by an unaccountable quango. Given that the majority of funding for the NHS is raised out of national taxation, it is unlikely that national politicians would wish to relinquish control. More likely would be the development of informal (but no less powerful) pressures on the NHS agency as ministers sought to control its activities. Parliament would also be concerned about the implications for accountability of an NHS corporation. Some form of direct accountability to Parliament would be needed to address these concerns (Dewar, 2003).

Alternatively, a model based on regional and local government might strengthen accountability in one sense, but would not deal with the issue of central funding – which underpins the demand for 'upwards accountability'. Moreover, the democratic credentials of local government are limited – as indicated by low turnouts at local elections. There is currently little appetite for regional government, seen as too remote from local people. Perhaps the best that can be hoped for in the present context is greater scrutiny at these levels, building on the newly created local authority overview and scrutiny committees (see Chapter 12).

There are broader problems associated with greater devolution. The NHS is based on a universal principle. This does not sit easily with efforts to encourage devolution and diversity. The political implications are that central government will be held responsible for any inequities and failings that result from devolution, creating pressures to recentralise. The history of the NHS has been that of central government trying to delegate responsibility to the NHS, being held responsible for failure and seeking tighter control. Indeed, it has been pointed out that it is extremely difficult to devolve in the context of a centralised and hierarchical system such as the NHS, and that efforts to simply import policies from countries that have weak hierarchies may not work (Kumpers et al., 2002).

Moreover, there is the fundamental issue of politicisation. As many commentators – including health service managers and politicians – have acknowledged, the contemporary health service is unavoidably political (see Edwards, 1993, p. 181; Lawson, 1992, p. 613). The reasons for this are succinctly expressed by Douglas Black (1987, p. 38): 'it is not possible, as some wish, to take the health service out of politics – both the amount of money involved and the sensitivity of anything to do with health will keep the health service a major political preoccupation'. It is therefore naïve to think that the NHS can be depoliticised by simple administrative restructuring, or that policy and management can easily be separated. Indeed, in some ways it is perhaps good that the NHS is politicised. It focuses attention on those managing and working in the service and their political masters, and it strengthens their demands for resources.

Conclusion

The NHS is bedevilled with confusion about different types of accountability in the context of health services (see Day and Klein, 1987; Ferlie et al., 1996), and many of these conflict with each other. There is the managerial accountability of the NHS to Government, the political accountability of Government to Parliament and the public, and the clinical accountability of professionals to patients. Centralisation has not resolved these tensions, nor has it produced a satisfactory balance between central and local responsibilities. But it also remains difficult to decentralise the service in the face of the pressures faced by central government. As long as the NHS continues to be perceived as a national service, is centrally funded out of taxation, and remains high on the political agenda, ultimate responsibility for the service will remain focused at the centre.

_____ *Further Reading*_____

Day, P. and Klein, R. (1997) *Steering but not Rowing – The Transformation of the Department of Health* (Bristol, Policy Press).

Dewar, S. (2003) *Government and the NHS: Time for a New Relationship* (London, King's Fund).

Ham, C. (2000) *The Politics of NHS Reform 1988–97 – Metaphor or Reality?* (London, King's Fund).

Hutton, W. (2000) *New Life for Health: The Commission on the NHS* (London, Vintage).

Klein, R. (1995) *The New Politics of the NHS* (London, Longman).

Palfrey, C. (2000) *Key Concepts in Health Care Policy and Planning – An Introductory Text* (Basingstoke, Macmillan).

Wall, A. and Owen, B. (1999) *Health Policy: Health Care and the NHS* (Eastbourne, The Gildredge Press).

Access to Health Care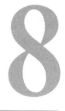

Over the lifetime of the NHS, debates about fair access, waiting lists and delays in treatment have been ever-present. These issues have became even more prominent in recent years in view of Government commitments to promote equitable access, reduce waiting lists and waiting times, and introduce greater choice and convenience for patients. This chapter begins by exploring the meaning of access in health care. It moves on to consider the problems of access within the British health care system. This is followed by an analysis of policies in this field. Finally, the related issues of priority-setting and rationing, and their implications for access, are considered.

What is Access?

Access is a notoriously complex concept (see Gulliford et al., 2001; Rosen, Florin and Dixon, 2001). It can be interpreted as any of the following:

- a service available for use when needed

- using a service

- having available or using a service that is responsive to clinical needs (both in terms of urgency and severity)

- having available or using a service that is responsive to individual choices and circumstances, and is convenient to use

- having available or using a service that provides care of high quality (both in terms of the process of delivery and the outcome).

To complicate matters further, there are two ways of analysing access, and the factors which impede it. First, one can explore the general experience, such as the problems faced by all citizens or service users, irrespective of social background, condition, location or circumstances. The second approach is to examine the situation faced by different subgroups within the population and how this compares with the general experience. Rosen, Florin and Dixon (2001) have defined the former as '*absolute* access', and the latter as '*relative* access'. These different aspects are now examined.

Absolute Access

Problems associated with absolute access can be divided into four related issues: non-entry to a service; delays in diagnosis, care or treatment; lack of convenience and choice; and failure to access high-quality care.

Non-entry

With regard to absolute access, non-entry is where individuals, irrespective of their location, circumstances or socio-economic factors, do not access a service. This may be due to problems of 'supply'. For example, people may have difficulties in registering with a GP as a result of shortage of trained professionals, or it may be that professionals are unwilling to supply a service for some reason. For example, many people across the country have found it increasingly difficult to register as NHS patients with dental practices, because many dentists have chosen to expand their private practice and reduce or abandon their NHS work. Problems can occur on the demand side too. Individuals may be reluctant to seek help from health service providers for their particular condition, or could be unaware that they have a health problem.

Delays

Delays are most commonly associated with waiting lists, a perennial feature of the NHS. Waiting lists appear an obvious indicator of poor access to health care. Their sheer size makes them difficult to ignore (940,000 people waiting for hospital admission in England in November 2003). Yet they are neither an accurate nor a useful indicator of access (Harrison and New, 2000). Waiting lists are inaccurate because they include people who may never receive treatment, such as those inappropriately referred for treatment, or who die on the waiting list (Tudor Edwards, 1997, p. 15). Waiting lists exclude people who may need treatment, but who have not been admitted on to the list. This may happen because they have not sought a diagnosis or have not been appropriately referred. It can also result from deliberate manipulation of the waiting list figures.

Although waiting lists continue to occupy the attention of the media and politicians, waiting times are acknowledged as a better indicator. Waiting times in the UK are relatively long, compared with European Union countries and the United States (Wanless, 2001, p. 97). In November 2003, over 140,000 people had waited over six months for hospital treatment in England; over 30,000 had waited over nine months. However, waiting times are also regarded as a flawed measure. Armstrong (2000) observed that waiting-time calculations reveal how many people are waiting and how long those admitted for treatment have waited, but not the likelihood of admission by those currently waiting.

Furthermore, waiting times tell us little about the clinical needs of those await-ing treatment. Obviously, a lengthy wait for cancer treatment is likely to be of greater concern than for varicose veins. But, even in the field of cancer, the same waiting time can have different outcomes, depending on the stage and type of the disease. Such subtleties are obscured by overall waiting-time statistics. The focus on overall waiting times also obscures significant variations in the per-formance of different providers. One study found that a quarter of hospital trusts contribute between half and four-fifths of patients waiting six months or longer and argued that a more focused approach towards these providers is more appropriate (Martin et al., 2003). Finally, overall figures obscure specific 'bottlenecks' which affect the timing of other interventions. For example, one of the main causes of longer waiting times has been the build-up of patients awaiting diagnostic procedures. The Audit Commission (2002a) found that approximately half a million people were waiting for a CAT or MRI scan, with an average wait of five months.

Convenience and choice

Although waiting times remain the primary concern, access is not simply about prompt diagnosis, care and treatment, but about the convenience of services, the scope for choice and the availability of information about services (see Kendall, 2001; Henke, Murray and Nelson, 2002). It is now believed that patients want a more convenient service organised around their needs. Furthermore, it is argued that patients also want more information about health and health care. They want to be treated and cared for in comfortable surroundings. There is also an acknowledgement that patients now want a greater say in their care and more choice about the kind of care they receive and where they receive it. The issues of choice, convenience and information are discussed in the context of con-sumerism in health care in Chapter 12.

Quality

The final aspect of access relates to quality. It is obviously important to incor-porate quality into the notion of access. No one would want speedy access to a service that was poor. Similarly, choice and convenience have little meaning if the alternatives are all of low standard. Quality issues are discussed further in the next chapter.

What affects absolute access?

Absolute access is shaped by a range of factors (see Rosen, Florin and Dixon, 2001; Gulliford et al., 2001). First, the supply of services places a limit on what can be accessed. At the extreme there may be no service available for a particular condition. Usually though, the problem is insufficient resources to meet demand. Other supply-side problems include obstacles that block or inhibit access (for example, inadequate systems of referral, restricted opening hours, or distant location of services). There are also important demand-side factors. An individual's health-seeking behaviour can strongly influence whether they access health care and what kind of service they receive once in the system. Financial barriers are also important, particularly for low-income groups. For example, charges for health care can deter people. In addition, there are other costs which people incur when using health services, such as transport, telephone, and opportunity costs, including loss of earnings. Information, too, is a significant factor. Without information, people are limited in their ability to access services. Indeed, they may not know that a particular service exists.

Relative Access

The problems of relative access – experienced by people with different social backgrounds or with particular circumstances – are even more complex. This is because the idea of relative access is closely bound up with equity – itself a highly complex concept.

Equity and access

Equity in health can be defined in various ways (see Pereira, 1993). Essentially, equity of access to health care is about systematic variations in the experience of individuals and social groups that are regarded as unfair. This introduces an element of value judgement into an already-difficult field. To complicate matters further, there are several dimensions of equity, which are detailed in Exhibit 8. 1.

Other useful distinctions have also been made (see Gulliford et al., 2001; Goddard and Smith, 2001). *Equity of finance* is where contributions towards health care reflect variations in income, with the rich paying at least the same proportion of their income as the poor towards the health care system. *Equity of resource* refers to the distribution of resources within the health care system relative to need and is based on a premise that resources should be distributed according to the variations in need. *Equity of access* refers to the extent to which different groups have access to health care. *Equity of treatment* is concerned with how closely actual treatment reflects the different needs of various social groups. *Equity of outcome* focuses on how the benefits of health care interventions are distributed among groups with different levels of need.

Exhibit 8.1 Equity in Health Care

In the context of the NHS the following principles of equity have been identified:

1 *A universal health service*: the service should be available to all, irrespective of ability to pay. It should not be means-tested. The service should be open to those who make use of private facilities, ensuring that the system is not simply 'for the poor'.
2 *Sharing financial costs*: the service should be free at the point of use. Contributions to the cost of the service through taxation should be linked to the size of income.
3 *Comprehensive service*: all aspects of health care should be covered by the service and there should be no exclusions.
4 *Geographical equality*: services should be of the same quality and accessibility in different parts of the country.
5 *Selection on the basis of clinical need*: people should receive services on the basis of their needs, not their financial situation or because of social position or connections.
6 *The encouragement of 'a non-exploitative ethos'*: this involves the maintenance of high ethical standards and the removal or minimisation of economic incentives that might lead to exploitation of patients.

Sources: M. Whitehead, 'Who Cares About Equity in the NHS?', *British Medical Journal*, p. 1285 Cmnd 7615 (1979); *Report of the Royal Commission on the NHS*

Despite this complexity, most studies do not adopt a clearly defined approach to measuring equity. This is partly due to the absence of an agreed conceptual framework in this field. It can also be attributed to the difficulties of distinguishing between the various dimensions of equity in practice. Indeed, many of the factors affecting these different aspects are common. In the remainder of this section, these factors are examined more closely.

Socio-economic factors

As discussed in Chapter 1, there has been controversy over the relationship between socio-economic factors and health. If anything, the relationship between socio-economic factors and access to health care is even more problematic, largely owing to difficulties in estimating the relative needs of different social groups (see Goddard and Smith, 2001).

Most studies that have adjusted for different levels of need between socio-economic groups suggest that lower income groups and social classes make greater use of services. GP consultation rates, for example, are higher for deprived and lower socio-economic groups, even when their higher levels of need are taken into account (McCormick, Fleming and Charlton, 1995), though consultations for preventative care tend to be lower among these groups. There is a similar pattern in children's GP consultations; higher for social classes IV and V than for classes I and II, but again lower rates for consultations about prevention (Saxeena, Majeed and Jones, 1999). Utilisation of in-patient care has been found to be higher among unskilled manual workers compared with professional groups after controlling for need (Haynes, 1991). Also, studies of health care expenditure have found a slight 'pro-poor' distribution for NHS care (O'Donnell, Propper and Upward, 1991; Propper and Upward, 1992; Propper, 1998).

Drawing conclusions from these studies is hazardous. While the pro-poor, pro-working class bias suggests a degree of equity, there are two reasons why this may not be the case: first, the relative needs of these social groups may be greater than estimated; secondly, affluent groups and higher social classes have greater access to non-NHS services, reducing the poor and working-class share of total services.

Location and access

It has long been argued that deprived areas have poorer-quality health services. This is the kernel of Tudor-Hart's (1971) famous 'inverse care law': that the 'availability of good medical care tends to vary inversely with the need for it in the population served'. The law is predicted to hold more strongly in market systems, though state health care systems are not immune, particularly, as in recent years, when they have embraced market mechanisms and commercial provision.

The inverse care law has been criticised (Powell, 1990), both conceptually (strictly speaking it is a hypothesis not a law) and empirically (a lack of solid evidence in support). However, data has since emerged that lends support to the hypothesis. For example, areas with high needs tend to have fewer doctors, who in turn have higher workloads (see Appleby and Deeming, 2001). While area deprivation was found to be a key factor in explaining variations in GPs' medical referrals to hospital, the association between deprivation and *surgical* referrals is weak, suggesting that those with greater needs are under-served (see Hippisley-Cox et al., 1997). The variable impact of deprivation on surgery rates has been further indicated by other studies. Chaturvedi and Ben-Schlomo (1995) found discordance between GP consultation rates and surgery rates among people in deprived areas for some conditions (hernia, gallstones, osteoarthritis). In other words, for these conditions, consultations increased with greater deprivation but operations ratios did not. Meanwhile, specifically with regard to heart disease, people living in deprived areas have a lower likelihood of receiving coronary artery revascularisation, despite their higher levels of need as indicated by symptoms of angina (Payne and Saul, 1997). Another study found that patients from the most socio-economically deprived areas were given lower priority for surgery and had to wait longer for treatment (Pell et al., 2000). With regard to cancer, one study found that proportionately more acute services were used by affluent groups (Graham, Normand and Goodall, 2002).

This may partly explain differences in survival rates from cancer between people from different socio-economic groups (Coleman, 1999).

Geographical variations in access may be related to other factors as well as deprivation. For example, some areas may have different policies on access to specific treatments. Indeed, one of the main criticisms of the NHS in recent years has been the so-called 'postcode lottery', where the availability of treatments varies, often between neighbouring areas. This issue is considered later, along with policies aimed at reducing variations in the availability of treatments.

Another geographical factor is the distance of some communities from health care services, notably acute services. This is particularly the case in some rural communities, which also contain significant socio-economic deprivation. Distance from services, and the additional costs of access (particularly travel costs), seems to inhibit access (Haynes et al., 1999; Gregory et al., 2000). These problems are particularly acute in isolated areas (particularly in Wales and Scotland), but are increasingly faced by other rural communities and even small urban settlements, given the trend to concentrate health services in larger hospitals based in major cities (see Mohan, 2002). Indeed, proximity to specialist services has been identified as an important factor in access to coronary revascularisation services (Black and Langam, 1995; Gregory et al., 2000) and renal replacement therapy (Roderick et al., 1999), and could also apply to other services (Christie and Fone, 2003).

Ethnicity

It is difficult to come to firm conclusions about the impact of ethnicity on access to health care, largely because of the variation between and within ethnic groups, and the interaction with other factors such as location, social class and income (not to mention gender and age, discussed below). Certainly, there are possible reasons why ethnic groups may not get the services they need. There may be language barriers which inhibit communication and understanding, cultural barriers which impede the take-up of services, and even racial discrimination by health care providers.

The evidence, however, is limited. Smaje and Le Grand (1997) did not find strong patterns of inequity between ethnic groups in their use of the NHS after adjusting for their greater needs and other possible confounding factors. The only exceptions were the Chinese population, which displayed consistently lower levels of utilisation, and the low use of GP services by Pakistani women. The same study found that use of GP services by ethnic groups was at least as high as the white population, but use of out-patient services was lower. In some services, rates of usage are higher in areas with large ethnic populations (notably renal replacement therapy in areas with large Asian and Afro-Caribbean populations–Roderick et al., 1999), reflecting the underlying disease pattern in these groups. However, there is evidence that some ethnic minorities may not get access to the best secondary care, even when their needs are relatively higher. For example, a study of Asian heart patients found that they were less likely to be admitted early to a coronary care unit and less likely to be given thrombolysis–'clot-busting' drugs (Lear et al., 1994). Such variations are usually attributed to a reluctance to seek care. However, in one study, some ethnic groups (Hindus and Sikhs) were more likely to seek immediate care for chest pain compared with Europeans (Chaturvedi, Rai and Ben-Schlomo, 1997), suggesting that further investigation of service-related explanations (such as difficulties of diagnosis or differences in the management of conditions) is necessary.

Gender and access

Although women use health services more then men, it is possible that they may have greater needs that are not being met. There may be specific factors that discourage them from consulting with health professionals when in need. Moreover, once in the system they may not get access to the best care.

There has been an assumption that women are more likely than men to consult a doctor, given the same underlying extent of illness. According to Hunt and colleagues (1999), women are no more likely than men to consult a GP when experiencing five common conditions, nor are they more likely to consult at a given level of severity of illness (except for mental health problems). In terms of specialist care, men are more likely than women to undergo non-invasive investigations and renal transplants, and there is some indication that women have poorer access to heart and vascular surgery and hip replacement (Raine, 2000). Other studies have found disparities in the treatment of heart conditions (Clarke et al., 1994), and a recent study found that, at the same levels of need, men with hypertension were nearly twice as likely as women to have rehabilitation treatment after acute cardiac admission (Raine, Hutchings and Black, 2003).

However, women do get greater access to some treatments. They are more likely to receive a liver transplant or a cataract operation (Raine, 2000). Moreover, some categories of men appear to make insufficient use of services relative to their needs. Young men, for example, have been identified as a group that underutilises services (Hayes and Prior, 2003).

In summary, the issue of gender and access is complex. Some disparities may be due to discrimination. But there are other factors, in particular the design of services and their appropriateness, that may have an important bearing on access and the quality of care for the respective sexes. Three examples illustrate this. The treatment of heart disease is strongly shaped by the perception that it is a male disease (Raine, Hutchings and Black, 2003). Women's specific needs may, therefore, not be adequately catered for, and this may explain some of the disparities above. Breast cancer, on the other hand, though overwhelmingly a female disease, affects a small number of men (around two hundred and fifty a year in England and Wales). Services are geared to the needs of women, and men may be reluctant to seek help. This is likely to undermine both access to services and the survival chances of those unfortunate men who develop breast tumours. Finally, mental illness, though affecting both sexes substantially, is managed differently in women compared with men (see Payne, 1998). This is unhelpful if mental health problems are not properly managed as a result. For example, it has been suggested that there is a failure to acknowledge addiction problems in women, and that they have greater difficult in getting help. It is also claimed that, compared with men, women are more likely to be referred for coercive treatment for mental health problems.

Age

There has been growing concern about discrimination against people on the basis of their age. There are many possible reasons why older people may not get appropriate access to the care they need. It is believed that they tend to be more deferential, and less likely to complain. Because they are older, and in general less healthy than younger people, they may be regarded as a low priority for treatment. Given the focus on efficient use of resources, funds spent on elderly people might be regarded as poor value for money, particularly if they are frail and there are doubts about their quality of life after treatment. As we shall see later in this chapter, such beliefs are reinforced by the use of cost-benefit analyses in determining who gets treatment.

There is much anecdotal evidence about elderly people's difficulties in access and many examples of poor-quality services. But hard data about the extent of inequalities in particular services is thin on the ground (Gilchrist, 1999; Health Advisory Service, 1998). However, one study did find that the likelihood of receiving statins for people with coronary heart disease was greatly reduced for older age groups (Reid, Cook and Whincup, 2002). There is evidence of processes that underpin discrimination (Royal College of Physicians, 1994; Roberts, Robinson and Seymour, 2002). These include the isolation of older people into units where access to other specialist services is impeded; the use of admission and treatment policies that refer to age restrictions; the low priority of the elderly as a client group; and negative attitudes among staff which could lead to discrimination.

Key factors affecting access

Although the specific factors affecting access vary, there are some recurring themes. These can be summarised as follows. Access is influenced by factors operating on both the demand and the supply side. Factors on the supply side include location of services, their organisation and coherence, the consistency and appropriateness of their approach to all different types of patient, the attitude of health professionals towards specific groups of people, and clinical judgements about need and how illnesses should be managed. Factors on the demand side include patients' attitudes and beliefs about seeking help for conditions, their information and knowledge about services, and financial and cultural factors.

What Has Been Done to Improve Access?

As problems of access to health care are wide-ranging and complex, no single intervention can fully address this issue. Rather, a combination of initiatives is needed, some aimed at improving absolute access, others focused more on problems of relative access. This section examines the policies that have been pursued in this area, focusing mainly on England.

Improving Absolute Access

The current approach dates back to the *Patient's Charter*, introduced by the Major Government during the early 1990s. Before this, a piecemeal approach prevailed, where regional health authorities were given specific targets within a framework of national priorities. These included targets to treat more patients in areas such as cardiac surgery and renal dialysis, for example. Waiting list initiatives were also introduced, with specific earmarked funds to reduce the longest waiting lists.

The *Patient's Charter* (DoH, 1991, 1996a) set overall standards of access, which were modified and extended throughout the 1990s. These included a guaranteed maximum waiting time for admission (initially of two years, then 18 months) and a range of 'expected' standards that included a maximum 30-minute wait in out-patients, and later maximum waiting times of 26 weeks for a hospital appointment (with nine out of ten people having a hospital appointment within 13 weeks). Performance review focused strongly on the waiting-time targets, and health authorities were expected to deliver continuous improvements in these indicators. The *Patient's Charter* also contained a number of rights, some of which had implications for access (the right to be registered with a GP, for example). But these were not enshrined in law, and some were not clearly specified and therefore difficult to measure. Given the emphasis on measurable targets, it was 'standards' rather than 'rights' which drove the performance review process.

Initially, the Blair Government moved away from this approach. Its version of the *Patient's Charter* was less specific about standards, but equally vague about patient rights (see Chapter 12). However, the Government's commitment to reduce waiting lists – the key health pledge by the Labour Party at the 1997 general election – ensured that emphasis on the quantitative access indicators remained. The Blair Government continued its predecessor's commitment to a maximum 18-month waiting time for in-patients. It also introduced specific waiting times for patients with cancer, beginning with a two-week maximum waiting time for an out-patient appointment for patients with suspected breast cancer, urgently referred by their GP. This was later extended to all suspected cancers.

This was followed by a range of commitments to improve access, set out in the NHS Plan (see Exhibit 5.3). The Plan set out ambitious targets for maximum in-patient and out-patient waiting times (six and three months respectively by 2005), as well as waiting times in primary care and accident and emergency. In addition, 'milestones' were identified for the intervening period (for example, no in-patient should have been waiting more than 15 months by March 2002). Other specific commitments emerged out of the National Service Frameworks (NSFs – see Exhibit 7.4) and the Cancer Plan. The Coronary Heart Disease NSF specified a two-week wait for specialist assessment of suspected new cases of angina, a three-month maximum wait for bypass surgery (DoH, 2000d) as well as a target of three-quarters of eligible patients to receive thrombolysis within 30 minutes of hospital arrival by April 2002 (and within 20 minutes by April 2003). Meanwhile, the Cancer Plan (DoH, 2000e) set a goal of a one-month maximum wait for treatment for people urgently referred by a GP with some suspected cancers (including children's cancers). A target of a two-month maximum wait from referral to first treatment for all cancers was set for 2005.

The Blair Government sought to achieve these ambitious targets in a number of ways. First, earmarked funds were allocated to local health authorities to reduce waiting lists. Central funding was also available to implement the NSF and Cancer Plan standards. In addition, from 2000 more generous financial settlements for the NHS increased the overall resources available to tackle waiting times (see Chapter 6). Secondly, access was identified as a key aspect of the Performance Assessment Framework. Three components of the framework – 'effective delivery of appropriate health care', 'patient carer experience' and 'fair access' – incorporated indicators of access. Indicators of absolute access initially included surgery rates associated with national priority targets, the percentage of patients waiting 12 months or longer for treatment, out-patients seen within 13 weeks of GP referral, and maximum waiting times for admission through accident and emergency (DoH, 1999c). Fair access indicators included surgery rates and the size of in-patient waiting lists per head of population (weighted). These were used to assess the performance of health authorities and subsequently PCTs and to support the assessment of trust performance. Changes in the performance assessment process, coupled with the new national targets in the NHS Plan, brought changes in some indicators. New access indicators were added (for example, access to a GP within 48 hours) and others altered ('percentage of patients waiting less than 6 months for an inpatient admission' replaced the previous indicator). Waiting times also formed part of the cluster of indicators that produced the 'star rating' of trusts, and subsequently PCTs (see Chapter 7). Thirdly, new ways of providing more accessible care were introduced. These included nurse-led primary care services, 'walk-in' clinics and NHS Direct. The NHS Plan also announced an expansion of 'one stop' primary care centres which, by combining primary and community health practitioners in one place, could speed up cross-referral and diagnosis (see Chapter 10).

In addition, efforts were made to improve the movement of patients between primary and secondary care. The introduction of booking systems – where a GP is able to give a specific out-patient or in-patient appointment – is one example. All patients are expected to receive pre-booked appointments by 2005, according to the NHS Plan. Others include an expansion of out-patient services in primary care settings, such as minor surgery, outreach clinics and diagnostic tests. Other developments include efforts to redesign health care systems, particularly with regard to the management of conditions such as cancer and heart disease. The development of care pathways and efforts to improve the network of services for particular conditions have important implications for the reduction of unnecessary delays and improving access to services. For some conditions, 'rapid access' centres were developed to improve the speed of diagnosis and treatment (such as chest pain clinics, for example). In addition, an expansion in diagnostic and treatment centres for surgery was announced, focusing on routine surgery with the longest waiting times (see Chapter 6).

Finally, there was a commitment to improve information about local services and to facilitate greater choice. The NHS Plan stated that patients would be given more information about GP practices, including list size and performance against National Service Frameworks. Meanwhile, trusts were required to produce a prospectus setting out information about local services, patient-satisfaction ratings, and performance against national standards. Broader developments in the field of health information technology were also highlighted (see Chapter 9). The introduction of the Patient Advice and Liaison Service (PALS) and changes in public and patient involvement mechanisms were heralded as increasing information about services while improving the responsiveness of health services to patients' needs. Finally, patients were promised greater choice of providers, which was expected to bring greater competitive pressures to bear and thereby reduce waiting times (see Chapter 12).

What effect?

It is extremely difficult to assess the impact of these various initiatives, largely because there are so many of them and most are relatively recent. Most of the evidence available so far is quantitative, relating to waiting times and lists (see Appleby and Coote, 2002, ch. 3). This shows that the Blair Government was successful in fulfilling its manifesto pledge (to reduce waiting-lists by 100,000 by the end of the first term in office). However, there was considerable variation in waiting-list sizes between different areas (18 per cent of health authorities saw an increase in waiting lists 1997–2000 – Appleby and Coote, 2002, p. 27). By March 2002, the number of in-patients and day cases waiting over six months in England was around 250,000, with over 22,000 waiting 12 months or more (Yates, 2002b). The 'two-week waits' for cancer patients had not been achieved on time, though over 90 per cent of patients were referred within this timeframe. Since this time, official waiting times have fallen further, with only a few people waiting over 12 months by November 2003. At the same time, over 98 per cent of patients with suspected cancer were given first out-patient appointments within two weeks following an urgent referral by their GP.

Even where targets are met, this does not mean that access has improved. As Appleby and Coote (2002, p. 27) have noted, reclassification of some patients as 'planned cases' led to some being removed from the waiting list. There are also other reasons why people may be removed (Tudor Edwards, 1997) – if they cannot accept an admission date or if the procedure they need is no longer funded by the relevant commissioning body. Moreover, in a minority of hospitals, evidence of inappropriate adjustments to waiting-list data was uncovered where managers and staff deliberately manipulated figures to conceal their failure to hit government targets. 6000 patients were affected, and some had their treatment delayed as a result (Public Accounts Committee, 2002). Further investigation of a sample of trusts by the Audit Commission (2003c) found deliberate misreporting of waiting-list information at three trusts, reporting errors in a further 19. In only three trusts did spot checks reveal no significant problems. In the remaining 15 that provided information, weaknesses were found that increased the risk of errors.

Improving Relative Access

Policies on equity in health care

Little was done to address the problems of relative access during the 1980s and 1990s. The Thatcher Government did not regard health inequalities as a serious issue. The Major Government took a slightly different line, urging the NHS to explore ways of reducing 'health variations' (the terms 'inequities' or 'inequalities' had been removed from the official discourse – Exworthy and Powell, 2000). This was followed by NHS guidance to reduce 'variations in health status by targeting resources where needs are greatest' (DoH, 1995b, p. 3). But this aside, little else was done. Indeed, the Conservatives' internal market and reluctance to align resource allocation more closely with needs (see below) arguably worsened the situation, as did their approach towards social inequality generally (see Chapter 13).

Equity received far more attention from the Blair Government, in its first White Paper on NHS reform (Cm 3807, 1997), in its Performance Assessment Framework, and in guidance to the NHS, where 'fair access' to health services was clearly stated (DoH, 1998d). The Blair Government was ready to acknowledge the broader issue of health inequalities – which included other factors affecting differences in health between social groups, in addition to poor access to health care. It established an inquiry into health inequalities under former Chief Medical Officer, Donald Acheson, which made a series of recommendations about how health and health care inequalities should be addressed (Independent Inquiry into Inequalities in Health, 1998). This is discussed further in Chapter 13. With specific regard to access to health care, the report stated that equitable access to effective care in relation to need should be a governing principle of NHS policies. It recommended that reducing inequities in access should be a priority at every level in the NHS and should be included in local plans. It also stated that priority should be given to a more equitable allocation of NHS resources and called for changes in the resource-allocation mechanism to achieve this. Subsequently, national targets for reducing health inequalities were set and a cross-governmental review renewed the commitment to tackle health inequalities across Government (see Chapter 13). With regard to health care, commitments to tailor services to overcome cultural, linguistic and social barriers were outlined. It was also emphasised that local health organisations must identify groups and areas not receiving services according to need (DoH, 2003b).

National Service Frameworks also identified the extent of inequalities in care and how this should be tackled. The Older People's NSF included a standard on eliminating age discrimination, which required audits of age-related policies in health and social care. The NSF for coronary heart disease mentioned reducing inequalities in treatment. It set out standards of care related to need and risk, and included performance indicators to identify variations in access to treatment between different areas.

Meanwhile, the establishment of the National Institute for Clinical Excellence (NICE) provided a national, evidence-based approach to the availability of treatments (see Exhibit 8.2). The aim was to reduce and eliminate variations in access to different treatments on the basis of where one lived. Subsequently, NICE guidance became mandatory for NHS organisations, producing greater pressures to reduce local variations.

Exhibit 8.2 The National Institute for Clinical Excellence (NICE)

NICE was established in 1999 and given three main roles: to appraise and produce guidance on the cost-effectiveness of new and existing technologies; to develop clinical guidelines for the treatment of different conditions; and to assist the NHS with clinical audit.

⟶

Exhibit 8.2 continued

→

A further role has since been added. In 2003 NICE acquired the responsibility for checking the safety and efficacy of new interventional procedures. The main reason for establishing NICE was to provide clear, evidence-based guidance for the NHS in England and Wales about the cost-effectiveness of interventions. NICE has been very active, publishing 62 technology-appraisal reports between 2000 and 2003 (Bosanquet, 2003).

NICE has faced considerable controversy. One of the most controversial issues concerned Beta Interferon, used in the treatment of multiple sclerosis. In 2001 NICE stated that, on the basis of current evidence, the drug could not be recommended on cost-benefit grounds. However, patients' groups and the drug manufacturers argued that the decision was based on limited data and did not take into account the drug's impact on the quality of life. Subsequently, the Department of Health agreed to a scheme whereby patients could receive the treatment on an experimental basis with funding related to outcomes.

Critics of NICE have argued that its credibility is undermined by several factors, including a failure to work with other agencies that have a role in monitoring clinical and cost effectiveness (such as the British National Formulary, for example). Others have suggested that it has changed initial guidance in response to political pressure (notably in the case of the flu drug, Relenza, where an initial decision not to recommend was reversed following a hostile response from the drug industry).

NICE is constituted as a Special Health Authority. Its board consists of a chairman and non-executive members appointed by the Secretary of State for Health and the National Assembly of Wales, along with executive members. The DoH and the National Assembly for Wales, advised by a Technologies Advisory Group, determines NICE's programme of work, and sets the key criteria for health technology appraisal and clinical guidelines. Topics for investigation can be provided by professional, patient or NHS groups, though most arise from 'horizon scanning' undertaken by a research centre, and from 'specialty mapping'–in-depth analysis of the need for guidance in the main areas of clinical activity. A web-based system to encourage people to suggest topics has been promised. Other changes in the pipeline include an enlarged Technologies Advisory Group to include a wider range of stakeholders, and further clarification of the criteria for selecting topics.

According to some observers, the credibility of NICE has been undermined by flawed processes. There has been particular criticism that it has failed to include all stakeholders and sources of expertise in its appraisals. Doubts have been expressed about how it has selected participants. However, NICE has attempted to include patients' organisations, as the voice of the user. It may have been less effective in incorporating views of NHS professionals who have a key role in implementing guidelines. NICE established a Partners' Council consisting of a range of stakeholder (including patients' groups) to advise it. A further body, the Citizens' Council, comprising members of the public, was subsequently established to inform value judgements relating to its work.

NICE processes have been criticised for lacking openness and transparency in the way decisions are made and with regard to the availability of evidence. This is partly the result of 'commercial confidentiality', which drug companies insist upon with regard to data submitted about product costs and effectiveness. However, NICE publishes summaries of its appraisals of technology, and independent assessments of the literature. In addition, NICE is explicit about the ground rules for appraisal.

It was believed that NICE guidelines would simply be ignored by health authorities and practitioners. While its impact has been variable, NICE appraisals are now incorporated into

→

Exhibit 8.2 continued

→

the clinical monitoring process of the Commission for Health Improvement, and its recommendations on medicines and treatments have been mandatory since 2002. This may create yet another set of problems. The removal of discretion about whether or not to implement NICE guidance could impact negatively on other services, including those which have not yet been evaluated. It is crucial that NICE considers treatments in their wider context, in particular their impact on the whole system of care for a particular condition. However, Government rejected a recommendation from the Bristol Inquiry that NICE be responsible for co-ordinating all action relating to setting, issuing and keeping national clinical standards under review. Some also believe that NICE's concern with specialised technological innovation has been misplaced, and more could be achieved by focusing on the cost-effectiveness of intervention in prevention, primary care, and infrastructure (such as IT) (Bosanquet, 2003).

Other problems include 'NICE blight', where NHS bodies save money by refusing to support a new intervention that is under investigation, thereby preventing or delaying access to it. There is also concern that the guidance produced by NICE reduces clinical discretion. Although evidence on cost-effectiveness may not justify interventions across the broad range of cases, it may be justified in specific cases. Finally, the health care environment is dynamic and the evidence on which NICE makes decisions dates quickly. It must alter recommendations when technology (and other factors) changes the balance of costs and benefits relating to an intervention.

Source and further reading: Health Committee (2002c) (HC 515-I) *2nd Report* 2001/02. National Institute for Clinical Excellence; Consumers Association (2001) National Institute for Clinical Excellence.

Developing services

NHS organisations are expected to implement national policies and standards relating to equity. Primary care groups were given explicit responsibility to address health inequalities in their community and ensure that local services met local needs (DoH, 1998d). Subsequently, these responsibilities passed to PCTs, which, along with local strategic partnerships (see Chapter 13) are expected to undertake local equity audits in relation to the health inequalities targets. Strategic Health Authorities, meanwhile, are expected to co-ordinate action on reducing health inequalities and ensuring that the National Service Frameworks and other standards are implemented in an equitable way.

Other initiatives encouraged local NHS bodies, and their partners in local government and the voluntary sector, to respond proactively to problems of relative access in health care. Health Action Zones (see Exhibit 10.2) were created in areas of high need. Their brief included the reduction of health inequalities and the promotion of equality of access to health services. HAZ projects have tended to focus on deprived areas, and on the needs of groups such as ethnic minorities, the elderly and women. Other relevant developments in primary care include PMS contracts which enabled a more flexible approach to meeting the needs of citizens in their area through the appointment of salaried GPs and nurse-led primary care services. They are particularly of value to inner-city areas that have greatest difficulty in recruiting GPs, and where the obstacles to access primary care services are greater (see also Chapter 10).

Funding and resource allocation

Another way of improving access to health care is to alter the way in which resources are allocated. Resources could be reallocated to areas and population groups with relatively high needs, such as economically deprived areas, ethnic groups, or areas with a large concentration of elderly people. As noted in earlier chapters, successive Governments have shifted the allocation of resources towards areas of higher need, beginning with RAWP in England and Wales, and equivalent systems in other parts of the UK .

Changes to the allocation formula followed, based on factors indicating variations in needs. However, other policies operated in a different direction. The Conservatives 'internal market' was widely seen as making the system less equitable (Mohan, 1995; Marks, 1995). Despite a commitment to resourcing purchasers on the principle of 'weighted capitation' (i.e. equal resources for equal needs), in practice, purchasers had very different leverage in the local health care market. Allegations of a two-tier system emerged, particularly with regard to GP fundholding. Efforts to produce a fairer system of resource allocation were hampered by technical and political factors. With regard to the former, the search for a formula that captured the actual variation in needs proved elusive. But even when improvements to the allocation formula were proposed, those areas that were likely to lose out (London and the south-east) were able to oppose changes, limiting the impact of needs-based factors.

The Blair Government was prepared to add greater weight to such factors. It altered the funding formula for primary care trusts, introduced a health inequalities adjustment to the allocation formula, benefiting areas where need was highest, and gave greater weight to indicators of need in the allocation of resources to general practice. Even so, the speed at which funding will be reallocated in order to reflect needs more closely is crucial (Hacking, 2003). Other parts of the UK also reviewed their resource-allocation mechanisms, placing greater weight on deprivation indicators and other problems of access. In Scotland, for example, a new index was developed to reflect the need for health care based on indicators of deprivation (unemployment rate, percentage of elderly people on income support, households with two or more indicators of deprivation) and mortality rates.

Impact

It is even more difficult to assess the impact of initiatives to improve relative access than absolute access. There are anecdotal examples of how local schemes, particularly those associated with Health Action Zones, have made it easier for particular social groups to access services. But there is no systematic evidence on the impact of policies and initiatives on relative access to health care.

Access, Priority-setting and Rationing

Access to health care is affected by the overall capacity of the health care system, and its priorities. If one treatment or condition is given priority, this will impact on the resources available for others. Attempts to 'ration' health care – by excluding certain treatments, or by less explicit means – also have an impact on access. This section explores priority-setting and rationing in this context.

The term 'priority-setting' is reserved by some for decisions about overall budgets and their distribution, with 'rationing' being associated with resource decisions about individual treatment (Klein, Day and Redmayne, 1996). Irrespective of which term is used, the object is basically the same: to identify treatments or services that will receive a favourable distribution of resources and those that will not (and in some cases may receive nothing at all). Such decisions have implications for individuals and have interpersonal distributional effects. These may be compounded by specifying individual circumstances when making decisions about priorities and rationing (such as treatment of elderly or disabled people, or people with particular types or stages of a condition), which, as noted earlier in the context of the elderly, can exacerbate problems of access.

What is Rationing?

Various forms of rationing have been identified (see Harrison and Hunter, 1994; Klein, Day and Redmayne, 1996, p 11). These are *deterrence* – obstructing the demands for health care (such as charges for services), *delay* – as indicated by waiting lists, *deflection* – diverting demand to other services (provided by other agencies, such as social services) or discouraging demand (by giving patients more information about the side-effects of treatment, for example), *dilution* – reducing the amount of service offered (including reductions in quality), *denial* (where services are explicitly excluded), *selection* – where service providers identify clients who are most likely to benefit from intervention, and *termination* – where treatment is actually stopped.

Another distinction is between implicit and explicit rationing, which, as Locock has observed (2000, p. 93), operates along a continuum. In explicit rationing there is 'a clear attempt to distinguish who will receive what; the decisions are understood and agreed by a group of people, not just the individual clinician'. The first four types of rationing above are implicit because they tend not to have clear criteria for excluding services, such as measures of need, benefits and costs of treatment. All have been practised within the NHS since its inception, and have enabled the 'myth' of a comprehensive service to persist. However, in recent years there has been a greater acknowledgement of explicit rationing, such as selection and denial based on overt criteria.

The Rationing Debate in Britain

Several factors encouraged the debate about explicit rationing. Arguments that the NHS cannot meet the demands placed on it, owing to technological advance and other factors (see Chapter 1), have been influential. The availability of so-called 'non-essential treatments' on the NHS accentuated the debate, notably the controversy surrounding the impotence drug, Viagra.

The Department of Health sought to limit the availability of Viagra, first by trying to prevent GPs prescribing the drug (later ruled unlawful), then by issuing guidance on who should receive NHS prescriptions (i.e. only people currently being treated with impotence drugs or becoming impotent due to a specific conditions such as diabetes, for example) and the maximum weekly amount for each patient. The controversy raised a number of key issues. First, it is difficult to draw the line between deserving and undeserving cases – in fact the Department of Health subsequently extended the range of conditions eligible for a GP prescription and referral to a specialist for those in severe distress. Secondly, the issue showed that there was no consensus about where the boundaries of the NHS lay. While most acknowledged that Viagra was on balance a beneficial treatment, opinion was divided on whether it should be funded by the NHS.

Another factor fuelling the rationing debate has been the media coverage of cases where treatment has been denied. Attention has focused on cases where patients have faced exclusion from treatment because of their age, disability or lifestyle. Examples include a young woman who, having taken ecstasy, was allegedly refused a liver transplant, though doctors were later adjudged to have acted on medical criteria not moral grounds. There have also been instances where smokers, heavy drinkers and overweight people have cited discrimination on the basis of their condition. People with disabilities also claim to have been refused treatment. In one high-profile case in 2000, a mentally and physically disabled baby girl was refused heart surgery by one NHS trust on medical grounds. Subsequently, she was successfully treated by another trust, prompting allegations of discrimination on grounds of her disabilities. As noted earlier in this chapter, there have been similar allegations that patients are discriminated against because of their age.

One of the most high-profile cases in recent memory, however, turned on the issue of cost-effectiveness rather than discrimination. This was the case of 'Child B', later revealed as ten-year-old leukaemia patient Jaymee Bowen (Price, 1996; Ham and Pickard, 1998). In 1995 legal action was brought by the child's father before the High Court following the refusal of the health authority to pay for a second bone marrow transplant. The treatment was not covered by existing service contracts with providers and represented a substantial cost to the health authority, estimated at £75,000. Moreover, the health authority received clinical advice that further treatment was not in the child's best interests and argued in court that it would not be an effective use of resources. Although the action failed on appeal, Jaymee did receive further treatment (but not the bone marrow transplant), paid for by a private benefactor and provided by a private practitioner. Initially this appeared to be successful, but a relapse followed and she died the following year.

Cases such as 'Child B' have exposed rationing decisions to public scrutiny. Coupled with growing demands for public accountability, this makes it more difficult to use implicit forms of rationing, as increasing scrutiny of clinical decisions makes it more difficult to deflect and divert demands in the traditional way. Meanwhile, the scope for delay, the familiar tactic used by clinicians and doctors to manage demand within the NHS, has been reduced in line with Government commitments on waiting lists and waiting-times (see above).

A further stimulus to the rationing debate has been the development of techniques for assessing the cost-effectiveness of various treatments and interventions. These have caused unease among the public, who tend to recoil from the idea of putting a price on someone's life. Nonetheless, interest has been attracted by lessons from other countries (Coulter and Ham, 2000; Honigsbaum, 1995; Hunter, 1997), in particular, the Oregon case in the USA (see Exhibit 8.3). The introduction of health care commissioning was intended to add further pressure to scrutinise budgets and ration health care accordingly. In theory, potential investment for 'health gain' would be identified and there would be a withdrawal of funds from services that were relatively cost-ineffective. In practice, things were less straightforward.

Another factor behind the rationing debate was the adoption of evidence-based clinical practice (see Chapter 9), which placed budgetary pressures on treatments that are shown to be less effective.

Rationing in Practice

Research on the impact of rationing indicates that commissioners of health care were slow to examine priorities and reluctant to rule out treatments. By the mid-1990s only a quarter of health authorities actually specified services that they would not fund (Redmayne, 1996), the list usually including breast augmentation, tattoo removal, reversal of sterilisation, gender reassignment. However, a greater proportion identified services that they were reluctant to fund and cited evidence of clinical effectiveness in support of this position (Klein, Day and Redmayne, 1996). To refuse to fund a treatment risked

---

Exhibit 8.3 The Oregon Experiment

In the late 1980s Oregon, like many other states in the USA, faced two main health care problems: rising health care costs, and large numbers of uninsured people. The state government decided to try a different approach towards the allocation of health care resources (see Honigsbaum, 1992). Plans were outlined to alter the coverage of Medicaid, the state-run system for funding the care of poor people (and also blind people, the disabled, and children in foster care). The idea was to extend Medicaid to a larger proportion of those on low incomes without private health insurance, while at the same time restricting the range of treatments it funded. The state began collecting cost–benefit data with respect to the various treatments available. An initial ranking of treatments was produced but was subsequently withdrawn after criticisms of the data-collection process. A second list was produced and the public were consulted about the benefits of healthcare. The final ranking reflected public values, costs, duration of benefit from treatment and quality of wellbeing.

The Oregon legislature approved the funding for the first 587 treatments listed (out of a total of 709). Had the plan gone ahead at this stage, the Medicaid system would have been extended to an additional 120,000 individuals currently excluded from the programme. At the same time, public funding for the treatment of many 'low-priority conditions' (including varicose veins and treatment for terminal-stage HIV), would have ended.

However, the necessary approval from the Federal Government in Washington was initially withheld following pressure from patients' and disabled peoples' organisations. Further negotiations between state and federal officials produced concessions (including an agreement that treatment for HIV/AIDS patients would not be withdrawn). Subsequently, permission was granted which enabled Oregon to introduce its plan for a five-year trial period, beginning in 1994. In 1999 a new list of 743 conditions was created, with 574 covered by the Oregon Health Plan.

Judgements about the impact of the Plan have varied. Some saw it as a great success, having facilitated health care coverage to a further 130,000 people, decreased the percentage of uninsured people (from 18 to 11 per cent), reduced the use of hospital emergency rooms (by 5 per cent) and reduced the shifting of costs on to the commercially-insured population (Leichter, 1999). However, others believed that the achievements attributed to Oregon were exaggerated (Jacobs, Marmor and Oberlander, 1999). They argue that there has been no widespread rationing of services and that the benefit package of the new scheme is more generous than that which existed previously. The expansion of coverage occurred not by rationing but by raising additional revenues for health care and by introducing managed care schemes for Medicaid recipients. It has also been noted that many Medicaid recipients continued to receive services that were meant to be excluded. The efficiency improvements of the new scheme were small – only 2 per cent of what the previous system would have cost over the five-year period. From this perspective, Oregon's attempt to create a set of priorities based on cost-benefit analysis has had little effect. Subjective judgements and political pressures have proved more influential than economic analysis, though, on a more positive note, the process has been credited with encouraging both public support and raising revenues for expanding health care cover for the poor.

---

opposition, notably from doctors, who complained of infringement of clinical autonomy, and from patients. A more effective strategy was to set criteria for eligibility in co-operation with the medical profession. Hence 'denial' was replaced by an approach that emphasised 'selection' based on medical criteria.

Locock (2000) confirmed that explicit rationing grew in the latter part of the 1990s. She attributed this in part to the internal market reforms, and, more specifically, the division between purchasers and providers. Other factors were influential, especially the desire to control rising expenditure. Like Klein and colleagues, Locock found that commissioners increasingly used a selective approach based on medical criteria, rather than outright denial. This was not simply a return to the older implicit forms of rationing, because the criteria for intervention were now more clearly stated. This new approach relied on a combination of explicit criteria (set out in guidelines and protocols, for example) set collectively by professionals, and individual discretion by clinicians operating within set budgets.

The abolition of the Conservative Government's internal market did not produce any significant departure. This is hardly surprising in the light of Locock's observation that it was the division between commissioners and providers that provided the impetus for change, rather than the contracting process itself. The retention of this divide in England and Wales has maintained the emphasis on prioritisation and the development of explicit criteria. Other developments were important. First, the focus on national priorities was maintained by the four key priorities in the White Paper of 1999, *Saving Lives* (see Chapter 13): cancer, heart disease and stroke, mental health, and accidents. Although this followed on from an earlier Conservative policy to target the major causes of illness and mortality (see Chapter 13), the Labour Government's approach appeared to be more directive than that of its predecessor, reflected in its Performance Assessment Framework (see Chapter 7). Secondly, the Government set out National Service Frameworks for the major-condition areas (coronary heart disease, mental health, and a national plan for cancer) and for certain population groups (children, older people). As noted, NSFs identify the main principles on which services should be based, along with the standards of service that should be provided at each stage of a particular condition and each aspect of care of a particular client group. The NSFs also contained targets for service improvement to meet these standards and made other recommendations about how they can be achieved. Thirdly, the creation of the National Institute for Clinical Excellence (see Exhibit 8.2) was a clear attempt to eliminate less effective treatment while placing more emphasis on cost-effectiveness. Its guidance – which is now mandatory – covers the appraisal of new technologies and guidance on the cost-effectiveness of treatments for particular conditions.

Improving Rationing

According to some commentators, further improvements to the system of allocating resources within health care are needed. Such arguments are not confined to the UK (Coulter and Ham, 2000; Ham and Robert, 2003). In exploring these arguments, one can find several positions. First, the NHS should specify more clearly what it will do and what it will not do (National Economic Research Associates, 1994). According to this perspective, there should be a clear menu of services which the NHS would provide free of charge; the remainder would have to be paid for privately (directly or with insurance) or by charitable contributions. However, this is fraught with problems, in particular the practical difficulties of dealing with complex patients' needs and the uncertainties posed by medical technology (Klein, Day and Redmayne, 1996, p. 133, see also Health Committee, 1995a; Lenaghan, 1996). Mindful of the difficulties of establishing a 'core' service, New and Le Grand (1996) argue that the whole range of services relevant to the health care system should be specified and that all health authorities would have to ensure the provision of at least some level of these services. However, this should be combined with clear criteria on how access to these services should be allocated.

Others have demanded greater transparency in how health care decisions are made. Research into rationing decisions has found that although decision-making has been evidently strengthened, with commissioning bodies giving careful consideration to choices, taking independent advice and testing out options through internal debate and discussion, 'the NHS still lacks clear and consistent processes for making priority-setting decisions' (Ham and McIver, 2000, p. 77). In this context New and Le Grand (1996) have called for improved systems of monitoring so that the criteria for access to publicly-funded health care are properly implemented and clinicians held to account for their decisions. At national level, a National Council for Health Care Priorities has been suggested (Royal College of Physicians, 1995), to undertake the task of improving priority-setting, examining the evidence relating to resource allocation and reviewing the basis for determining allocations. This body would exercise these functions in an open and comprehensive manner. Others have made similar recommendations, such as a National Health Commission to aid the development of a fair and transparent decision-making process in the NHS that would include the consideration of distributional issues (Lenaghan, 1996). Those at local level have also been exhorted to make decision-making more systematic and transparent. Some health authorities have responded, as in Oxford, where a priorities forum was established in an attempt to ensure a reasonable and evidence-based process of decision-making (Hope et al., 1998).

There are those who question the wisdom of relying on technical approaches to rationing (see, for example, Hunt, 1997; Klein, Day and Redmayne, 1996). This is not simply a critique of health economics (see Chapter 3). Rather, there is an acceptance that rationing decisions are complex and heavily value-laden and cannot be solved by a technical fix. Hunter (1997), for example, argues for a more subtle, incremental approach which seeks to balance various interests (of patients, professionals, managers), which he calls 'muddling through elegantly'.

This approach accepts that rationing is 'an unavoidably messy affair and always will be' (Hunter, 1997, p. 147). Similarly, Klein, Day and Redmayne (1996) argue that the notion of an 'ultimate solution' provided by a rational scientific analysis is illusory. The best that can be hoped for is to improve the process of decision-making, so that competing values, interests and concepts can be reconciled, improving the prospect of socially acceptable solutions. Others go even further and argue against explicit rationing on the grounds that it can damage patients' confidence in the system and place burdens upon them to make decisions that they are unwilling to make (Coast, 1997). But perhaps the scope for rational and directive decision-making in health care allocation has been exaggerated anyway. McDonald and Baughan (2001) found that most decision-making was reactive and that health authorities had limited capacity to engage in explicit rationing.

Finally, others argue that there should be greater public involvement in priority-setting and rationing (Health Committee, 1995a). Public and user involvement in the NHS is discussed further in Chapter 12, but there has been much effort in recent years to gauge public views on priorities, though debate continues about the most effective method of doing this. Others, however, are more cynical about public involvement. Klein, Day and Redmayne (1996, p. 131) argue that there is no strong case for pursuing greater public involvement, because opinion is often divided and inconsistent. They note that most people believe that doctors should make these decisions. Hunter (1997), too, is critical of public involvement on the grounds that 'participation is inherently inegalitarian' (p. 129). He also expresses doubts about the ability of the public to make informed decisions, and rightly argues that proper attention must be given to preparing them for such a role, particularly with regard to information. The danger of public involvement is that they will merely confirm prejudices or legitimise decisions made by others (see also Coast, 1997; Mullen, 2000).

Conclusion

Issues of access, priorities and rationing in health care are closely interlinked. Access to care is often determined by systems of rationing and prioritisation. Access, priorities and rationing all raise issues about equity in health care. It is perhaps strange that these concepts are rarely brought together when designing health care processes. There are exceptions. Score-based waiting systems, as found in New Zealand, for example (see Harrison and New, 2000), give patients scores reflecting the severity of their condition in relation to priority thresholds for both clinical and financial factors (so it is possible a patient may score enough in terms of clinical need but not enough for the operation to be funded). Another approach is the development of local policies on clinical priority which define 'bands of time' within which priority patients must be seen (Audit

Commission, 2002b). These approaches make explicit the links between access, rationing and resources, raise important questions about whether the primary problem is one of access (due to excessive demand) or under-resourcing of health care (Mullen, 1998; Best, 1997). Others acknowledge the link between under-resourcing and access (Green and Irvine, 2001; Redwood, 2000) but view it as an intrinsic problem of state health care systems such as the NHS. Their remedy is not to increase public funding but to encourage diversity in funding sources to extend individual choice and improve overall access to health care.

Greater reliance on private funding is likely to have adverse implications for equity (see Chapter 6). But even with a state health care system there are trade-offs between relative and absolute access. Promoting better access overall might create greater problems for relative access, if patients with greater needs are disadvantaged. Improved access can also conflict with other desirable aims, such as efficiency. According to Sassi and Le Grand (2001), for example, there are significant trade-offs between the equity of access and efficiency and there is no consistency in judgements made in this field. Indeed, there has been little evaluation of the cost-effectiveness of different methods of improving overall access. Increased choice may conflict with fair access, as some individuals are less willing or able to make choices (for further discussion see Chapter 12). Finally, as Doyle (2001) has observed, the evidence-based approach to health care can conflict with perceptions of fair access by patients and carers. People who have contributed to the NHS may feel entitled to care and treatment, even if, on the basis of the evidence, there is little benefit from intervention.

In Summer 2004, the Blair Government published an NHS Improvement Plan, which echoed many of the themes of the NHS Plan of 2000. It made several commitments on access including greater choice and convenience for patients and a guaranteed maximum waiting time from GP referral to treatment of 18 weeks by 2008.

Further Reading

Coulter, A. and Ham, C. (eds) (2000) *The Global Challenge of Health Care Rationing* (Buckingham, Open University Press).

Ham, C. and Robert, G. (2003) *Reasonable Rationing: International Experience of Priority Setting in Health Care* (Buckingham, Open University Press).

Hunter, D. (1997) *Desperately Seeking Solutions: Rationing Health Care* (London, Longman).

Managing Quality and Standards

This chapter examines issues surrounding the quality of health care in the UK. Its main focus is upon hospital care, though much of what follows is also relevant to primary care (discussed further in Chapter 10) and social care (Chapter 11). It begins with a discussion of the concept of quality improvement. This is followed by a review of policies and initiatives introduced in recent years to improve quality and standards. The implications for health service management and for interprofessional relationships are then explored.

Quality Improvement

Organisational and Cultural Approaches

Ovretveit (1992) defined quality in health services as 'fully meeting the needs of those who need the service most, at the lowest cost to the organisation, within limits and directives set by higher authorities and purchasers' (p. 2). He outlined the 'quality approach', a systematic and scientific approach to quality improvement, which could be achieved by changing organisational processes. This included changing relationships (between managers and staff, staff and patients) and introducing new systems of specification and measurement.

Over the past two decades, the NHS has been strongly influenced by ideas from management experts, particularly drawing on private sector practices. For example, general management (see Chapter 5) was based on principles adopted extensively in business organisations. Similarly, corporate board structures introduced into the NHS in the early 1990s (see Chapter 7) were based on the strategic decision-making bodies in the corporate sector. Total Quality Management (TQM), which seeks to embed a philosophy of continuous improvement within the culture of an organisation (Joss and Kogan, 1995), was also imported from the business sector. It is rooted in four principles: that organisational success depends on meeting customer needs, that customer-defined quality is achieved by the production process, that most employees are motivated to work hard and perform well, and that simple statistical methods can reveal faults in production processes and identify ways of continually improving quality (Berwick, Enthoven and Bunker, 1992). Criticism that such an approach is not appropriate to health care (Freemantle, 1992) – because of the difficulties in evaluating the quality of a highly personal service – did not inhibit its application. While there have been difficulties in implementation (Joss and Kogan, 1995; Marnoch, 1996, p. 82), TQM has nonetheless exerted influence over the general approach taken to quality improvement, reflected in the use of accredited quality systems in the NHS (such as BS5750 and ISO 9000, which set standards for effective quality-management systems), clinical governance (which is based on continuous improvement) and the increasing emphasis on consumer evaluation. It is also evident in efforts to 're-engineer' service-delivery processes and to develop 'learning organisations'.

Hospital re-engineering is based on business process re-engineering, which focuses upon ways of improving organisational processes to improve quality, reduce costs and improve profitability (Buchanan, 1996). In the context of the NHS, it comprises projects where staff pool knowledge and experience to identify improvements in services, such as greater patient-satisfaction, better outcomes, or improved cost-efficiency. Strong claims have been made about the potential benefits of re-engineering (Hammer and Champy, 1993). It may facilitate changes which improve patient care, such as better co-ordination of out-patient clinics for people with multiple conditions, or by improving the availability of test results, enabling quicker diagnosis and treatment. However, there are problems associated with re-engineering, which are exacerbated when leadership, staff co-operation, good-quality data, and skills are lacking (Ho, Chan and Kidwell, 1999; Walston, Burns and Kimberly, 2000; McNulty and Ferlie, 2002; Packwood, Pollitt and Roberts, 1998). A balanced view is that while 'the re-engineering perspective does not deliver clear solutions, it may form part of a broader change management strategy, that identifies and develops new designs or approaches' (Buchanan and Wilson, 1996).

Re-engineering methods can be applied to interorganisational processes as well. For example, the NHS collaboratives (see Exhibit 9.1) have been used as a vehicle to improve the quality of care for patients served by different health care organisations. An important aspect of both re-engineering and collaboratives is harnessing the knowledge and experience of staff, and helping them to identify solutions to problems. The development of 'learning organisations' takes this further, enabling staff to acquire and develop skills and knowledge in order to bring about improvements (Davies and Nutley, 2000). However, there are considerable obstacles for learning organisations in the NHS, not least of which are the difficulties of achieving cultural change (Davies, Nutley and Mannion, 2000), including greater openness, a willingness to learn from mistakes, greater trust, and breaking down 'tribal' barriers between professional groups.

Exhibit 9.1 Collaboratives and Beacons in the NHS

Collaboratives vary, but their essential principles are the same (see Bate, 2000). Based on an idea from the US Institute for Health Care Improvement, they seek to challenge existing ways of delivering services by identifying problems and implementing solutions through the involvement of various stakeholders. They pool knowledge from a variety of perspectives and then spread this in order to improve practice in a particular area of provision. The collaboratives operate at local and regional level, but are part of a national initiative. They have been developed by the Modernisation Agency, though in the light of its proposed abolition, much more responsibility will fall on Strategic Health Authorities in the future.

So far the collaboratives have been centred on key service areas, primary care, cancer, heart disease, orthopaedic services, and accident and emergency care. They focus on issues such as improving access to services, improving the quality of care for the patient, and ensuring that different professionals and organisations work together to optimise the care of the patient, including the identification of appropriate care pathways and protocols (De Luc, 2001). The projects vary considerably between specialties, their content being determined to a large extent by the relevant national targets and standards (as set out in National Service Frameworks, for example). In coronary heart disease, for example, the key areas – secondary prevention, acute myocardial infarction, angina, heart failure, revascularisation and cardiac rehabilitation – reflect the content of the NSF. The collaborative projects involve local clinicians and managers, so there is scope for developing local clinical networks (see Chapter 7) and identifying 'bottom up' solutions to service improvement. Good practice in one area can be disseminated to others.

Systematic evaluations of collaboratives have found that though many positive outcomes are evident, their impact could be stronger. This may be partly due to the way in which they have been introduced, and the role of the centre in setting the framework for change (see Bate, Robert and McLeod, 2002). It remains to be seen whether the commitment to 'shift the balance of power' will lead to more freedom and greater local ownership of service-redesign initiatives.

Collaboratives are an important way of harnessing knowledge about how to improve services. Another has been the 'beacons' approach, which also enables the identification and dissemination of innovative practice in various health care and health improvement settings. NHS practitioners and organisations are encouraged to submit case-studies of innovation in areas such as teamworking, improving access, building effective interagency partnerships, and reducing delays, among others. Exemplary activities are accorded beacon status and others are encouraged to learn from these experiences by contacting and visiting beacon sites.

It is difficult to assess the impact of beacons (SHM, 2002). Good practice may be spread by other means, notably through professional networks and other processes (such as collaboratives, for example). It is difficult to measure the overall cost-effectiveness of the scheme. However, the beacons themselves have seen financial benefits, improved morale, enhanced opportunities for learning, leadership and professional development. The beacons have also been credited with creating a favourable climate for change and improvement, as well as a culture of sharing ideas. Visitors to beacon sites are able to identify benefits from their experiences, including strengthening their efforts to improve services in their own institutions.

Criticism of the beacons initiative centred on significant costs associated with the programme. This included the time and resources involved in applying for beacon status, and disseminating good practice. Although beacons received additional resources, many felt this did not recompense them fully for their increased workload. Other criticisms include

$\longrightarrow$

Exhibit 9.1 continued

→

the lack of patient focus in many service-improvement schemes, and the fact that the scheme was a competition, and this could inhibit the collaborative ethos. The selection process was considered opaque and clearer criteria needed to safeguard its credibility. Perhaps beacons also needed to be more closely integrated with other initiatives promoting systematic improvement in services.

The importance of the beacons and collaboratives lies in their potential to change the culture of the NHS. Much lip-service has been paid to changing the culture of the NHS, particularly in pursuit of improvements in quality. However, policies, structures and processes must be conducive to the development of such a culture. Politicians have tended to view NHS staff as part of the problem not part of the solution, and this has brought a more interventionist approach, rather than one which enables these staff to improve services (Ham, 1999b). Also relevant here is Bate's (2000) observation that the potential of clinical networks to improve services will only be fully captured with corresponding and dramatic changes in culture, relationships and skills, part of an overall effort to develop and change organisations. In particular, the hierarchy has to 'let go' and allow local solutions to thrive. By the same token, policy-makers at national level must be more sensitive to the local culture when introducing reform (Atkinson, 2002) and should not seek to impose blanket solutions which are inappropriate.

Evidence-Based Practice

An important aspect of quality in health care has been the emphasis on evidence-based practice (EBP), which arose from several concerns (see Grayson, 1997; Harrison, 1998; Muir Gray, 2001): first, that clinical practice was not currently informed by accurate and up-to-date research findings; secondly, that ineffective and inappropriate interventions wasted resources that could be used more effectively; thirdly, that variations in the use of effective treatments created unacceptable inequities, with some people failing to get access to the best care.

A formidable coalition of support underpinned efforts to improve evidence-based practice. Health professionals saw evidence-based practice as preserving the scientific credibility of health care and enabling them to retain control over their work. Politicians and health service managers believed that it made the health budget go further and gave them greater influence over the allocation of resources. Patients' representatives welcomed it as a means to improve and universalise the quality of care.

The emphasis on evidence-based practice led to several initiatives, including a new approach to Research and Development (R & D). In the 1990s, following the Culyer report (DoH, 1994b) a single R & D budget was introduced with national and regional research priorities. Following a further review (see DoH, 2000f), separate streams of funding were introduced for NHS priorities and needs and for the NHS contribution to the science base. NHS R & D funds are now targeted on the main research priorities: cancer, coronary heart disease and mental health. Efforts have also been made to strengthen performance management of NHS research funds, promote R & D partnerships (within the NHS and between the NHS, researchers and users) and improve the governance of R & D in the NHS (DoH, 2001f). Three national research programmes are particularly relevant to evidence-based practice: the Health Technology Assessment Programme (HTA) commissions research into the cost, effectiveness and broader impact of health technologies; the New and Emerging Applications of Technology Programme (NEAT) promotes the use of new technologies to enhance the quality, efficiency and effectiveness of health care; the Service Delivery and Organisation Programme produces evidence about how organisation and delivery of services can be improved to increase the quality of patient care.

Other initiatives to strengthen evidence-based practice include continuing professional development (see Exhibit 2.4) and the dissemination of information about effective practice to professionals and managers. Important bodies in this field are the Cochrane Collaboration (and the Cochrane Centre at Oxford), which reviews the results of RCTs, and the NHS Centre for Reviews and Dissemination at York University, which reviews results of research and disseminates findings. Another organisation is InterTASC, a collaboration of research organisations that provides commissioning bodies with information about cost-effectiveness of interventions. Systematic reviews can be found in publications such as *Evidence Based Medicine, Bandolier, Clinical Evidence*, and *Effective Health Care* Bulletins. There is also a variety of Internet-based resources on clinical effectiveness (see Muir Gray, 2001). The National Electronic Library for Health (NELH) is also being developed to meet the needs of managers, clinicians and patients for access to evidence.

Those *commissioning* health care are expected to do so on the basis of evidence. Under the Conservative Government of the 1990s, guidance was issued to promote investment in effective treatments and disinvestment in those of doubtful effectiveness (NHSE, 1996). Increasingly, clinical guidelines and National Service Frameworks are included in the specification of service agreements. This has been reinforced by a *duty of quality* on NHS organisations, and the introduction of systems of clinical governance, discussed in a moment. This built on earlier efforts to audit clinical practice and to identify problems and recommend how these should be addressed. The national confidential enquiries into perioperative mortality, stillbirths and infant deaths, maternal deaths, and suicides and homicides by mentally ill people were supplemented by a system of medical audit in 1989 (Marinker, 1990; Pollitt, 1993b; Packwood, Kerrison and Buxton, 1994; Black and Thompson, 1993) and a move towards more integrated systems of clinical audit in the 1990s.

Finally, the Blair Government established new institutions to oversee clinical effectiveness and service quality: a National Institute for Clinical Excellence (see Exhibit 8.2) to produce guidelines on clinical and cost effectiveness of services; and a Commission for Health Improvement (now the Commission for Healthcare Audit and Inspection) to promote improvements in clinical services (see Exhibit 9.2). In addition, new bodies were established to protect patient safety and improve poor performance among professionals, such as the National Patient Safety Agency.

Why Evidence-Based Practice?

Moves to promote EBP have been controversial (see Hurwitz, 1999; Harrison, 1998), particularly when they appear to limit the availability of treatments, or constrain practitioners' discretion (Haycox, Bagust and Walley, 1999). Others have argued that EBP reinforces dominant professional and political perspectives, and call for a more eclectic approach (Colyer and Kamath, 1997). Some point out the additional costs arising from research, improvements in dissemination and the setting of guidelines (Jankowski, 2001). EBP has been criticised for giving greater weight to particular types of evidence (RCTs, large-scale quantitative studies) at the expense of others (small-scale qualitative studies), even though the latter may indicate effectiveness. Another issue is the updating of guidelines, which must be undertaken in the light of technological change, health care resources and the changing values placed on evidence (Shekelle et al., 2001).

There is no guarantee that practice will change as a result of issuing guidelines and disseminating evidence. Previous initiatives were not systematically implemented (Clinical Standards Advisory Group, 1998a), and there was much room for discretion at local level. Furthermore, there is weak evidence that such isolated interventions are effective in promoting change among practitioners (Haynes et al., 1997; Halladay and Bero, 2000). Indeed, in general practice a wider range of factors shape the process of implementing clinical evidence, including the personal and professional experience of the doctor, the doctor–patient relationship, knowledge of the particular circumstances of the patient, and the more pragmatic approach of GPs compared with specialists (Freeman and Sweeney, 2001; Armstrong, 2002). Even when practice changes following the dissemination of evidence, this may be due to other factors (such as pre-existing concern or publicity about particular treatments – Mason, Freemantle and Browning, 2001). It might be expected that the acute sector would be more responsive to the implementation of EBP. Despite the lip-service paid to EBP, NHS trusts have not given high priority to implementation (Wallace and Stoten, 2002).

Clinical Governance

Central to the Blair Government's approach to improving quality in the NHS was *clinical governance* (Scally and Donaldson, 1998; Lugon and

Secker-Walker, 1998). Clinical governance built on earlier efforts to audit, monitor and improve practice. It has been defined as 'a framework through which NHS organisations are accountable for continuously improving the quality of their services and safeguarding high standards of care by creating an environment in which excellence in clinical care will flourish'(DoH, 1998b, p. 33). Clinical governance comprises the following processes (see DoH, 1999d; Scally and Donaldson, 1998; Swage, 2000, pp. 5–6):

1. *Clear lines of responsibility and accountability for clinical care*: NHS trusts (and PCTs) have a duty of quality whereby the chief executive is ultimately responsible for the quality of services, and each trust has a designated senior officer to ensure that systems of clinical governance are effective. There are also formal reporting responsibilities in the form of a clinical governance committee which reports to the trust board, and an annual, public report on clinical governance.
2. *A comprehensive programme of quality improvement*: this includes participation in clinical audit and confidential inquiries. It also includes a commitment to evidence-based practice, and to the implementation of clinical standards in National Service Frameworks and NICE recommendations. There must be a commitment to ensuring that workforce planning and continuing professional development is consistent with the pursuit of improvements in services.
3. *Procedures for identifying and remedying poor performance*: this includes complaints procedures, incident-reporting and clear policies for reporting of concerns by staff.
4. *Clear policies for identifying and minimising risk.*
5. *Clinical governance arrangements for each trust*: these were examined by the Commission for Health Improvement (now the Commission for Healthcare Audit and Inspection – see Exhibit 9.2).

It is difficult to argue with these broad principles and requirements. However, because clinical governance is such a comprehensive concept, there have been concerns about actual implementation. A study of acute trusts (Walshe et al., 2000) found that clinical governance had not proceeded beyond the production of strategies and making key appointments. At this stage there was little evidence of trusts trying to promote the kind of cultural change required for clinical governance to develop fully, though most had sought to raise awareness of the clinical agenda among staff and managers. In primary care too, initial efforts mainly took the form of building the infrastructure for clinical governance. This was followed by a number of developments with considerable potential to improve quality. These included programmes of education to support professionals, incentives to promote improvements in care and better information about the quality of care (Campbell, Roland and Wilkin, 2001).

Exhibit 9.2 From the Commission for Health Improvement to the Commission for Healthcare Audit and Inspection*

The Commission for Health Improvement (CHI) was established by the Health Act 1999 to monitor and help improve the quality of patient care in the NHS in England and Wales. Scotland has its own regulatory body, *NHS Quality Improvement Scotland* (see Exhibit 7.1). CHI was given four functions: (1) clinical governance reviews of all NHS provider organisations; (2) monitoring NHS organisations against standards set by NICE and the National Service Frameworks; (3) undertaking investigations into serious service failures in the NHS; (4) leading, reviewing and assisting health care improvement and sharing good practice in the NHS.

CHI was established as a non-departmental public body, with commissioners appointed by the Secretary of State of Health and the Welsh Assembly. Changes arising from the NHS Reform and Healthcare Professions Act 2002 strengthened its independent status: it was required to present an annual report on the state of services to Parliament and the Welsh Assembly, and its director was no longer subject to ministerial endorsement. CHI responsibilities were also extended. It was given a clearer remit to monitor hospital cleanliness and the patient environment. It also acquired powers to inspect NHS organisations and premises, and could recommend closure or suspension of services, and franchising for poorly-performing services. CHI was required to publish information on performance, including the star rating system. It was also responsible for the commissioning of national clinical audits and the management of national patient and staff surveys.

In one survey, undertaken by the NHS Confederation (2002), the majority of trusts were positive about their experiences of the CHI review process, though there was criticism that reviews lacked clarity of purpose. There was also believed to be a lack of consistency in the approach of review and methodologies adopted (see also Day and Klein, 2004; Benson, Boyd and Walshe, 2004). There was also concern that CHI reports accentuated negative findings and did not give sufficient credit where due. In a subsequent survey, fewer trusts reported a positive experience (NHS Confederation, 2003).

In 2002 it was announced that the audit and inspection functions of CHI, along with the national value-for-money functions of the Audit Commission, the responsibilities of the Mental Health Act Commission, and the National Care Standards Commission's responsibilities for regulating the health care sector would be brought together under a new body – the Commission for Healthcare Audit and Inspection (CHAI). From 2004, this will assess the performance of NHS organisations, promote improvements in healthcare provision, report on the state of health care and act as the leading inspectorate in this field (Dewar and Finlayson, 2002). It will also have responsibility for the second stage of the NHS complaints process in England (see Chapter 12). CHAI will be run by a board appointed by the NHS standards appointments commission. This indicated considerable independence, though much will depend on how it can exercise its powers independently of government (Walshe, 2002a). CHAI will continue to carry out functions in Wales, though a new Health Care Inspectorate has been established there to undertake local reviews and inspections.

There is considerable uncertainty about the style of the new regulatory body. CHI tried to allay suspicions that it was a punitive body by emphasising its role in assisting service improvement (Day and Klein, 2001). But the new body seems more aggressively interventionist than its predecessor, more focused on exposing and rooting out 'poor practice' than encouraging improvement. It remains to be seen whether this will be the case.

*From 2004 the Commission for Healthcare Audit and Inspection will be known as the Healthcare Commission.

A review of CHI reports from 175 trusts sheds further light CCHI, 2002). Although noting examples of good practice, the report found that the majority of NHS organisations had responded to problems rather than trying to anticipate and avoid them. It found a lack of organisation-wide policies, poor implementation of policies, and variation between different departments. A failure to share learning across and between organisations was noted, as well as poor communication, especially between strategic and operational levels. The report expressed particular concern about poor management of risks. It noted that trusts had poor workforce planning and very few routinely involved patients and relatives in policy and service development. It identified many barriers to staff and patients wishing to make a complaint, and it was critical of information systems (see Exhibit 9.3). These themes were developed further in a later Commission for Health Improvement report (CHI, 2003b). A report from the NAO (2003b) noted that there had been several beneficial impacts – notably that clinical-quality issues had now become mainstream. The report also noted greater or more explicit accountability for clinical performance, and a move towards more open, collaborative and transparent ways of working in professional cultures. However, the NAO also observed that implementation varied between and within trusts, and between the different aspects of clinical governance (see also CHI, 2003b).

It was assumed by Government that clinical governance would be cost-neutral, though opportunity costs arising from the new system were highlighted (Dewar, 1999), alongside additional costs in research and development, and information technology (Bloor and Maynard, 1998). The NAO (2003b) estimated the annual cost in secondary and tertiary care to be at least £90 m per annum, excluding clinical and managerial staff time and the cost of running the national bodies supporting clinical governance. Others warned of the dangers of underfunding quality-assurance systems (Campbell, Roland and Wilkin, 2001) and their impact in damaging rather than strengthening public confidence in the NHS (Bloor and Maynard, 1998).

A further problem lay in the quality of the evidence-base for decisions about clinical effectiveness. There were concerns about the accuracy and timeliness of data on the outcomes of care. A Scottish study found that although published clinical outcomes data helped to raise the level of awareness of quality issues among trust staff, they were not regarded by clinicians as being of sufficient quality or relevance to assess performance or improve quality (Mannion and Goddard, 2001). Poor dissemination of information was also a concern (see Clinical Standards Advisory Group, 1998a). In primary care, these problems were complicated further by a weak research base and specific problems of collecting, accessing and sharing information (McColl and Roland, 2000).

Clinical governance has the potential to duplicate other systems of quality-improvement and regulation. Despite official commitments to work with existing processes such as professional self-regulation, audit and complaints, it is unclear

Exhibit 9.3 Information and Communication Technologies (ICTs)

An effective information system can improve efficiency, planning, performance management, accountability, access to services and patient choice. Above all, it can affect the quality of care. Professionals need information about their patients, in the form of accurate records. They require information about the latest research on the effectiveness of treatments in order to implement 'evidence-based' practice. They need to be able to exchange information with each other, and with other agencies, in order to produce a coherent service.

However, the UK's record in promoting ICTs in the health sector has been poor. The Wanless (2001) report noted that the level of expenditure on health care ICT in the UK (at 1.5 per cent of health care spending) was markedly less than that of other countries, notably the USA (6 per cent of health care spending). The Foresight Health Care Panel (2000) stated that ICT development in the NHS was at least a decade behind the commercial sector in the UK. Meanwhile, the Bristol Royal Infirmary Inquiry (2001b) was critical of patient-information systems and called for an independent body to assess the adequacy of data and to evaluate systems of data collection and analysis. Its view was reiterated by an Audit Commission report (2002c), which found that non-clinical data collection – such as waiting lists and waiting times – was unreliable (ten or more areas of data collection were unreliable in one in five trusts). Furthermore, CHI (2002) observed that doctors and nurses often did not have access to the information needed to treat patients effectively.

ICT policy has too often been focused on generating information for policy-makers at the centre to monitor performance, rather than on supporting health care commissioners and providers in meeting health care needs. It has tended to be dominated by financial factors. Yet, ironically, there has been considerable financial mismanagement and waste in the procurement of ICT facilities and services, including several major scandals. One of the most serious occurred in Wessex Regional Health Authority in the 1980s when £20 million was wasted on a computer integration scheme (Public Accounts Committee, 1993). There were problems with implementing integrated hospital information systems (Public Accounts Committee, 1996b) and computer coding systems (Public Accounts Committee, 1998). A strategy had been introduced, but was criticised for not setting clear and measurable objectives (NAO, 1999). Local health bodies tended to develop their own systems and, as a result, there was little coherence. For example, the NHS intranet network (NHSnet), was bedevilled by low take-up, poor access, high cost, concerns about security, and unreliability (Keen, 1999; Bolton, 2000).

One of the major features of ICT in the NHS has been fragmentation, with individual decisions producing incoherence and lack of progress on key policy objectives. A new strategy *Information for Health* (DOH, 1998e), which was updated in the light of the NHS Plan, focused on several key initiatives: the extension of NHS Direct to an on-line service; electronic health records and patient records, which can be accessed by different agencies and professionals; the introduction of hospital-appointment booking systems; the National Electronic Library for Health (NELH), to provide access to the latest knowledge on health care (Muir Gray and de Lusignan, 1999); and electronic prescribing. A special health authority – the NHS Information Authority – was created to develop products and standards and to support local implementation of the strategy. Increased funding was also announced for ICT in the NHS. But dissatisfaction with progress continued (Majeed, 2003; de Lusignan, 2003). This heralded more centralised control over the procurement and management of ICT, prompting further changes, such as the replacement of NHSnet with a system of regional broadband used by all public bodies, and national contracts for providing key elements of the ICT programme.

in practice how this is achieved. According to Dewar (1999), clinical governance confuses rather than clarifies accountabilities by exacerbating tensions between accountability to central government, local clinical governance and the local public. This point will be returned to later in this chapter.

Finally, there is confusion about the ethos of clinical governance. Although it has been portrayed as a means of improving quality in an open and inclusive way, there are fears that it is intended to constrain clinical autonomy and punish 'non-conformists' (Davies, 2000). Others see it as empty rhetoric which does not inspire actual improvements. For them, quality is a product of good working relations rather than new processes of measurement and accountability (Goodman, 1998). The persistence of these views amongst clinicians, whether well-founded or not, is likely to be damaging to the implementation of clinical governance, as it is they who ultimately implement the system (Dewar, 1999; Taylor, 1998; Bloor and Maynard, 1998).

Improving Quality by Preventing Adverse Incidents

The Extent of Adverse Incidents

An adverse clinical incident is defined as an unintended injury caused by medical management of an illness rather than the disease process. Such incidents not only cause unnecessary harm to patients, but have important resource implications, given the rising cost of meeting compensation claims due to negligence. The National Audit Office (NAO, 2001c) estimated that the NHS in England faced a bill of almost £4 billion from future clinical negligence claims, then approximately a tenth of its annual budget, a sevenfold increase since 1995. There are additional costs arising from both unnecessary and corrective treatment.

Estimates of adverse incidents vary, owing to different methodologies (Weingart et al., 2000). The Harvard Medical Practice Study (1990) found that just under 4 per cent of admissions to hospital in New York experienced adverse incidents. In a quarter of cases, doctors had been negligent, in 7 per cent disabilities caused were permanent, and in 14 per cent they led to death. A further American study found that almost one in five hospital patients had experienced at least one adverse event leading to longer hospital stays and increased costs (Andrews et al., 1997). A study of health care quality in Australia found adverse events in over 16 per cent of cases (Wilson R.M. et al., 1995), half of which were considered preventable. Researchers in the UK found that around 11 per cent of patients suffered from adverse incidents, and that a third of these involved moderate or greater disability, or death (Vincent, Neale and Woloshynowych, 2001).

Weingart et al. (2000) found that the key factors behind these errors were inexperienced clinicians and the introduction of new procedures. Errors were more common among the oldest patients, those needing complex and/or urgent care, and those having prolonged hospital stays. Meanwhile, reports from the National Confidential Enquiry into Perioperative Deaths (NCEPOD) have revealed evidence of inappropriate operations, poor pre-operative management, a failure to apply knowledge, and, in some cases, operations being undertaken by inexperienced and underqualified doctors (see Buck, Devlin and Lunn, 1987). Subsequent NCEPOD reports have detailed how organisation, management, information and resources can affect both death-rates and the quality of care (see Campling et al., 1992, 1995; National Confidential Enquiry into Perioperative Deaths, 1998). For example, reports have been highly critical of record-keeping, and the role and quality of post-mortem examinations (National Confidential Enquiry into Perioperative Deaths, 2001). Other specific confidential inquiries have detected serious problems. A confidential enquiry into maternal deaths found evidence of avoidable deaths as a result of substandard care, including failure of junior staff and GPs to diagnose and refer to senior colleagues, failure of consultants to attend births or inappropriate delegation, lack of teamwork, failures to identify and seek advice about diseases that did not commonly occur, and the failure of some units to have a clear policy on the prevention of life-threatening conditions (DoH, Welsh office et al., 1998).

Autopsies can yield information about adverse incidents (Lundberg, 1998). Studies have found that autopsies do not always confirm diagnosis. In one study, clinical diagnoses were confirmed in only 61 per cent of cases (Cameron and McCoogan, 1981). Another found that doctors had failed to diagnose treatable diseases in 13 per cent of cases (Mercer and Talbot, 1985), while an American study found undiagnosed causes of death in almost 45 per cent of autopsies and identified two-thirds of these conditions as treatable (Nichols, Aronica and Babe, 1996). Reviews of diagnoses have also revealed shortcomings. For example, a study of the diagnosis of PVS (persistent vegetative state) discovered that 43 per cent of patients had been misdiagnosed (Andrews et al., 1996). Cases of medical negligence have revealed much about adverse incidents. A quarter of medical negligence cases won by patients against GPs were directly related to errors in prescribing, monitoring or administering medicine (Mihill, 1996). Finally, inquiries into service failures (Walshe and Higgins, 2002) and associated court proceedings can reveal much about the nature of adverse incidents – see Exhibit 9.4.

Errors of diagnosis or management of illness are not the only cause of adverse incidents. In some cases, a design fault in diagnostic or treatment technologies, or mistakes in the delivery of clinical procedures or medicines, are key factors. As a result, incidents are repeated. For example, in the past 15 years ten cancer patients have died and four have been paralysed as a result of the chemotherapy drug Vincristine being wrongly injected into their spine. More generally, errors

Exhibit 9.4 Medical Scandals in the 1990s

A succession of high-profile cases in the late 1990s raised important questions about the adequacy of medical regulation. At the forefront were allegations of poor standards of surgery at the Bristol Royal Infirmary (Bristol Royal Infirmary Inquiry, 2001b), where cardiac surgeons continued to perform operations on children despite evidence of adverse outcomes for some procedures and criticism from colleagues. Other cases included Rodney Ledward, a gynae-cologist struck off the medical register in 1998 for serious professional misconduct (Ritchie, 2000). It was revealed that Ledward lacked essential clinical judgement and skills, and engaged in inappropriate delegation to juniors, yet had continued to work in the NHS and private sector for many years. But the most notorious individual case in recent times was Harold Shipman, a general practitioner convicted of murdering 15 elderly patients in 2000. A subsequent inquiry estimated that he had probably killed 215 people (The Shipman Inquiry, 2001). There was also the issue of illegal and unethical organ retention, raised by the Bristol case (Bristol Royal Infirmary Inquiry, 2001a) and subsequently at the Alder Hey Hospital in Liverpool (The Royal Liverpool Children's Inquiry, 2001) and elsewhere (DoH, 2001g).

All the above cases were seen as much as failures of the system of regulation as of individuals. Moreover, the official inquiries into these events identified key lessons and made recommendations about future regulation and how to secure high-quality health services. The Bristol inquiry (Bristol Royal Infirmary Inquiry, 2001b), in particular, was a landmark investigation which took almost three years to complete and made 198 recommendations, most of which were accepted in full or part by Government. These included (*denotes recommendation not accepted):

■ The notion of partnership between patients and professionals, whereby they are regarded as equals with different expertise, must be adopted by all health care professionals.
■ The quality of information for patients should be improved and tailored to the needs, wishes and circumstances of the individual. Information should be given to enable patients to participate in their care.
■ Tape-recording facilities should be available to enable patients, if they wish, to record discussions with clinicians.*
■ Obtaining patients' consent should be regarded as a process, not just the signing of a form. The process of consent should involve all clinical procedures and examinations that involve any form of touching. Patients should be given sufficient information to enable them to make a choice (including information about the performance of the trust, the specialty and the consultant unit).
■ All those working in the NHS have a duty to tell patients if an adverse event has occurred. When things go wrong patients have a right to an acknowledgement, an explanation and an apology.
■ Complaints systems should have a strong independent element (not part of the trust board or management). An independent advocacy service is needed to help patients and carers.
■ The Department of Health roles in relation to the NHS must be more explicit. Its two roles should be to operate as the headquarters of the NHS; and to establish an independent framework of regulation for health care.
■ A Council for the Quality of Health Care to bring together all the agencies involved in regulating health care standards and institutions and a Council for the Regulation of Healthcare Professionals to bring together professional self-regulatory bodies. These overarching bodies should together co-ordinate standard-setting, performance monitoring,

→

Exhibit 9.4 continued

→

inspection and validation. The various bodies involved in assuring quality of NHS care and professional competence should be independent of and at arm's length from the Department of Health. They must also involve and reflect the interests of patients, the public, and health care professionals, as well as the NHS and government.

- Professional codes of practice should be incorporated in contracts of employment for doctors, nurses, professions allied to medicine, and managers (who should be subject to a regulatory body and a code). Trusts should be able to deal with breaches of the relevant code independently of the professional body. (The Government rejected the recommendation to incorporate the code in medical contracts.)
- The notion of professional competence should be broadened to include communication skills, teamwork, shared learning across professional boundaries, clinical audit/reflective practice, leadership, and education about NHS principles and organisation, about how care is managed and about skills needed for management. Competence in these areas should be formally assessed as part of the process of obtaining an initial professional qualification. Periodic appraisal and revalidation should be compulsory for all health care professionals and part of the contract of employment. The public should be involved in the revalidation process.
- The NHS must learn from adverse events and every effort should be made to create an open and non-punitive environment where it is safe to report 'sentinel events' (defined as 'any unexplained occurrence involving death or serious physical or psychological injury, or the risk thereof'). There should be a national system for reporting such events. Staff should receive immunity from discipline if they report a sentinel event within 48 hours (except where they have themselves committed a criminal offence).
- The National Patient Safety Agency should be independent of the Department of Health and the NHS.*
- One body should be responsible for co-ordinating all action relating to the setting, issuing and review of clinical standards. This should be NICE, restructured to give it independence and authority.*
- The current system of inspecting trusts and PCTs should become a system of validation and revalidation. The system should be supportive and flexible and undertaken by Commission for Health Improvement. The validating body should be able to withdraw, withhold or suspend a validation if standards threaten the quality of care or patient safety. Standards of validation and revalidation should be made public.*
- Clinical audit should be compulsory for all health care professionals providing clinical care and should be included in employment contracts.
- The monitoring of clinical performance should be brought together and co-ordinated by an independent Office for Information on Healthcare Performance. Performance indicators should be fewer, of higher quality and comprehensible to the public as well as health care professionals. Improvements should be made in information collection and data processing, including investment in 'world-class' IT systems.
- In a patient-centred health care service, patients must be involved wherever possible in decisions about their treatment and care. Trusts and PCTs should publish periodic reports on patients' views and suggestions, and action taken as a result. The involvement of the public in the NHS must be embedded in its structures. The perspectives of patients and the public must be taken into account wherever decisions affecting the provision of health care are made. The processes of involving patients and the public must be transparent and open and should be routinely evaluated.

in the administration of medicines are common. One study found a 49 per cent error rate in intravenous drug doses (Taxis and Barber, 2003). Hospital-acquired infections, which may affect as many as 9 per cent of those in hospital (NAO, 2000b), are linked to factors such as low standards of hygiene (see also Office of Health Economics, 1997, which found that 5000 people a year die from HAIs) as well as clinical factors (such as over-prescribing of antibiotics). There is also the wider issue of harmful therapies, which include the adverse effects of drugs such as Opren and Thalidomide (Collier, 1989), and contaminated blood products. In addition, complex issues arise where a therapy has an adverse effect on a particular group of patients (such as vaccine-damaged children, and long-term users of steroids and tranquillisers). Both adverse clinical incidents, which are about incorrect but unintentional management and diagnosis of illness, and harmful therapies, where diagnosis and treatment may have been properly administered by clinicians, are part of what Illich calls 'clinical iatragenesis', discussed in Chapter 3.

Reducing Adverse Incidents

Health care systems have attempted to reduce adverse incidents. This is based on a shift in thinking away from blame and punishment and towards the need for a better understanding of errors and causes of harm (see Rosenthal, Mulcahy and Lloyd-Bostock, 1999). In the USA, for example, the Federal Government announced a programme to reduce the number of deaths due to adverse incidents – estimated at between 44,000 and 98,000 a year (Kohn, Corrigan and Donaldson, 1999). This included the mandatory adoption of error-reporting systems by all states, the creation of a national Centre for Quality Improvement and Patient Safety, and programmes for reducing medical errors in hospitals treating Medicare patients (the state health insurance scheme for elderly people).

In the UK, a House of Commons Inquiry (Health Committee, 1999c) found that a culture of blame dominated the NHS, inhibiting openness and the reporting of errors. It recommended that there should be a culture of organisational responsibility, as well as individual responsibility within the service for dealing with adverse incidents and poor outcomes. The Chief Medical Officer established an inquiry in the late 1990s in an effort to devise a new strategy. Its report, *An Organisation with a Memory* (DoH, 2000g), acknowledged that health care was a high-risk activity, where adverse events were inevitable. It drew parallels with the aviation industry, which has a highly developed system of reporting and investigating critical incidents and 'near misses'. The report recommended a new system of early warnings to alert the NHS to adverse incidents. The aim was purportedly to create a 'blame-free' culture where future errors could be identified and prevented. This was followed up with a further document which set out the Government's plans (DoH, 2001h), which included a new, national, mandatory system for reporting adverse events and 'near misses' (where an adverse outcome following an error was avoided); a means of analysing patterns, clusters or trends and disseminating appropriate guidance to NHS organisations at local level; the creation of a National Patient Safety Agency to implement and operate the system with the purpose of improving patient safety by reducing the risk of harm through error; and, in cases of serious dysfunction, service or system failure, a new streamlined procedure for investigation involving either an independent inquiry commissioned by the Department of Health or by the Commission for Health Improvement (now CHAI, see Exhibit 9.2). In cases where there is major national concern, a public inquiry may be established.

In addition, four targets were set: to reduce to zero the number of patients dying or being paralysed by maladminstered spinal injections by the end of 2001; to reduce by a quarter by 2005 the number of instances of harm in obstetrics and gynaecology which result in litigation; to reduce by 40 per cent by 2005 the number of serious errors in the use of prescribed drugs; to reduce to zero by 2002 the number of suicides by mental health patients (as a result of hanging from a non-collapsible bed or shower curtain rails on wards).

The patient-safety initiative is one of several that may improve the standards of care; others include those already discussed, such as improved clinical audit, clinical governance, better and more accessible research on interventions, clearer standards for care and treatment and controls on new techniques. Patient safety is also likely to be enhanced by other efforts and initiatives, such as improvements in medicines management which can reduce adverse reactions and improve efficiency (Audit Commission, 2001b), and improved packaging and labelling (NAO, 2003c). Another area of activity has been hospital-acquired infections. New guidelines on the prevention and control of such infections were issued (DoH, 2000h), relating to the formulation, implementation and monitoring of infection-control policies, the establishment and functioning of infection-control committees and control teams, ensuring appropriate hygiene and cleanliness levels through the contracting process (with infection-control teams involved in service specification), and ensuring proper surveillance of infection. There have also been efforts to strengthen infection control within the system of clinical audit and governance, alongside more specific initiatives to control the prescribing of antibiotics (Arason et al., 1996; House of Lords, 2001; DoH, 2000i), which have been held responsible for the spread of antibiotic-resistant bacteria. Further attempts have been made to improve standards of hygiene in NHS hospitals. Targets were introduced, forming part of the performance indicators package discussed in Chapter 7. These are based on 'unannounced' inspections from the Patient Environment Action Team, which rates trusts in relation to national cleaning standards. Additional funding was given to trusts in Autumn 2000, and by April 2001, 94 per cent were adjudged to have good or acceptable standards of cleanliness. The remainder were publicly named. Eleven were put on 'special measures' and given some additional funds for improvement. In 2002, the quality of the patients' environment – which includes hygiene – was included in the remit of Commission for Health Improvement. Ensuring cleanliness was also part of the new responsibilities of 'modern matrons' heralded by the NHS Plan. Further guidance on hospital-acquired infections was introduced in 2003 (DoH, 2003c).

Another element in identifying adverse events is the protection of 'whistle-blowers'. As the Bristol case (see Exhibit 9.4) indicated, staff who highlight shortcomings in services need protection. Despite the importance of 'whistle-blowing', those who raise concerns face considerable obstacles (Hunt, 1995), and as a result of their actions often suffer severe and long-lasting health, personal and financial problems (see Lennane, 1993). During the 1990s, the culture of secrecy appeared to become stronger within the NHS (Craft, 1994; Crail, 1995). The Conservative Government introduced guidance on the raising of legitimate concerns in the public and the media in 1993, but this did not protect staff.

The Public Interest and Disclosure Act 1998 now gives some protection to staff who identify problems within their organisations (including the NHS) or to regulatory bodies. Other disclosures (i.e. to the media) have to meet the test of being both reasonable and justified. The Act provides for compensation for genuine whistle-blowers adversely affected by their actions, and controls the use of so-called 'gagging clauses' in contracts. The legislation was followed by NHS guidance that required that such clauses be dropped. Each trust should have a designated senior manager or non-executive director with whom staff can raise issues outside the usual management chain, guidance for staff on raising concerns, and a guarantee of protection from victimisation. Much depends on implementation. Formal rules mean little if the organisational culture remains antagonistic towards whistle-blowers. Indeed a BBC survey in 2002 revealed that over half of NHS senior managers felt unable to raise concerns about the service for fear of recrimination (BBC, 2002), while Commission for Health Improvement (CHI, 2002) found that staff were reluctant to report problems for the same reason and that there were significant barriers (to staff and patients) to making complaints.

Dealing with Poor Professional Performance

Efforts to improve the quality of care and avoid adverse incidents inevitably raise questions about the poor performance of individuals. Even in a 'blame-free' culture, this must be addressed, and indeed a range of formal and informal controls impinge on medical workers and other health professionals (Allsop and Mulcahy, 1996; Allsop and Saks, 2002).

Professional Bodies

Traditionally, regulation has been in the hands of the professional bodies. All healthcare professions, and some practitioners of complementary therapies, have systems of self-regulation. At the time of writing there are eight statutory professional self-regulatory bodies in Britain: the General Medical Council, the Nursing and Midwifery Council, the General Dental Council, the General Optical Council, the Royal Pharmaceutical Society, the General Osteopathic Council, the General Chiropractic Council and the Health Professions Council. These organisations identify and promulgate principles of good practice, maintain registers of those who are qualified and fit to practice, discipline those professionals who fail to uphold these principles, and respond to complaints from the public and from other authorities (such as the police, for example) about the conduct or performance of a professional. The professional regulatory bodies also have an important role in relation to standards of education and training of professionals. However, there are important differences, both in the way these organisations operate and in their powers. For example, there has been a considerable variation in the extent to which these bodies involve lay people and the degree to which they are able to exercise their functions without interference from other bodies (National Consumer Council, 1999; Allsop and Saks, 2002).

In recent years, professional regulatory bodies have been under pressure to reform themselves, following a lack of public confidence in procedures for dealing with incompetent and dangerous practitioners, concern about the insular nature of these bodies, suspicions that they act mainly in the interests of the professionals rather than the public, and a desire to promote a more efficient, co-ordinated and integrated system of professional regulation. The media, politicians and pressure groups have articulated such views. Moreover, there has been discontent from professionals themselves, who have criticised their own institutions for being aloof, unresponsive to their views, and ineffective in maintaining their professional standing.

The doctors' regulatory body, the General Medical Council (GMC), has been at the forefront of public criticism for a number of years (see Stacey, 1992; Klein, 1998). Following a major inquiry in the 1970s (Cmnd 6018, 1975), new procedures for dealing with sick doctors were introduced and the composition of the GMC was changed, giving more seats to members elected by the profession. But this did not allay criticism that the GMC could only punish doctors for 'serious professional misconduct', which usually concerned matters of a criminal or sexual nature rather than serious clinical errors. The standard punishment, removal from the medical register, was rarely used. The GMC could do little about doctors whose clinical practice was poor or dangerous, until 1997 when it acquired powers to investigate complaints regarding seriously deficient practice. If substantiated, the doctor could be prevented from practising medicine or could have certain restrictions imposed (such as not being allowed to undertake a particular procedure, or practising it only under supervision) until certain remedial action had been taken, such as counselling or retraining. In addition, GMC complaints processes and hearings were infused with a greater level of lay involvement than had previously been the case.

These steps were regarded as minimal, a view confirmed by the subsequent scandals in the late 1990s. In the Health Act of 1999, the Government introduced new powers to make it easier to amend the legislative basis for professional bodies' powers in areas such as regulating standards and performance, discipline, education and training. Further change was heralded by the NHS Plan of 2000, which proposed a new body to oversee the system of professional regulation, as recommended by the Bristol inquiry. Subsequently, the UK Council for the Regulation of Healthcare Professionals was created. This new body was established with a lay majority and a lay chairperson. Its main tasks are to promote the interests of the patient and public in the way the professional regulators carry out their functions, to identify principles of best practice and to promote them among the regulatory bodies, and to promote co-operation between them. It cannot intervene in cases currently being heard by the regulatory bodies but can appeal against their decisions. It also has reserve powers that may be used in exceptional cases to require other professional regulators to make new rules.

In the meantime, there have been important changes to other professional bodies. The Nursing and Midwifery Council (NMC) has replaced the UK Central Council of Nursing, Midwifery and Health Visiting, though, despite its name change, it retains responsibility for health visitor regulation. The Health Professions Council has replaced the former Council for Professions Supplementary to Medicine. Both these new bodies are expected to focus more in future on standards of conduct and performance, professionals' fitness to practice and remedial measures for those whose practice is deficient. For example, the NMC is able to strike off or suspend those found to have committed serious errors and misdemeanours, but may also attach conditions to a registrant's practice, or can issue a caution.

Meanwhile, other individual regulatory bodies have continued to introduce reforms. The GMC may now restrict a doctor's practice immediately when allegations of a very serious nature are made, for example a serious alleged criminal offence or evidence of serious, on-going risk to patients. The GMC can suspend a doctor immediately following a finding of misconduct or unfitness to practice and can also impose conditions on a doctor's practice immediately where impairment of fitness to practice has been found. It can take into account convictions overseas and disqualification by another country's professional body, which it could not do before. Procedures relating to the restoration of doctors to the register have also been strengthened, extending the minimum period before an application to rejoin the register can be made, and introducing more rigorous readmission procedures. The GMC was reduced in size to 35 members, and lay membership increased to 40 per cent(from a quarter). It pledged to introduce new procedures to speed up the investigation of complaints against doctors, and promised more lay involvement in disciplinary processes. The GMC also agreed to implement a revalidation process. Every five years every doctor must demonstrate that he or she is adopting the standards of practice set out by the GMC. For doctors working in the NHS, this will be linked to an annual appraisal. Doctors who cannot provide sufficient evidence for revalidation will not be granted a licence, which will be necessary in order to practice from 2005.

NHS Disciplinary Systems

Professionals who are NHS employees are subject to its disciplinary procedures, and may be suspended or dismissed, irrespective of what action their professional body takes. A new national disciplinary procedure has been promised, to provide a consistent and quicker approach. It is expected that in future doctors being investigated for personal conduct will be subject to the same procedures as other NHS employees. It has been proposed that consultants' right of appeal on disciplinary issues to the Secretary of State for Health be removed. A review of suspension procedures, to form part of the new national disciplinary process, is also being undertaken. Disciplinary procedures are supplemented by procedures for doctors whose practice is causing concern (DoH, 1999e, 2001i). A new body, the National Clinical Assessment Authority (NCAA) was established to advise NHS employers on poor clinical performance. Lay and medical assessors assess and report on the doctors' clinical practice. A course of action is then recommended, though the employer remains responsible for taking action.

There is also a system of 'alert letters'. These are sent on a confidential basis by employers who believe that a former employee or contractor poses a serious threat or risk to the safety of staff, patients or carers, or if their conduct has seriously compromised the functioning of a clinical team or primary care services. These letters are an important mechanism, but depend on employers checking the registration of professional staff. In practice, this is surprisingly lax, complicated further by an increased reliance on agency and locum staff. Indeed, a report from Commission for Health Improvement (CHI, 2002) found that there was poor management of such staff and a widespread failure to check professional registration. New guidance, introduced in 2002, attempted to strengthen the system of pre-and post-appointment checks for health services employees, and included a requirement to check registration.

Regulatory Overload?

Stronger regulation was introduced to reassure the public about the quality and safety of health care. However, these developments have occurred in a haphazard way. There are several regulatory agencies, whose functions overlap considerably (Walshe, 2002b; NAO (National Audit Office), 2003b). To some extent, this reflects the tradition of fragmented self-regulation in Britain (Baeza, 1999; Salter, 2000). Although the Council for the Regulation of Healthcare Professionals can be seen as an attempt to reduce fragmentation, it does not incorporate other state regulators. Notably, the Bristol inquiry called for better co-ordination within a single overarching body, a Council for the Quality of Healthcare, which was accepted by Government, but became subsumed in the creation of CHAI (see Exhibit 9.2). In a further move to improve joint working, GMC drew up 'memoranda of understanding' with Commission for Health Improvement and NCAA to clarify the position of each body and their working relationships (including cross-referrals and information sharing).

The style of the new regulatory regime has been centralist, with the emphasis on setting national standards, frameworks and processes (Davies, 2000; Walshe, 2002b). This may be understandable, given the political pressures arising from the scandals of the late 1990s. It is certainly consistent with the 'command and control' approach adopted by the Blair Government in relation to performance management. However, most observers believe that regulators need independence to maintain credibility (see Patterson, 2001; Walshe, 2002b). This sentiment was also expressed in the Kennedy Report: 'the various bodies whose purpose it is to assure the quality of care in the NHS... and the competence of Healthcare professionals... must themselves be independent of and at arms length from the Department of Health' (Bristol Royal Infirmary Inquiry, 2001b, para: 41).

Commentators also argue that, despite the apparent shifting of balance towards state regulation, self-regulation remains important. This is because the involvement of professionals in maintaining quality and protecting patients is crucial. Professionals play a vital role in peer review and assessment, in identifying poor practice by colleagues, and in giving support to fellow professionals. Any system of regulation that is unable to carry the support of professionals with it will ultimately fail (Davies, 2000; Bloor and Maynard, 1998).

The Management of Professions

Managing Professionals

Central government has attempted to exert stronger control over the quality of health care, as well as other aspects, such as access and cost-efficiency. Indeed, a recurring theme of reform has been to improve the management of doctors, nurses and other professional groups, with the aim of controlling the cost and quality of professional work. This was reflected in changes to management structures and processes, and efforts to integrate professionals within the corporate decision-making structures of the NHS. The impact of these changes on professionals will now be explored, focusing particularly on doctors and nurses in the acute sector.

The Medical Profession

The contemporary relationship between doctors and managers was shaped by initiatives introduced in the 1980s and 1990s. The Griffiths report of 1983 (see Chapter 5) attempted to strengthen line management and clarify accountability in the NHS. General managers, appointed at every level in the service, were held accountable for the performance of their organisation, while having more discretion over their own management structures. Griffiths also recommended that doctors be more closely involved in management, taking more responsibility for the resource implications of their work.

Although general management was perceived as a threat to medical power, the medical profession resisted efforts to limit its autonomy and externally monitor its performance (Strong and Robinson, 1990). As Harrison and Pollitt (1994, p. 50) observed, most managers avoided issues where the medical profession was likely to raise strong objections, and the relationship between the two remained to be renegotiated (Harrison et al., 1992). Where zealous recruits (usually from the minority drawn from outside the NHS) did overtly challenge the local medical establishment, they were invariably and ignominiously defeated. In some hospitals, overt conflict between doctors and managers was evident (Blackhurst, 1995), but many of these already had a troubled history. By the mid-1990s, according to one survey, only one in eight senior doctors believed that their trust management style was 'very or extremely confrontational' (*Health Service Journal*, 1995).

Managers, in theory, had more leverage. Annual job plans for consultants were introduced. However, this was not fully implemented (Health Committee, 2000a). In practice, it was difficult for managers to influence the work of senior doctors. One of the main reasons was the inflexible nature of the consultants' contract (see Health Committee, 2000a). However, dissatisfaction with the contract was not confined to Government and health service managers. Even consultants' representatives accepted that revision was long overdue. Eventually, after protracted negotiations and a rejection of the draft contract by consultants in England and Wales, a new contract was agreed in 2003. This attempted to clarify the nature of consultants' NHS commitments and workload, introduced mandatory job plans and annual appraisals.

Trust status, introduced in 1991, appeared to strengthen managers' authority by giving them freedom to develop their own management structures. Meanwhile, the purchaser – provider split, as Harrison et al. (1992) noted, placed additional levers of power and persuasion into their hands. Certainly, the need to secure contracts and generate income added weight to their arguments for changes in service organisation and delivery, improved monitoring of service quality, and the matching of workload to resources. The system of planning and service level agreements, which replaced the Conservatives' internal market, was unlikely to give managers the same leverage.

It could be argued that the introduction of clinical governance and performance ratings strengthened the position of managers to tackle quality issues. However, their actual influence over the quality of health care remains limited. The increased surveillance of medical work in the 1980s and 1990s, did not threaten autonomy (see Flynn, 1992). Indeed, medical audit was introduced in the late 1980s (Marinker, 1990). Doctors accepted the need for this, but only under certain conditions: that the process remained under their control, that it was confidential, that participation was voluntary, and that there would be no compulsion to alter practice. They resented attempts by outsiders to use audit as a tool to challenge clinical autonomy. The Department of Health agreed that the process should be managed by the doctors themselves. As a result, medical audit did not directly challenge the clinical autonomy of the profession and was 'inwardly-focused' (Pollitt, 1993b; Packwood, Kerrison and Buxton, 1994; Black and Thompson, 1993). Indeed, the history of medical audit in England, and in other countries, indicates that the profession is capable of maintaining its autonomy through 'renegotiated mechanisms of self-control' (van Herk et al., 2001). There was also evidence of poor implementation and outcomes: A sizeable minority of doctors did not participate in audit, the scheme was costly, and there was insufficient monitoring of the benefits accruing to patients (Public Accounts Committee, 1996c).

In the second half of the 1990s there was an attempt to shift the focus towards a multidisciplinary approach, focused on overall quality of service. The move towards comprehensive *clinical audit* aimed to integrate the audit processes of all the professions involved (i.e., medical audit, nursing audit, and the audit of professions allied to medicine). In 1996 health authorities were given the responsibility for developing clinical audit. It was expected that they and other commissioners of care would specify in greater detail the quality of service they expected from providers. As a result it was expected that clinical audit would have a larger role in ensuring that standards were actually met.

There is now greater specification of service standards, as well as a reliance on evidence-based practice and the measurement of outcomes. Moreover, participation in audit is now compulsory for doctors. But it still remains firmly in the hands of the medical profession, largely because service standards continue strongly to reflect medical criteria, values and methods. There may be opportunities for managers and others to exert more influence over the definition of quality in future. This could happen as performance standards and clinical governance begin to reflect other considerations, such as patient perspectives and the wider healthcare environment.

Doctors in Management

Another way in which Government has tried to strengthen the management of doctors is by involving doctors in NHS management. Medical involvement in management is not new. Psychiatric hospitals had medically qualified superintendents up to the 1970s (Harrison, 1999), and Medical Officers of Health were responsible for managing a range of health services until 1974. The important contribution of doctors was recognised in management changes in the 1970s, with the introduction of consensus management (see Chapter 5). But this did not deal with a fundamental problem – the inability to incorporate doctors within a coherent system of management. Griffiths, as noted earlier, recommended that doctors become more active in management and, in particular, the management of resources.

The resource management initiative (RMI), following on from a Griffiths recommendation, was introduced in 1986 to relate workload to resources. Resource management involved the development of information systems about cost and activity, and management systems that explicitly involved clinicians and gave them responsibility for budgets. These schemes faced considerable problems: they were expensive and produced little evidence of improvements in care (Packwood, Keen and Buxton, 1991; Health Services Management Unit, 1996b). Nonetheless, they appeared to produce greater participation by clinicians in management.

Resource management encouraged restructuring within hospitals. This was accelerated by trust status, introduced in 1991, which established the post of medical director with a seat on the trust board. The role of medical director was not clearly defined by Government (see Miu, 1997), but encapsulated the following functions: advising on overall clinical policies, monitoring medical performance, overseeing medical audit, managing contractual arrangements with consultants, leading on restructuring arising from initiatives on junior doctors' hours, facilitating and supporting clinical directors (see below), and being involved in strategic planning (British Association of Medical Managers, 1996).

The job of medical director is a challenging one. The difficulties of managing medical staff, especially consultants, are well known (it has been likened to 'herding cats' – Mui, 1997, p. 67; Fitzgerald and Reeves, 1999, p. 17). The medical director can only influence his or her fellow-doctors; there is no effective line management function. The workload is heavy, largely because most medical directors wish to retain a clinical role, and there is a lack of administrative support (Newman and Leigh, 1996). The continuation of clinical activity is vital in maintaining credibility with medical colleagues, though the latter may still be suspicious of medical directors, seeing them as managers first, and medics second. Medical directors believe that clinical practice is useful in helping to keep open their options in the future should they wish to leave management and go back to full-time practice (Millar, 2000; Mui, 1997).

As well as appointing medical directors, trusts created new management structures below board level, known as clinical management teams (CMTs). Although there are a variety of models, the most common is the clinical directorate which itself takes a number of forms (see White, 1993; British Association of Medical Managers et al., 1993; Austin and Dopson, 1997). Clinical directorates are focused on the main areas of a provider's activity. In hospital units they are organised according to the main specialties such as medicine, surgery, specialist surgery, obstetrics and gynaecology, and other clinical services (for example, pathology, radiology and anaesthetics). In practice, groupings vary considerably and may be subdivided further into associate directorates based on departments. Some directorates, particularly in non-acute units, are focused around client groups, such as the elderly.

Although clinical directorates are usually headed by a consultant, some clinical directors (particularly of community health services and non-medical therapies) have a non-medical background. The clinical director is usually part-time, maintaining some professional practice. Working with the clinical director and responsible to him are a nurse manager and a business manager. In some directorates, these roles are combined into a single post. There are other models, including the specialty directorate model, where a full-time specialty manager, usually from a non-medical background, holds the budget. He or she agrees activity levels with clinicians and with trust management. In this model, clinicians are less directly involved in the management process.

The clinical director has a number of responsibilities which he or she undertakes with the assistance of the other members of the clinical management team (CMT). These include management of the budget, staff, workload and, increasingly, overall quality of service. Clinical directorates produce a 'business plan' and monitor performance against this. Finally, clinical directors represent the directorate within the trust, for example by participating on management boards and committees. Clinical directors can also channel views through the medical director, who sits on the trust board and has overall responsibility for monitoring medical performance.

Despite the difficulties of getting doctors to participate in management activities, the experience of the clinical management systems has been broadly positive (Marnoch, 1996, p. 25). Certainly they represent a more coherent structure than the haphazard arrangements they replaced. But a number of obstacles to progress have been identified. Clinical directors (like medical directors) seem to be overloaded (Simpson and Scott, 1997; Buchanan et al., 1997), partly because of continuing clinical duties. They lack training (Buchanan, et al., 1997; Bristol Royal Infirmary Inquiry, 2001b), though this may be improving (Simpson and Scott, 1997). The career options are limited; most take the job for negative reasons, and aim to return to full-time medicine (Simpson and Scott, 1997; Buchanan et al., 1997).

At best, clinical management teams work in a consensual way. But team-building can be undermined by a refusal to share decision-making (Walby and

Greenwell, 1994) which usually strengthens medicine and undermines the position of other professional groups (see Fitzgerald and Reeves, 1999). Even so, there are strong arguments in favour of medically-qualified clinical directors. According to Buchanan and colleagues (1997), they can play a valuable role in bringing clinical issues to bear on trust decision-making and can emphasise a patient-centred approach, they have credibility with medical colleagues, as well as a high level of skills and education, and are well networked. However, as he goes on to argue, this does not mean that other configurations should not be experimented with, including opening up directorates to non-clinical staff and collective responsibility models.

Although clinical directors operate within a devolved management system, they have been perceived by some staff as part of a mechanism of control (Fitzgerald and Reeves, 1999). Meanwhile, flexibility has been frustrated in practice by the failure to devolve budgetary responsibilities to clinicians (British Association of Medical Managers, 1996). Yet, in practice, clinical directors have limited influence over their colleagues and cannot be held responsible for their performance (Orchard, 1993; Buchanan et al., 1997). Doctors still retain a high level of autonomy, especially over technical matters (Fitzgerald and Dufour, 1997). They are particularly suspicious of line management, and may ultimately refuse to co-operate with the plans agreed by the clinical director at unit level. Case-studies have shown how doctors can resist and limit the impact of internal reorganisation, for example (see, McNulty and Ferlie, 2002).

By the mid-1990s, most clinical directorates remained devices for managing budgets and balancing the books (Audit Commission, 1995c; Marnoch, 1996). More recently, they have begun to focus more on clinical quality and performance (Fitzgerald and Dufour, 1997). Even so, there was little evidence that clinical directors could secure improvements in service quality (Marnoch, 1996). Other researchers detected a reluctance among clinical directors to tackle difficult issues (Fitzgerald and Reeves, 1999) or to take on management responsibility for sensitive matters, such as consultant performance (Buchanan et al., 1997). Although there have been cases where doctors have resigned following allegedly poor performance, such cases remain comparatively rare. Moreover, there is a suspicion that clinical management could be used to block improvements. In extreme cases, clinical management can end up in the hands of the very people whose performance is a cause for concern, as happened in both the Bristol and Ledward cases.

Clinical governance is having some impact on these structures, according to some researchers (Fitzgerald and Reeves, 1999). The number of directorates in some trusts is being reduced; in some cases clinical director roles are changing, becoming more interventionist, and taking greater responsibility for operational issues. It is too early to say whether this trend is general or will lead to stronger line management, though history would suggest that this will be fraught with difficulties. The lesson of previous efforts to improve quality (Joss and Kogan, 1995; Marnoch 1996; Hadley and Forster, 1993) is that managers must engage with clinicians closely in this process. Failure to do so leads to greater alienation, distrust of management and poorer levels of performance. The current ethos to shift the balance of power to front-line professionals sits uneasily with the strengthening of central regulatory systems.

It is difficult to assess the impact of these initiatives on the hospital doctors' power and autonomy. As Harrison (1999) notes, the evidence is equivocal, and it is more likely that a redistribution rather than a reduction of autonomy has taken place. Doctors are increasingly governed by standards set by other doctors (with input from others, including patient groups), such as clinical guidelines and national service frameworks. There may also be a shift in the balance of power between different parts of the profession, notably from consultants to GPs given their role in commissioning. Clinical governance may produce further shifts in the balance of power towards doctors who organise and oversee clinical activity.

Another scenario portrays a different relationship between doctors and managers, one that is characterised more by co-operation than conflict. This agenda is actively encouraged by government, stressing the importance of collaboration, co-operation and partnership values in NHS management (DoH, 2002h). According to some, trust managers and senior doctors are finding common agendas and objectives in terms of maintaining and improving services (Fisher and Best, 1995; Loveridge and Starkey, 1992; Ong, Boaden and Cropper, 1997). This is because of the growing interdependence between them, arising from the need to meet national targets and standards, and to respond to the demands of commissioners who control most of their income. The future of a trust, therefore, will increasingly depend on the perceived quality of its services and how it meets patients' needs. In seeking to respond to these challenges, managers and doctors cannot do it alone, but must work together more effectively to meet organisational objectives, the former by facilitating change and the latter by improving practice. This could encourage strategic alliances between doctors and managers within a trust (see Wood, 1989 for a case-study of a US hospital) and legitimise stronger line management of clinicians. However, one should perhaps not be over-optimistic. Research by Davies, Hodges and Rundall (2003) found a divergence of views about the doctor–manager relationship, with chief executives being the most optimistic and clinical directors the least. They pointed out that the most obvious divide was not between doctors and lay managers but between senior and middle managers. Clinical directors were the most disaffected group, holding negative views about managers' capabilities and the balance of influence between doctors and managers.

Nurses and Management

The reforms of the 1980s and 1990s diminished the role of nurses at senior levels in the management structure. Following the Griffiths management report

(DHSS, 1983), few nurses were appointed as general managers (less than a tenth had a nursing background). Moreover, the new management structures post-Griffiths often changed in ways unfavourable to nursing, especially at district level where nursing officers began to disappear from the management boards. The impact of Griffiths's reforms, particularly upon senior nursing staff, has been viewed in extremely negative terms (Ackroyd, 1995; Walby and Greenwell, 1994; Robinson, 1992; Wells, 1999; Traynor, 1999; Fatchett, 1998).

Shrinking opportunities for nurses at senior levels were compounded by reorganisations, which led to senior nursing posts being abolished at regional level and reduced at health authority level. Further down the hierarchy, the situation was more complex. The internal market was generally regarded as having a negative impact on nurses, subjecting them to tighter control by lay managers. This was in part because nursing represented a major cost element which had to be closely controlled in order to remain competitive (Fatchett, 1998; Traynor, 1999). The main issue was cost-control not care, and nurse managers were regarded as managers rather than nurses (Wells, 1999). There is evidence that at least some of those with a nursing background began to adopt a managerialist rather than a nursing perspective, though they rationalised such changes in clinical terms (Traynor, 1999).

Nevertheless, the creation of trusts increased opportunities for some nurses to contribute to management. Trust boards had to include a senior nurse. In addition, the development of clinical management teams in some situations enabled the representation of the nursing perspective below board level – though much depended on local personalities and conditions (Jones, 1994; British Association of Medical Managers et al., 1993). Also, the introduction of clinical governance enhanced the position of those nurses who had acquired management responsibilities for the quality of care (Wells, 1999).

One should also consider the impact of management reforms on nurse management at ward level. The devolution of budgets to ward level was believed to have increased the financial and management role of nurses (Alaszewski, 1995). However, this development seems to have been double-edged, shifting ward managers away from clinical management towards financial management responsibilities (Wells, 1999, 73–4). Although placing more management responsibility on nurses at this level, these changes did not improve their ability to affect change (Keen and Malby, 1992). This was confirmed by research into the stress levels of ward sisters and charge nurses, which revealed that such staff shouldered a heavy burden of responsibility with very little support (Allen, 2001). They felt increasingly accountable to a range of other stakeholders, while losing control of their own clinical territory. In addition, they were cynical about their power to influence change, and believed that they had little influence over management decisions.

Further reforms were introduced to address some of these issues. At the ward level, sisters (and charge nurses) were promised new budgets. These included ward environment budgets to improve essential care and the patient environment. It was also proposed that sisters would be supported by ward housekeepers responsible for laundry, catering and other support services. They are also expected to have a greater say in future over standards of cleanliness and quality of food, as set out in cleaning-contract specifications. In addition, modern matron posts have been established to act as clinical leaders and care co-ordinators (DoH, 2002j). Each post covers a group of wards and their brief is to ensure that the fundamentals of care are provided. Modern matrons will be expected to ensure that administrative and support services contribute to the achievement of high standards of care. It was proposed that they will be able to withhold payment to cleaning and catering providers where standards are not being met. They also have a clinical leadership role, in theory strengthening the voice of nurses above ward level.

It is too early to predict the impact of these changes (Cole, 2002b). However, other developments may also strengthen the position of nurses in management processes. Improvements in leadership training for nurses, and the creation of consultant posts in nursing, midwifery and health visiting, could lead to a new cadre of high-profile nurse leaders (DoH, 1999a). Also important will be the greater emphasis on 'team working' between the different professions, which may give nurses an enhanced role in co-ordinating and managing care.

Nurses, doctors and teamwork

Nurses have historically played the supporting role to doctors, and have been regarded as having less influence over health care practice, policy and management. Although medical hegemony is still intact, one must be aware that the relationship between doctors and nurses is quite complex. Nurses are not always and everywhere subservient to doctors, and are able to influence the care and treatment given to patients. Moreover, as we shall see, the simple relationship of 'dominant doctor – handmaiden nurse' is complicated by the emergence of new modes of provision based on teamwork.

The power relations between doctors and nurses are variable, and much depends on the particular situation, on the grades of staff concerned, and on personalities (Mackay, 1993; Porter 1999). In trying to make sense of this, one can draw on different models of medical-nurse relations (see Porter, 1999 for further discussion), as follows.

1. *Subservience model*: doctors are the masters; nurses carry out their instructions (see Freidson, 1988; Gamarnikow, 1978).
2. *The doctor-nurse game*: the subservience of nurses is an appearance in an attempt to minimise open disagreement (see Mackay, 1993). Nurses are influential but their influence is hidden, largely because their opposition and

recommendations are coded, so that from an outsider's perspective they are not seeking to influence the doctors' judgement (see Stein, 1978).

3. *Opportunistic model*: nurses can take the opportunity offered by particular circumstances to exert direct influence on care and treatment. This might include, for example, situations where nurses' greater knowledge of the trust or departmental culture gave them an advantage over doctors. (Hughes, 1998).

4. *Negotiated Order*: nurses have resources which they may use to influence decisions. These include their practical assistance and their knowledge of the patient. They can use these resources to negotiate openly over boundaries of work (Svensson, 1996).

5. *Informal power model*: nurses exercise independent judgement and work beyond their formal boundaries in order to maintain the continuity of care, which is accepted on practical grounds by the doctors rather than openly negotiated (Allen, 1997).

6. *Nursing power model*: nurses are given the freedom to make decisions about care and to evaluate the outcomes without medical 'interference'. This is the principle on which Nursing Development Units are based – see Exhibit 2.5).

Rather than one model being 'correct', the reality is that there are elements of truth in all these, depending on the circumstances (Porter, 1999; Lockhart-Wood, 2000; Manias and Street, 2000). Nurses are certainly not subservient and indeed have, in some respects, strengthened their claims to professional status both through educational reforms and by taking on more specialist clinical roles (though, as earlier suggested, this has not always been straightforward and has not been without costs – see Exhibit 2.5). Indeed, as Wicks has observed, the relationship between doctors and nurses is not only variable, but dynamic. She argues that the voice and active resistance of nurses to medical domination has been ignored. This means that in some situations doctors may be able to subordinate nurses, but that in others nurses can be successful in challenging medical authority, and in yet others an accommodation or common ground will be achieved (Wicks, 1998). Others too have noted that, while nurses are generally reluctant to challenge doctors' authority, some questioning of decisions did occur, particularly where justified by the nurses' role as 'patients' advocate' (Snelgrove and Hughes, 2000).

Towards better teamwork

The current reform agenda is very much about overcoming divisions between professional groups and creating a more flexible and responsive health service. For example, the NHS Plan aimed to break down the old demarcations between staff, by extending the roles of non-medical staff. There has also been greater interest in developing the roles of professionals and workers in the health service, to enable greater flexibility (Buchan, 2002). Policies have also been introduced to clarify the different roles which staff can play in relation to diagnosis, care and treatment through the use of protocols. In addition, reform of the pay system for NHS staff (known as *Agenda for Change*) was proposed in order to foster new and more flexible ways of working. It has also been recognised that a common approach is needed to certain aspects of professional work, notably education and training, regulation and audit. Hence the Council for the Regulation of Healthcare Professionals may bring some consistency to professional regulation; the education and training of professionals is expected to become more integrated, with doctors and nurses sharing courses at pre-registration level and continuing professional development activities. Meanwhile, clinical governance seeks to bring together the separate forms of audit undertaken by each clinical group, and has widened the focus to include basic care as well as clinical interventions.

Shared decision-making and improved team-working are increasingly emphasised. These themes are found not only in the acute sector but also in community and primary health care settings, where models of interprofessional teamworking have a longer history. Improved interprofessional working has been encouraged, particularly in new organisational forms of service provision, such as hospital re-engineering projects and, more recently, collaboratives. The rationale for this is fairly clear; poor teamworking is linked to poor-quality services and even increased mortality of patients. (see Baggs et al., 1999, Larson, 1999; National Confidential Enquiry into Peri-operative Deaths, 2002).

Nonetheless, attempts to break down professional barriers and produce better team working have a mixed record (see Soothill, Mackay and Webb, 1995). Professional rivalries and the desire to preserve territory are often very strong. Often this is justified. Flexibility can mean deskilling, increased workload and lower status and pay (see Corby and Mathieson, 1997). The problem is not simply that individual practitioners are opposed to more inclusive forms of teamworking, but that organisational and professional structures militate against more inclusive forms of collaboration. There are also often legal issues, notably the overall accountability of doctors for patient care. Financial factors that militate against collaborative working include different systems of remuneration and performance management, so that individual professionals are rewarded and evaluated individually rather than as a team.

Conclusion

Everyone agrees that improving the quality of health care is a good thing. But there is disagreement about the best way of achieving this. There are different interpretations of the meaning of quality in health care. There are also different views on what motivates service providers. Pressures to strengthen the accountability of the NHS have led to the development of a 'top-down' approach to quality assurance. New regulatory institutions have been created at national level. Self-regulatory bodies continue, but are more closely tied to the objectives of central government. National frameworks and institutions are important. They can promote consistency, set minimum standards and play a role in disseminating evidence of good and harmful practice. However, too great a reliance on central bodies is counterproductive. There are too many bodies, they duplicate each other, and make heavy demands on service providers. Rationalisation is, therefore, a positive step, one which government is now taking. (Note: In May 2004, the Department of Health announced that the number of 'arm's length' bodies, including regulatory bodies, would be halved by 2007/8. This is likely to lead to mergers between these organisations in the next few years.) It has also recognised that the system of quality improvement must carry the professions with it, and must allow for experimentation and innovation, Above all, systems of regulation have to promote and reinforce cultural changes that are conducive to improving services.

The Council for the Regulation of Healthcare Professionals is now known as the Council for Healthcare Regulatory Excellence.

Further Reading

Leatherman, S. and Sutherland, K. (2003) *The Quest for Quality in the NHS* (London, Nuffield Trust).

Muir Gray, J. (2001) *Evidence Based Healthcare: How to make Health Policy and Management Decisions* (Edinburgh, Churchill Livingstone).

Ovretveit, J. (1992) *Health Service Quality – An Introduction to Quality Measures for Health Services* (Oxford, Blackwell Scientific).

Ovretveit, J., Thompson, T., and Mathias, P. (eds) (1997) *Interprofessional Working for Health and Social Care* (Basingstoke, Macmillan).

Ovretveit, J. (1998) *Evaluating Health Interventions* (Buckingham, Open University Press).

Walshe, K. (2003a) *Regulating Healthcare: A Prescription for Improvement?* (Buckingham, Open University Press).

Primary Health Care 10

Primary care organisations and professionals have a crucial gate-keeper function, regulating access to other services. They play an important role in assessing the health needs of patients and populations, and ensuring that services are available to meet these, either through direct provision or by commissioning from other parts of the health care system. Primary care agencies also have great potential for ensuring the provision of co-ordinated and comprehensive services, particularly for people with complex health and social care needs, such as chronically ill and disabled people. Furthermore, they are in a position to promote health in a wider sense, by engaging with other agencies to address the underlying social, environmental and economic factors that impact on the health of the population. This chapter explores the main policy developments in primary care over the past two decades and assesses their impact. It analyses the Conservative reforms of the 1980s and 1990s, and those of the Labour Government since 1997. Before this, however, there must be a further examination of the concept of primary care, which, as Peckham and Exworthy (2003) have noted, is vague and ambiguous.

What is Primary Care?

Broadly speaking, primary care is a philosophy that emphasises the movement of health care out of large institutions into community-based settings, bringing it closer to the people and making it more responsive to their needs. The World Health Organisation (WHO, 1978) defined primary health care in these terms, and set out a number of practical ways in which policy should develop, including the promotion of self-help, the integration of medical care with other social services, environmental improvements, the promotion of good health as well as good-quality health services, greater efforts to meet the needs of underprivileged and under-served groups in the community, and allowing greater community participation in the planning and delivery of health services.

The WHO also identified primary care as 'the first level of contact of individuals, the family and community with the national health system'. The concept of primary care as a 'level' in the management of illness can be traced back to the Dawson report (Cmd 693, 1920), which identified three levels of service: primary health centres, secondary health centres and teaching hospitals. This approach has also been taken by others, including Starfield (1998, pp. 8–9), who defined primary care as 'that level of a health service system that provides entry into the system for all new needs and problems, provides person-focused (not disease-oriented) care over time, provides for all but very uncommon or unusual conditions, and coordinates or integrates care provided elsewhere or by others'.

Alternatively, primary care has been defined in relation to specific services provided, such as health maintenance, prevention of illness, diagnosis and treatment, rehabilitation, pastoral care, and the certification of illness (Pritchard, 1978). It has also been defined with regard to the services provided by specific professional groups, such as GPs, dentists, pharmacists, opticians, district nurses, midwives, health visitors, chiropodists and speech therapists (see Boaden, 1997).

The various definitions of primary care reflect different ambitions about the possibility and desirability of changing the focus of health care. The more traditional definitions, particularly those rooted in notions of professional territory and specific services, contrast with more radical approaches that emphasise health promotion and community empowerment. Each definition is therefore underpinned by a different set of assumptions and values (Peckham and Exworthy, 2003).

The Conservatives' Reforms

According to Peckham and Exworthy (2003, p. 72), 'the 1980s witnessed a shift in health policy which increasingly placed attention on primary care'. There were several reasons for this. The Royal Commission on the NHS noted that, while the demand for primary care would increase during 1980s, improvements were needed in several areas, including interprofessional working and the education and training of GPs (Cmnd 7615, 1979). The Royal Commission was particularly concerned about the difficulties of meeting the health needs of declining urban areas, sentiments echoed by a report highlighting the poor state of primary care in inner London which was commissioned by the London Health Planning Consortium (Acheson, 1981). Although specific to London, the latter contained lessons for other inner-city areas with similar problems, such as high numbers of GPs working alone, poor-quality premises, high workloads and underdeveloped primary care teams.

In the early 1980s, the Thatcher Government realised that primary care reform could be used to promote wider changes in the NHS. It recognised the importance of the 'gate-keeper' role of the primary care services, in particular GPs, in regulating access to hospital and other services, and as a means of controlling costs and promoting efficiency throughout the NHS. At the same time, it was recognised that primary care expenditure was itself difficult to control and could jeopardise efforts to tackle the rising costs of the NHS. Spending patterns largely reflected the clinical decisions of general practitioners and were not subjected to the strict cash limits imposed elsewhere in the health service. Government feared that efforts to contain costs in the hospital sector would be offset by increased expenditure on primary care. Primary care was an area where management practices were poor and accountability weak. The Family Practitioner Committees (FPCs) – the NHS bodies in England and Wales which at the time were responsible for primary care provided by the independent contractor professions such as GPs, dentists and pharmacists – in reality had little leverage (Allsop and May, 1986). The story was similar in Scotland, though – in theory – a more integrated approach was possible here, as the health boards were responsible for hospital, community and primary health care services.

In short, primary care provided a challenge to a Government committed to improving the management of the NHS. It was also seen by the Thatcher Government as fertile ground for its market philosophy. GPs and other independent contractors were perceived as small businesses, competing for patients. There was already an element of choice in this field, albeit limited, and services were based on contracts, though these were nationally negotiated. These mechanisms, however, held considerable potential for the market zealots in Government and could be reformed to increase choice and competition and to provide greater incentives to meet particular needs and priorities. Finally, the Government saw primary care as an area where private payment and individual responsibility could be extended. It believed that charges in this field were less controversial than elsewhere in the NHS and that important precedents existed, in the form of fees for dental treatment and prescription charges. The Government also argued that, by extending and increasing charges, individuals would have a greater incentive to take responsibility for their health and would be deterred from using health services unnecessarily.

Promoting Better Health

In the Thatcher era, primary care reforms began in a piecemeal way with greater competition in the supply of spectacles, the introduction of a limited list of medicines available on NHS prescription (which meant that more medicines had to be paid for 'over the counter') and the raising of prescription charges substantially above the level of inflation. However, it was not until 1986 that comprehensive plans were outlined, in the form of a Green Paper on primary care (Cmnd 9771, 1986), which was based on several principles: the introduction of greater competition, more incentives, clearer accountability, stronger management, and increased charges.

This was followed by a White Paper, *Promoting Better Health* (Cm 249, 1987), which discarded some controversial measures, while retaining these essential principles. Even so, the White Paper was heavily criticised (Marks, 1988), one of the most contentious issues being the imposition of charges for sight tests and dental checks. Opponents of this measure argued that it would discourage attendance and inhibit the early detection of serious diseases such as glaucoma and oral cancer. The Government responded by extending exemptions from the charge. Following the introduction of the charge, the percentage of the population having annual eye and dental checks fell, but later increased, suggesting that the impact was short-term. Moreover, the overall number of sight tests was higher in 1998 compared with a decade earlier, before the charges were imposed. Even so, research by the Royal National Institute for the Blind suggested that the sight test had a different impact. Among people aged over 60, a larger proportion of people left longer intervals between tests, and those in the wealthiest groups were more likely to have regular tests (Grindey, 1997). Subsequently, in 1999, in response to pressure from blind people and older people's groups, the Blair Government reintroduced free sight tests for people over 60. In Wales, however, free sight tests were also extended to groups at high risk of developing eye diseases, while free dental checks were introduced for people aged over 60 and those under 25.

Promoting Better Health sought to extend the role of FPCs in the management of primary care, despite concerns that they were ill-equipped for this (Allsop and May, 1986). They acquired new financial powers, including discretionary funding for GP staff and premises. General managers were appointed to FPCs, which were later reconstituted as Family Health Service Authorities (FHSAs), run by smaller boards with fewer professional representatives. The FHSAs were given an important role in the monitoring of independent practitioners' contracts, service quality, and GP drug budgets. They also forged a closer relationship with the District Health Authorities, prompted by the internal market, which led to the establishment of joint commissioning and planning arrangements between the two bodies. Eventually, in the mid-1990s, FHSAs merged with DHAs to form single commissioning organisations, known simply as health authorities.

Changes to professional contracts were proposed. Negotiations over dentists' and GPs' contracts attracted most attention (see Exhibit 10.3 for discussion of NHS dentistry). With regard to GPs, Government wanted them to derive a greater proportion of their income from capitation fees – the payment received for each patient, irrespective of services provided. It was believed that this would create an incentive to attract and retain patients, and, by making it easier to change GPs, would create greater competition between practices. In the event, the proportion of GPs' income derived from capitation fees did not rise as much as originally intended. However, other financial incentives were also introduced, including payments to encourage GPs to undertake screening, immunisation, health checks, minor surgery, health promotion and child health surveillance (Moon and North, 2000).

The 1990 GP contract was imposed on the profession, though some conces-sions were made by Government, including new payments for GPs working in rural areas and the inner cities. But the broad thrust of the policy remained, amid complaints that it would add significantly to workload and reduce the effectiveness of the service. As Lewis (1998) noted, not all fears were realised and GPs' income actually increased following the introduction of the contract. Moreover, the overall picture in the 1990s was one of improving quality of serv-ice in primary care. More practices became computerised, employed practice managers, employed practice nurses, and provided disease-management pro-grammes for patients with chronic diseases, while immunisation and cervical-screening rates rose. However, inequalities persisted between different areas, with inner-city and some rural areas continuing to offer a lower quality of serv-ice (see Leese and Bosanquet, 1995a, 1995b).

However, GPs' workloads increased after 1990 (Leese and Bosanquet, 1995a). General practitioners expressed particular concerns about time spent on administration – which also resulted from other reforms, such as the *Patient's Charter* and GP fundholding. In 1996 the Major Government responded by reducing reporting requirements and simplifying the system of claiming fees and allowances. Another contentious issue was 'out-of-hours' services. The 1990 contract placed more emphasis on GP availability. This, cou-pled with a rise in requests for visits outside surgery hours, added to GPs' work-load. Following a protest by family doctors, which threatened the future of out-of-hours services, night-call fees were increased and new arrangements per-mitted greater flexibility in arranging out-of-hours cover. This issue was to resurface again in the context of negotiations surrounding a new GP contract a decade later, discussed later in this chapter.

GP Fundholding and Commissioning

Changes in the GP contract coincided with the internal market and the intro-duction of the fundholding scheme. By choosing fundholding, practices received a budget for commissioning a range of health care services from hos-pitals, later extended to include community health services. Each practice also received a budget for running costs and drugs, and were able to retain savings. Fundholding expanded during the 1990s. More treatments were covered by the scheme and the eligibility criteria were relaxed, enabling smaller practices to join. By the mid-1990s, about half of the population of England and Wales was covered by the scheme, with fundholding GPs purchasing around 20 per cent of their patients' health care by value. After a slower start, fundholding was also implemented in Scotland and in Northern Ireland. As discussed in Chapter 5, the scheme was credited with giving GPs greater flexibility to meet the needs and choices of their patients, improving efficiency, giving more leverage to GPs over the providers of hospital and community health services, and creating incentives for the development of improved and new services, such as outreach clinics. However, also noted in Chapter 5, the extent of these improvements was disputed. Moreover, GP fundholding was also criticised for undermining equity – with fundholders' patients benefiting at the expense of non-fundholders in terms of quicker access and better quality of service. Furthermore, it was believed that fundholders could undermine the commissioning plans of health authorities, and had little incentive to collaborate with other practices and community-based health services.

During the 1990s, commissioning evolved in various ways, some of which addressed the above concerns (IPPR, 1995a; Shapiro, 1994; Balogh, 1996). Groups of non-fundholding GPs, concerned about losing influence over services, began to advise health authorities on commissioning decisions. In some areas, these commissioning groups included both fundholding and non-fundholding GPs. Because fundholding did not cover all services and treatments, even fundholders had an incentive to engage with the health authorities which had wider responsibility for commissioning services. Increasingly, health authorities decentralised these arrangements by establishing locality commissioning groups. Meanwhile, some GPs began to form multifunds – where individual practices combined into a single management structure. These arrangements were particularly useful for smaller practices, eligible to join a new variant of the fundholding scheme called community fundholding.

The evidence on locality commissioning and GP commissioning (see Mulligan, 1998) was that, compared with fundholding, they had lower transaction costs (though estimates did not include some costs, such as time spent on negotiations). These schemes demonstrated service improvements, though to a lesser extent than fundholding. However, they appeared to have a greater scope for promoting equity. They were also believed to improve accountability to health authorities and contributed to some extent to peer accountability among GPs.

Efforts to bring together practices into a single management structure arose from experiments to extend fundholding to a much wider range of services. These schemes, known as total purchasing pilots (TPPs), were introduced in the mid-1990s. Some were based on single practices, while others attempted to bring together fundholders to engage in joint commissioning. Evaluations suggested that multi-practice projects in particular required considerable organisational resources in order to achieve their objectives (see Goodwin et al., 1998; Mays and Mulligan, 1998). This held important lessons for the Blair Government, which brought local practices into commissioning groups. Although the success of TPPs varied, the overall picture was positive. There were several examples of how schemes promoted improvements in services by encouraging better integration between primary care and other health and community care services (see Mays et al., 2001). Evaluations found that more was achieved in primary care – by extending the functions of the primary care team and developing intermediate care services – than in shaping secondary care through the contracting process.

By 1997, the Conservative Government's approach to primary care had changed considerably. The dogmatic approach of the Thatcher years had yielded to a more pragmatic approach, where various forms of commissioning were tried out. As a result, policy development became more incremental and less directive (Boaden, 1997). In the mid-1990s, a further review of primary care took place, based on wide consultation. This led to further policy statements (Cm 3390, 1996; Cm 3512, 1996) that emphasised the importance of diversity and experimentation in this field. Proposals included: allowing trusts (and others, including the private sector) to develop primary care services; new contracts that allowed non-medical practitioners to hold practice contracts and variations in the terms of general practitioners; salaried GPs; and unified budgets for general medical services, prescribing, and hospital and community health services. This led to the NHS (Primary Care) Act 1997, one of the last pieces of legislation enacted by the Major Government, which allowed health authorites to contract with NHS trusts, doctors and other NHS employees to provide primary care services.

The Blair Government

The Blair Government continued to emphasise the importance of primary care. Although it abolished GP fundholding, aspects of the internal market remained. The division between commissioners and providers was retained, but with stronger requirements to co-operate and participate in planning, a greater emphasis was placed on appropriate standards and the quality of care, and commissioning was based on longer-term service level agreements rather than short-term contracts. All these developments accentuated current trends already evident in the NHS.

In England, primary care groups (PCGs) were created, bringing together clusters of general practices within each health authority area. In Wales, local health groups (LHGs), similar to PCGs, were created to undertake the task of commissioning and to promote co-ordination across the health and social care system. Meanwhile, in Scotland, Local Health Care Cooperatives (LHCCs) brought together local practices on a voluntary basis, under the auspices of primary care trusts, which had overall responsibility for primary care and community health services, as well as some hospital services, within a particular area.

The PCGs varied considerably in terms of the population they covered. The average population size was supposed to be 100,000, but, in practice, the requirement that they encapsulate 'natural communities' meant considerable variation (Peckham and Exworthy, 2003, p. 151). Unlike fundholding, membership of PCGs was compulsory and therefore introduced collective responsibility above the practice level (Lewis, Malbon and Gillam, 2000), though there were few sanctions over individual practices.

PCGs were given several challenging tasks: to promote the health of the local population, to commission health services, to monitor the performance of service providers, to develop primary care, to integrate primary care and community health services, and to contribute to the health improvement programme so that it reflected patients' experiences and the perspective of the local community. Acknowledging the variation in local circumstances, the Government envisaged that PCGs would operate at one of four levels: level one PCGs would have an advisory role in the commissioning process; at level two, PCGs would have devolved responsibility for commissioning but would remain part of the health authority; level three PCGs would become primary care trusts (PCTs), free-standing bodies in their own right but still accountable to health authorities for commissioning care; level four PCGs would have the additional responsibility of providing community health services.

PCGs were promised unified budgets to commission services, to cover prescribing costs, hospital and community health services and general practice infrastructure (including practice staff, premises and computers). However, the non-cash limited element paid to GPs (see Chapter 7) was initially excluded – to avoid provoking them at a time when the Government needed their co-operation. Changes did occur later, however, following the introduction of new types of contract for general practitioners, discussed later in this chapter. PCGs were also promised budgets based on their population's share of resources, which, because this involved considerable reallocation of resources, was implemented gradually.

Central guidance was issued on the governance of PCGs, which created a leadership role for GPs. Subject to the agreement of local general practitioners, PCGs would be run by a board containing a majority of GPs and a chair drawn from their ranks. Nurses were also represented on the board, along with a lay member, a health authority representative and a social services nominee. These board members were all part-time appointees. In addition, each PCG appointed a general manager to take responsibility for the running of the organisation on a day-to-day basis.

It was expected that PCGs would evolve into PCTs. The first wave of PCTs, in 2000, was small, indicating local reluctance to move quickly to acquire this status. However, in the following year over a hundred were created. This increased enthusiasm resulted partly from a desire to achieve greater integration of primary and community services, but was also due to a recognition of the lack of management capacity and resources among existing PCGs (Wilkin, Gillam and Smith, 2001). Pressure from central government was also important. In the NHS Plan of 2000, despite earlier assurances to the contrary, the Government announced that all PCGs would move to PCTs by 2004, by which time it was envisaged that PCTs would control 75 per cent of the hospital and community health services budget.

The English PCTs differed from PCGs in several ways. As well as being statutory bodies in their own right, they covered larger populations, and were around twice the size of PCGs. In most cases, PCTs were formed out of mergers between erstwhile PCGs. The management structures of PCTs also differed from PCGs. PCTs are overseen by a trust board with a majority of non-executive appointees drawn from the local community. The board has a lay chair and also includes executive members such as the Chief Executive and Finance Director. Day-to-day management responsibility of the PCT is held by an executive committee. This body has a professional majority, and is usually chaired by a GP. Together with the Chief Executive, who is responsible for the management team, the lay chair and the executive-committee chair form a powerful triumvirate known as the 'three at the top' (Robinson and Exworthy, 2001).

Some PCT functions were similar to the PCGs they replaced: improving, and addressing inequalities in, the health of their community; developing primary and community health services, through improvements in the quality of care and better integration of services; commissioning secondary care services. But PCTs were given additional responsibilities: to provide community health and primary care services. Moreover, following the NHS Plan and the subsequent abolition of health authorities, more responsibilities were delegated to them, such as leading service planning and redesign, public health functions, and the oversight of primary care contractors, such as GPs. They were also given responsibility for the management, development and integration of all primary care services in their area, and it was expected that they would take responsibility for securing the provision of all health services in the future. In addition, PCTs were to receive their revenue allocations direct. Government also promised greater freedom in the commissioning of health care, though PCTs remained subject to central government's performance assessment framework.

As the English reforms began to evolve, important changes began to take place in primary care organisations in Scotland and Wales. In Wales, it was decided to abolish health authorities and devolve their commissioning functions to new local health boards (LHBs). These bodies were given responsibilities for planning and commissioning primary and secondary care for their populations. In one case, Powys LHB, the board took over responsibility for the services provided by the local NHS Trust, to create a more integrated body. In Scotland, meanwhile, there was concern that the front-line organisations in primary care, the LHCCs, needed stronger leadership and greater organisational resources. At the same time, the Scottish Executive was committed to abolishing both primary care trusts and acute trusts in order to create unified health systems under a single health board in each area. Consequently, it was decided to create new organisations, Community Health Partnerships, which would bring together local health service planners and providers in both primary and secondary care, along with local authorities and the voluntary sector, in an effort to improve the health of the local population and to improve the co-ordination and integration of services.

The Impact of PCGs and PCTs

Health improvement

In England, PCGs and PCTs were given a key role in improving the health of their local communities (DoH, 1998a). PCG/Ts were charged with initiating a process of assessing and targeting local health needs (see Exhibit 10.1), alongside a requirement to establish primary care plans, while contributing to the health improvement programme (and subsequently the health improvement and modernisation plan) of the relevant health authority (see Chapter 7).

As Regen et al. (2001) found, health improvement became a higher priority for PCGs and PCTs as they moved beyond the early phase of their development. A majority of PCGs and PCTs actually developed their own action plan on health improvement. Most health improvement activities were focused on health care, though some primary care organisations pursued activities with a wider public health agenda. PCG/Ts also reported closer working relationships with other agencies, such as local authorities and some became involved in Health Action Zones (see Exhibit 10.2). These findings were echoed by the national tracker survey of PCG/Ts (Wilkin et al., 2002), which found that PCG/Ts had made significant progress in establishing an infrastructure for health improvement. Almost two-thirds of PCG/Ts had a health improvement subgroup, with nine out of ten having a designated health improvement lead. The vast majority of PCG/Ts had allocated resources to wider public health initiatives aimed at improving health, such as accident-prevention schemes, leisure, exercise or recreation programmes, and community development projects (Wilkin, Gillam and Toleman, 2001). On the negative side, research findings identified variable levels of involvement in health improvement activities, with some PCG/Ts having less involvement in, and less influence over, the local health improvement programme (Regen et al., 2001). Staff shortages in key areas, such as public health, also proved a hindrance (Gillam, Abbott and Banks-Smith, 2001). Despite the apparent enthusiasm shown for health improvement and interagency working by these new organisations, concern was expressed about their capacity to undertake this new role, about their relationships with local government and primary care practitioners (Meads et al., 1999), and about the relatively low importance of health improvement compared with other PCG/T functions such as primary care development and commissioning (Health Committee, 2001a).

As noted earlier, following the abolition of health authorities in England, PCTs acquired a much more substantial public health function. In order to fulfil this, they appointed public health directors and teams. Expanding capacity was necessary, for many primary care organisations were already stretched.

Nonetheless, some PCTs faced difficulties making these appointments (Moore, 2003b), leading to concerns that public health skills and expertise was fragmenting as a result of the reorganisation. Doubt was cast, therefore, on the ability of PCTs to achieve public health objectives and articulate the commissioning of services to the health needs of their populations (see also CHI, 2004). However, the picture was mixed. Researchers found strong commitment to health improvement among some PCTs, with the most successful having common characteristics, including strong support and leadership at senior levels of the organisation, a corporate recognition of local socio-economic inequalities, and the availability of development funding (Abbott et al., 2001).

Scottish and Welsh primary care organisations faced similar challenges to improve the health of their populations. In Wales, the Local Health Groups were expected to contribute to improved health, both through commissioning and by strengthening working relationships with local government and the voluntary sector. Subsequently, as mentioned earlier, new Local Health Boards were created, and these were given a more explicit public health role. Meanwhile, in Scotland, health boards, PCTs and LHCCs – as well as local government – all had a role in relation to health improvement. However, dissatisfaction with the fragmentation of these responsibilities was one reason why a new regime of community health partnerships, focusing specifically on health improvement and integrated services, was proposed.

Commissioning

The commissioning of secondary care was slow to develop following the creation of PCG/Ts (Regen et al., 2001; Baxter et al., 2002). This was particularly the case in Wales, where the LHG commissioning role was less well-developed (Audit Commission, 2000a). In Scotland, where a more integrated approach was pursued, the LHCCs and PCTs did not have the same commissioning role as their counterparts in England and Wales.

Although almost all English PCG/Ts were engaged in commissioning acute services, with a smaller majority commissioning accident and emergency and mental health services (Wilkin et al., 2002), they appeared to exert little leverage over NHS providers of hospital services. Only 17 per cent held long-term service agreements with providers, and very few had taken advantage of the commissioning process to change providers (Wilkin et al., 2002). However, more progress was evident in achieving change through the commissioning of community services and services at the primary and secondary care interface, according to Regen et al. (2001).

Commissioning was identified by Government as the key to meeting needs (see Exhibit 10.1) and improving services. As PCTs acquire control over the majority of the NHS budget, more responsive secondary services, integrated with primary and community services, are likely to emerge (NHS Alliance,

2003). That one-third of PCG/Ts have developed integrated care pathways for coronary heart disease (Wilkin et al., 2002) is perhaps an indication that PCT commissioning has encouraged integration (see also Audit Commission, 2004a). However, achieving integration across the whole range of patient care is very difficult. As Edwards (2000) pointed out, the transfer of resources from

---

Exhibit 10.1 Health Needs Assessment

Health-needs assessment is the systematic assessment of the health needs of the public, or of a particular section of it. It may be undertaken to improve the planning of services, to ensure that resources are allocated in such a way as to maximise benefit, to respond more effectively to the needs of the public, or to identify 'hidden' needs. It may also be undertaken as a means of legitimising decisions, building 'shared ownership' of problems (if assessments are undertaken with other agencies), or to get issues on to the agenda for action (Hensher and Fulop, 1999).

Interest in health-needs assessment was raised by the introduction of commissioning in the 1990s, coupled with other factors, such as the imperative to improve the cost-effectiveness of health care, and the rise of consumerism (Wright, Williams and Wilkinson, 1998). Commissioners were expected to identify health needs, to inform decisions about contracts and the allocation of resources. In reality, this did not happen to the extent envisaged, largely because of the principal focus on the contracting process itself, the lack of data on health needs, limited efforts to engage with patients and the public, and disagreements over which particular method of assessment to adopt.

There are many different approaches to health-needs assessment (Wright, Williams and Wilkinson, 1998; Foreman, 1996). The two main approaches are *population-based*, which examines the needs of populations, and *individual*, which focuses on the needs of service users (Stevens and Gillam, 1998). There are also different methodologies: those that emphasise clinical data on illness and service utilisation, and qualitative approaches that rely more on measures of underlying socio-economic status and people's experiences of illness and services. In the past these have been seen as in competition with each other, largely because they represent different perspectives on health and illness. However, some may be more appropriate to certain circumstances than others (see Stevens and Gillam, 1998). In practice, health needs assessments may be eclectic, drawing on multiple methods and sources of data.

Since the late 1990s, health-needs assessments seem to have increased (Gillam, Abbott, and Banks-Smith, 2001). This followed clearer guidance to health authorities on health improvement, and the identification of a key role in needs assessment for PCGs and PCTs. Health-needs assessment is also linked with other agendas, such as improving access and tackling inequalities. It is relevant to patient and public involvement, which is seen as an important channel for communicating needs and preferences. Furthermore, health-needs assessment is linked to initiatives to improve joint working between the NHS and other agencies, such as the voluntary sector and local government. Increasingly, health bodies seek to identify and assess needs in partnership with these bodies. However, problems remain. Health-needs assessments can be costly and yet may be sidelined in the decision-making process (Hensher and Fulop, 1999). There are concerns about the information base on which assessments are made, and agreement that improvements in IT are needed in this area (Godden and Pollock, 2000). Moreover, there are problems in accessing and sharing data, because of different information systems and confidentiality requirements.

Exhibit 10.2 Health Action Zones

Health Action Zones (HAZs) were established in 1998 to improve interagency collaboration in health and health care in areas with high levels of deprivation and poor health (Powell and Moon, 2001; Matka, Barnes and Sullivan, 2002). They have three aims: to identify and address the health needs of the area; to improve services, making them more responsive to needs; and to develop partnerships between various agencies at local level. HAZ projects were expected to focus on where needs were greatest and given a brief to reduce health inequalities. They were expected to plan services on the basis of need, promoting integrated services, and reorganising primary, hospital and community care accordingly. They were also required to promote public health, as well as improve health care, by empowering people, building on existing community strengths, and focusing on improvements in wellbeing and quality of life.

There was much variation in the approach taken by different HAZs. By 1999, following two competitive rounds, 26 Health Action Zones were created in England, covering 13 million people. Specific HAZ projects included: the provision of integrated services to specific client groups such as elderly people, teenage mothers, people with mental health problems, people with learning disabilities, and ethnic minorities; improved access to primary and community services; and health promotion projects, such as smoking cessation.

Because of differences between HAZ schemes, as well as their coexistence with other initiatives in primary care discussed in this chapter, comprehensive evaluation is difficult. An interim evaluation found that HAZs adopted various strategies (Matka, Barnes and Sullivan, 2002): a consolidation strategy, where there had been an attempt to take stock of progress and consolidate on this; a mainstreaming strategy, where the HAZ had been used to secure change within mainstream organisations; an emergent strategy, where a more eclectic approach was taken to try out different approaches to health improvement and health inequalities; finally, an innovation strategy, where a wide range of new projects had been introduced to challenge existing ways of service provision and decision-making. The study found that the partnership capacity of HAZs was shaped by: perceptions about the legitimacy of the HAZ, the nature of power relationships within the HAZ, the capacity of the partners to contribute to the HAZ, the extent to which the HAZ was seen as a free-standing body, and the development of wider collaborative relationships among the partners. The study also found some evidence of positive change promoted by HAZ, including specific initiatives prioritising particular groups or issues, changes in working relationships between different agencies, impact on other regeneration initiatives, and shaping mainstream services and policies.

There were concerns that HAZs would suffer the same fate of earlier efforts to promote area-based interventions, which were short-term and raised unrealistic expectations (though some believed that important lessons had been learned from earlier schemes – see Powell and Moon, 2001). There was also considerable overlap between other current area-based schemes such as Education and Employment Action Zones (Crawshaw, Bunton and Killen, 2003), with some areas having all three. The Government subsequently sought to improve co-ordination between such schemes by promoting the creation of local strategic partnerships between the NHS, local government and other agencies. Other criticisms related to the community-development aspects of HAZs, including varying degrees of satisfaction with the extent of community involvement in HAZ Plans and problems of capacity, as well as recognition of the burden which community involvement placed on local communities (Matka, Barnes and Sullivan, 2002; Crawshaw, Bunton and Killen, 2003).

Although funding was agreed until 2005/6, the future of HAZs was in some doubt following a decision to integrate them within PCTs. Although now subject to PCTs' decisions about resources and priorities, the Department of Health stated that HAZ aims, particularly with regard to tackling health inequalities, would be continued.

secondary to primary care is problematic, largely because of the high fixed costs of hospital care and the associated difficulties of realising financial savings from new patterns of service provision, particularly in the short term. One way forward is to strengthen collaboration between GPs and consultants, particularly on service design (Edwards, 2000), which could be achieved by aligning the commissioning processes more closely with clinical networks (James, Dixon and Sonanja, 2002).

The situation has been complicated further by shifts in policy following the NHS Plan. The Government made it clear that, in the context of stronger market incentives, it wanted PCTs to exercise greater discretion in commissioning care from a variety of providers, based on twin considerations of value for money and high clinical standards (DoH, 2002q). However, doubts have been expressed about the ability of PCTs to undertake such a role (Lewis, Dixon and Gillam, 2003a; Rowe and Bond, 2003; see also CHI, 2004), particularly in the light of foundation trusts (see Exhibit 7.6). The granting of foundation status for hospitals seems likely to weaken PCTs. If foundation trusts acquire greater autonomy and legitimacy, PCTs might find it even more difficult to influence the pattern and range of services provided. However, much will depend on the actual autonomy and perceived legitimacy of the foundation trusts, and whether PCTs acquire similar status in due course.

Primary care development and clinical governance

Research indicated that PCGs and PCTs had undertaken a range of activities aimed at developing and improving primary care (Regen et al., 2001). This included efforts to improve practice infrastructure, such as premises and information technology, though IT remained problematic, both according to this study and the national tracker survey (Wilkin et al., 2002). Nonetheless, many primary care organisations made advances in developing services in the late 1990s (Regen et al., 2001). Wilkin et al. (2002) found that almost all PCG/Ts had introduced incentives to encourage improvements. They also commented positively on the expansion of specialist services, including counselling, specialist nursing, minor surgery, specialist GPs, and specialist outreach clinics, as well as efforts to promote shared resources between practices.

PCGs and PCTs did not necessarily operate in isolation when seeking to improve primary care services. Indeed, several initiatives were established to enable primary care organisations to learn from each other and to encourage them to employ best practice. The NHS Beacons initiative (see Exhibit 9.1) was applied to primary care, and examples of good practice identified in areas such as patient-held records, the use of health care assistants in general practice, and establishing specialist clinics. In England, a primary care development team was established in 2000 (later subsumed into the NHS Modernisation Agency) to support service improvements. This led to the introduction of the national primary care collaborative later that year. As noted in Chapter 9, the collaborative approach involves the gathering of best practice, and its dissemination and adoption. In primary care, this has involved an exploration of how services can be improved in three areas: access to primary care; access to routine secondary care services by developing primary care services; and, more specifically, care for patients with coronary heart disease. Across these areas, efforts have been geared to improving access, reducing unnecessary delays in order to ensure patients get appropriate and timely treatment, and implementing systematic changes in the ways in which patients are seen, diagnosed, referred and treated.

Improving access became a key area of activity for primary care organisations during the late 1990s (Regen et al., 2001; Wilkin et al., 2002). Examples of schemes undertaken by PCGs and PCTs included extended surgery hours, reduced waiting times, and targeting poorly-served areas or groups. In so doing, primary care organisations drew on new initiatives (such as Walk-in Centres – see below) and recent legislation, in particular the 1997 Primary Care Act, which enabled them to establish primary medical services schemes. According to the national tracker survey (Wilkin et al., 2002), over four-fifths of PCG/Ts had such schemes in operation by 2002. The importance of access was maintained by the NHS Plan, which set targets for access to primary as well as secondary care (see Chapter 8). By 2004, patients could expect to see a primary care professional within 24 hours, or a GP within 48 hours. By March 2004, 97 per cent of people saw a GP within 48 hours, and 98 per cent saw a primary care professional within 24 hours, according to official figures. Meanwhile, primary care was seen as the key to improving waiting times in secondary care. Booked appointments, where the patient can be given an outpatient appointment by his or her GP, were identified as a key priority. In 1998, the national booked-admissions programme was launched. Subsequently, the NHS Plan for England announced that by 2005 all consultant appointments and elective admissions would be pre-booked.

Clinical governance was an important requirement, and PCG/Ts became engaged in a range of efforts to improve quality and standards of practice. Along with primary care development, organisations identified clinical governance as the means through which they could engage GPs and their staff (Regen et al., 2001). The national tracker survey also found significant achievements in clinical governance, with more than two-thirds of PCG/Ts implementing clinical guidelines across all practices (Wilkin, Gillam and Toleman, 2001). This study also found that four-fifths of primary care organisations were sharing information between practices on quality issues. On the negative side, 42 per cent of PCG/Ts were found not to have dedicated budgets for clinical governance, and just under a third had little or no professional support for this function.

Clinical governance was most evident in areas covered by the national service frameworks (Wilkin et al., 2002). Indeed, NSFs appeared to have a major impact on priorities, with almost nine out of ten PCG/Ts stating that heart disease was a priority. However, less than half identified other NSF areas, such as older people and mental health, as a priority. Priorities were determined through a combination of central government targets and local needs, though the former weighed particularly heavily following the NHS Plan and the subsequent introduction of 'star ratings' for PCTs, beginning in 2003. Indeed, in the 2002 tracker survey, 90 per cent of PCG board and PCT executive committee chairs stated that they wanted to focus more on local health needs and service development (Wilkin et al., 2002).

Prescribing was another key area of activity for PCGs and PCTs (Regen et al., 2001), and continued to be so as PCG/Ts acquired greater responsibility for this area (Wilkin et al., 2002). Three-quarters of PCG/Ts were using guidelines for prescribing and all had dedicated posts for supporting improvements in prescribing. According to the Audit Commission (2003d), the cost of drugs prescribed by family doctors increased by almost a third between 1998/9 and 2001/2. It urged PCTs to continue to explore ways of containing rising costs, including the development of clear strategies, explicit links with clinical governance and commissioning plans, clearer incentives for practices to improve the cost-effectiveness of prescribing, and the development of clear treatment protocols incorporating best practice and backed by training and support. The report also backed the appointment of GPs with a clear remit to improve prescribing among colleagues, coupled with the sharing of comparative data on prescribing between practices.

The requirement that PCTs must now comply with NICE guidance places them in a position where they have to take a more explicit approach on cost-effectiveness and rationing. This will apply not only to drugs, but to other interventions considered by NICE. Increasingly, PCTs will have to take a line on the availability of treatments, particularly in individual 'high-cost' cases, either by strengthening local guidelines or by restricting access to certain treatments through the commissioning process. It appears that PCTs are at a very early stage in developing such strategies and, equally important, communicating them (Austin, 2002).

Capacity, internal management and governance

Most PCG/Ts believed they had inadequate resources with which to manage change (Wilkin, Gillam and Smith, 2001; Regen et al., 2001). As noted earlier, many organisations merged prior to becoming PCTs to increase their managerial resources. On average, English PCTs have three times as many staff as PCGs (Wilkin et al., 2002). However, PCTs have more onerous responsibilities than the bodies they replaced, particularly since they acquired functions from the abolished health authorities. Their management costs are low relative to this workload (Wilkin, Gillam and Smith, 2001), and management capacity has been acknowledged as a major problem, with many PCTs identifying lack of capacity to undertake basic administration tasks (Higgins, 2001b). It has also been found that their leadership capacity is stretched because of difficulties filling senior posts and the extensive roles of senior staff (CHI, 2004). On the other hand, an assumption behind the creation of PCTs has been that they can cater more efficiently for a larger population because of economies of scale. This has been scotched by research, which found that increases in population size covered by organisations neither produced economies nor improved performance (Bojke, Gravelle and Wilkin, 2001). It appears that optimal size varies for different functions of primary care organisations. Bigger is not necessarily better, though it may be possible to achieve optimal sizes by devolving certain functions within the larger organisations, while pooling others for smaller organisations.

PCGs and PCTs had different governance arrangements. The key locus of power in the PCG was the chair/chief executive pairing (Regen et al., 2001). There is little to suggest that PCG boards were anything more than monitoring and ratification bodies. Unsurprisingly, the in-built GP majority on PCG boards (including, in most cases, the chair) raised concerns about their dominance of both agenda and proceedings (Regen et al., 2001). Public involvement in meetings was minimal, though many PCGs made considerable effort to consult with the public in other ways, discussed further in Chapter 12. There is less evidence regarding PCTs, which are larger and more complex organisations. However, as noted earlier, the key locus of power here is the triumvirate of chief executive, lay chair and executive committee chair. There are also two different committees (the board and the executive committee), between which tensions have been found (Regen et al., 2001).

Collaboration with other agencies

The history of collaboration between primary care and social care agencies has been problematic (see also Chapter 11). Along with Health Action Zones (see Exhibit 10.2), PCGs and PCTs were introduced in order to improve joint working. Early findings were optimistic, as PCGs established a range of contacts with local authority departments, the social services representative on PCG boards playing an active role (Glendinning, Abbott and Coleman, 2001). In general, relationships between the NHS and local government improved in the period following the introduction of PCGs, with a positive impact on collaboration (Banks, 2002; Local Government Association, 2000). However, it was believed that early gains could be limited by traditional professional inequalities between medicine and social work (Moon and North, 2000; Glendinning, Abbott and Coleman, 2001). In addition, the organisational upheaval caused by the shift from PCGs to PCTs was identified as a key factor in disrupting good relations with local government (Banks, 2002; Local Government Association, 2000; Glendinning, Abbott and Coleman, 2001). Other researchers found that partnership working was concentrated at the strategic level, though joint working on operational matters was increasing (Regen et al., 2001). Meanwhile, it was apparent that the impact of social services representatives on PCG/T boards depended largely on the seniority of their nominee and their commitment to joint working (Hudson et al., 1999; Glendinning, Abbott and Coleman, 2001). The presence of social services representatives was, on its own, a limited mechanism for collaboration. Compared to other participants, they had limited influence over PCG/Ts decisions (Glendinning, Abbot and Coleman, 2001). Indeed, some observers argue that PCTs record on partnership has been poor, largely because partnership has not been a major priority and because of boundary differences (Hudson, 2002).

Even so, subsequent research found that PCG/Ts were involved in partnerships at both strategic and operational levels (Wilkin et al., 2002). Almost three-quarters had appointed staff to develop partnerships with local authorities. Efforts to improve intermediate care (see Chapter 11) had been a major impetus to the joint appointment of staff to co-ordinate services. Two-thirds of PCG/Ts were involved in the joint provision of intermediate care along with social services. Almost nine out of ten PCG/Ts had undertaken joint staff training with local authorities and a similar proportion had participated in reorganisation of NHS and local authority staff to improve collaboration. PCG/Ts were working with a wider range of departments, not just social services. All had working relationships with community development and regeneration departments, and over three-quarters reported links with leisure services, housing and education departments. But problems were still reported, particularly from social services representatives on the PCG/Ts. One in seven claimed that there was no routine liaison with local authorities about PCG/T matters. Half mentioned the continuing problems caused by boundary differences, while a similar proportion stated that they had faced problems in trying to improve collaboration.

Efforts to improve collaboration were evident in other parts of the UK. The Welsh local health groups had greater voluntary and local government representation, and were aligned with local authority boundaries. The Audit Commission (2000a) noted that these organisations had prioritised collaborative relationships. Their successor bodies, the Local Health Boards, were also expected to play a strong collaborative role with partners in the voluntary sector and local government. Even so, it was evident that stronger alliances were needed between social services departments and the NHS (Audit Commission, 2002d). Meanwhile, in Scotland, as already noted, continuing problems with joint working led to a proposal to establish community health partnerships as a means of improving collaboration and producing more integrated services. Collaboration was an important theme in both Scottish and Welsh health service reform plans.

Meanwhile, in England, collaboration was a key theme of the NHS Plan, with the role of PCTs in co-ordinating the health and social care system strongly emphasised. According to some observers, these are now in a key position to influence service redesign in this field (Audit Commission, 2002e). Care trusts were heralded as a means of integrating health and social care. These multipurpose bodies would commission and be responsible for all local health and social care for particular groups, such as the elderly and mentally ill people (see Chapter 11). The NHS Plan promised an expansion in intermediate care services for older people to prevent unnecessary admissions to hospital, delayed discharges and 'bed-blocking', including schemes to provide health and social care in people's own homes, in nursing homes, or in residential homes, as well as specialist rehabilitation and recuperation facilities (see Chapter 11).

Existing powers under the Health Act 1999, which enabled the pooling of budgets, transfer of responsibilities for commissioning services and integrated provision between health and local government bodies, were endorsed by the NHS Plan, which suggested that they would become a requirement in areas where they had not hitherto been used. Incentive payments were proposed for demonstrated improvements in joint working, and a new joint inspection system for health and social care organisations. The implementation and impact of these policies are discussed further in the next chapter.

Other Key Developments in Primary Care

The introduction of PCG/Ts was undoubtedly an important development. However, this reorganisation was only one of several policy initiatives affecting primary care. To focus solely upon it would be misleading, so in the remainder of this chapter attention is given to these other reforms.

NHS Walk-in Centres

In England, Walk-in Centres have been introduced as a means of improving access to primary care. Based in the high street and in shopping centres, and in or near railway stations, bus stations and airports, they offer quick access to services, including assessment, treatment for minor injuries, and advice and information. No appointment is necessary and the centres are open outside normal surgery hours. The service is led and staffed by nurses working within protocols. Where appropriate, the centres refer patients to other services, including general practice, social services, and accident and emergency (see Patten and Brandreth, 2001).

Walk-in Centres were criticised for several reasons. It was suggested that some failed to assess patients properly (Edwards, 2001). Another criticism was that such centres undermine general practice, disrupting the continuity of care and the gate-keeper role of GPs (Chapple et al., 2000). This raises the prospect of higher costs, as referrals increase and services are duplicated (Mountford and Rosen, 2001). Evidence from Canada, which has had doctor-led Walk-in Centres for over 20 years, indicated a lack of continuity between Walk-in Centres and general practice (Jones, 2000). Despite these concerns, there is evidence that Walk-in Centres provide good-quality care, and perform safely and adequately (Grant et al., 2002). Referral rates are higher than general practice, but lower than for NHS Direct (see below).

NHS Direct

The NHS Direct service is a nurse-provided health care information and advisory service. It was introduced in England and Wales in 1998, initially as a telephone service and was later extended to the Internet, as NHS Direct Online. There have also been experiments with access via digital television. Scotland has its own system – NHS 24 – launched in 2002. NHS 24 was established as a Special Health Board within NHS Scotland, and at the outset is seeking to integrate with other parts of the NHS such as out-of-hours services, A and E departments and the ambulance service (NHS 24, 2002).

NHS Direct is heavily used, with around 6 million calls in 2002. The most commons symptoms people reported are fever, vomiting, rash, cough and diarrhoea. User-satisfaction is high, with over 90 per cent expressing satisfaction with the service (O'Cathain et al., 2000; NAO, 2002c). The service offered has been adjudged as good-quality overall, with few adverse events (CHI, 2003c). However, the consistency of advice has been criticised by some researchers (S. Williams, 2000) and there have been concerns about the ability of the service to deal with rare conditions. Call waiting times have been a problem, with one in five patients waiting more than 30 minutes to speak to a nurse (NAO, 2002c). There has been criticism that the service does not represent a good use of resources, costing £80 million a year in 2002. At around £18 per consultation, it is more expensive than the average cost (£14) of a GP consultation (*Hansard*, 2002). In general, it does not appear to reduce demand for health services (Munro et al., 2000), and fears have been expressed that it may simply encourage the 'worried well' to clog the health system, as they are referred on to GPs and to Accident and Emergency Services. Even so, NHS Direct may encourage more appropriate use of other services by reducing demand on them, may offset costs by encouraging more appropriate use of NHS services, and may add value by reassuring patients and reducing their anxiety (NAO, 2002c).

NHS Direct is accessed more by those sections of the population who generally enjoy better health (NAO, 2002c). Those groups that have the greatest health needs – some ethnic minorities, disadvantaged groups, people with learning disabilities and elderly people – make least use of the service. This may be exaggerated further by the Internet-based service, as poorer and elderly people are less likely to be online. However, this is offset to some extent by the establishment of NHS Direct information kiosks in public places, such as libraries and supermarkets.

By 2004, NHS Direct is due to be integrated with out-of-hours care, providing a single point of access. There are plans to integrate the service with ambulance services, taking over the management of 'low priority' 999 calls. The service is also expected to become more closely linked with pharmacy services' and dental practitioners' out-of-hours services. All these developments may encourage more appropriate use of services. The use of telephone and Internet-based services may have wider uses. In 2003, a pilot scheme enabled people to report adverse drug reactions, raising the possibility of using the service to identify adverse events and monitor the quality of care. Pilot schemes have been used to monitor people with chronic conditions in their own homes and alert a response from emergency and other services when required. Other schemes have involved NHS Direct in reminding patients about out-patient appointments, carrying out telephone assessments of patients prior to surgery, and checking patient transport arrangements (NAO, 2002c).

Personal Medical Services

As already mentioned, the Blair Government drew on legislation introduced by its predecessor to allow experimentation in the provision of primary care services in England. The Primary Care Act pilots, later renamed personal medical services (PMS) pilots, permitted practices, trusts and other NHS bodies to provide services in an area renowned for contractual inflexibility. Normal contractual arrangements between the NHS and primary care providers could therefore be replaced by new forms of service provision, such as nurse-led practices, salaried GPs, and special primary care centres.

The PMS pilots varied considerably in character (Lewis and Gillam, 1999) and were introduced in several phases – 83 sites participated in the first wave. By 2002, one in three GPs in England worked under a PMS contract and 1700 schemes were operational. The vast majority of schemes were in England, though PMS pilots were adopted in Scotland, but not in Wales or Northern Ireland. The NHS plan envisaged that the majority of GPs would operate under PMS contracts by 2004. At the same time the Government sought to alter the standard general medical services (GMS) contract, to place greater emphasis on quality of service, needs and outcomes. Having broken 'the monopoly of the independently contracted general practitioner' (Lewis and Gillam, 2002), the PMS created pressures to alter the GMS contract along similar lines.

Initially, take-up of PMS schemes varied widely, some areas having very low coverage (Audit Commission, 2003e). Two types of pilot scheme were identified: 'PMS' pilots which provided a broad range of general medical services under a cash-limited and locally specified contract, and 'PMS plus' pilots, which included both non-GMS services (for example, community nursing) and GMS services in a single contract (Jenkins, 1999).

The variation in the scope and coverage of the schemes, coupled with the introduction of PCTs and other reforms, made evaluation difficult (Audit Commission, 2003e; PMS National Evaluation Team, 2002; Sheaff and Lloyd-Kendall, 2000; Huntington et al., 2000; Lewis and Gillam, 1999). However, the main benefits of the schemes included increased recruitment of GPs to deprived and under-served areas, and improved services for disadvantaged groups. Meanwhile, salaried status for GPs was associated with greater productivity, increased job satisfaction and no apparent fall in the quality of service. The scheme also extended the role of nurses in providing clinics for particular client groups, triage and treating minor illness. In some schemes – the nurse-led PMS pilots – nurses developed important leadership and management roles (Lewis, 2001a; Jones, 1999; Roe, Walsh and Huntington, 2000; see also below).

There was apparently little difference in the quality of care offered by the pilots and by GMS services (Lewis and Gillam, 2002). Furthermore, PMS schemes were not as radical as some believed. Sheaff and Lloyd-Kendall (2000), in an analysis of first-wave pilots, found that contracts failed to link incentives with objectives, and that performance monitoring was diverse and underdeveloped. A tendency to relabel previous arrangements was also observed, with most first-wave PMS contracts differing little from their GMS predecessors (Lewis and Gillam, 1999). The level of experimentation with new services may have been exaggerated. Huntington et al. (2000) questioned whether the PMS providers were fully using their freedoms and flexibility, though acknowledged that in many cases change and innovation was stimulated by PMS pilots. Subsequently, guidance was produced by the Department of Health to encourage greater use of the flexibilities allowed by the PMS scheme. A national contractual framework was issued for later 'waves' of the scheme to ensure greater consistency in monitoring, performance management and accountability, while requiring a stronger focus on standards and quality of service (DoH, 2002k). Moreover, a PMS National Development Team was established to support the scheme, providing advice and ensuring appropriate facilitator networks and peer support. Nonetheless, the Audit Commission (2003e) continued to find poor performance management among many commissioners of PMS, and recommended investment in appropriate management capacity and expertise.

Premises and Finance

The NHS Plan announced a programme to improve primary health care premises. Under a scheme called LIFT (Local Improvement Finance Trust), a form of private finance initiative, it was expected that up to £1 billion would be invested in primary care facilities. This would involve refurbishment and replacement of existing premises, as well as the building of new 'one-stop' primary care centres – 500 promised by 2004. The idea of health centres was not of course new, and dated back to the Dawson Report, mentioned earlier. There was also a significant expansion of health centres in the late 60s and early 70s. Nonetheless, the NHS Plan represented a significant new commitment to bringing services under one roof, in some cases alongside other services such as benefits and housing advice, health promotion and social services. Some innovative centres have already been established by a combination of agencies, usually in the most deprived areas. In such cases, PCTs, local government, regeneration agencies and voluntary organisations have worked together to create integrated services and facilities for populations with high and complex needs. In some cases, centres have been created as part of the Government's Healthy Living Centre initiative, funded from the National Lottery. These programmes, which vary in design according to local need and circumstances, seek to bring health and social services together with a selection of other community services, such as crèches, counselling, youth services, fitness schemes, and even cafés and children's play areas, though not necessarily in the same building.

There is wide agreement that NHS primary care facilities are currently less than adequate. Primary care infrastructure has developed in a haphazard way, reflecting the 'small business ethos' of the sector. Modern joined-up services involving professionals and workers from a variety of backgrounds and agencies will find it difficult to flourish in accommodation – often a converted house or shop – that was not designed for the purpose. On the negative side, the Government's chosen vehicle – LIFT – has been criticised, largely for similar reasons as PFI in the hospital sector. It is argued that it is a means by which private investors will profit at the expense of tax-payers and service users. In fact, the increased dependence on private loans began much earlier, following the privatisation of the state body that provided loans to GPs (the GP Finance Corporation) in the late 1980s. In addition to worries about profiteering, there have been criticisms of the bureaucracy involved in LIFT schemes and the delays this entails. With regard to this, it is true that projects have initially been slow to get off the ground. There is little evidence that such schemes will in the long run be any more cost-effective than those funded wholly out of public resources (see Kings Fund/NHS Alliance, 2001; Godden, Pollock and Player, 2001).

The Primary Care Professions

One of the long-standing problems of primary care has been poor interprofessional relations and a lack of effective teamwork. Reforms of the 1980s and 1990s sought to resolve these problems by reinforcing GP dominance within primary care (Boaden, 1997). There were several elements at work. GPs had incentives to employ nurses in their practices, and the number of practice nurses in England doubled between 1990 and 1994. GP fundholding – and also, to some extent, GP commissioning – strengthened the leverage of GPs over the work of community nurses employed by the trusts (Sibbald, 2000; Williams, A., 2000). This enabled GPs to change the skill mix, to the detriment of health visitors and, to some extent, community nurses, who became concerned about encroachment from practice nurses (McDonald, Langford and Boldero, 1997; Williams, A., 2000). Finally, the creation of PCGs (and subsequently PCTs) reinforced the dominance of GPs by giving them stronger representation relative to other professions (Regen et al., 2001).

Nurses

Primary care nurses have often expressed frustration that their skills are not being fully deployed. In 1986 the Cumberlege report on neighbourhood nursing (DHSS, 1986) had offered the prospect of an enhanced role for such nurses. It argued for a more equal relationship between GPs and community-based nurses. Its main recommendation, which included the reorganisation of all community nurses into local units or 'neighbourhoods', managed by a nurse and planning services on the basis of needs, was not endorsed by Government. However, many health authorities, and subsequently the community trusts, began to reorganise their community nursing services along these lines (Martin, 1992; White, Leach and Christensen, 1996). Furthermore, although the report's immediate impact on policy was small, many of its recommendations – including its support for nurse practitioners and nurse-led clinics – have been implemented in other ways (through PMS pilots, for example). Moreover, another of its key recommendations, nurse prescribing, was introduced and has since been extended.

The number of nurses in primary care grew during the 1980s and 1990s, and their range of tasks expanded. For example, practice nurses took on delegated tasks from GPs, such as chronic-disease management and health promotion (Broadbent, 1998). Community nurses took on greater responsibility for the management of elderly and chronically ill patients in community settings, who in previous times would have remained in hospital (McDonald, Langford and Boldero, 1997). As noted earlier, PMS pilots enabled nurses to extend their role as practitioners, and in some cases they became involved in leadership and management roles. Other reforms, such as NHS Direct and Walk-in Centres were also based on enhancing the role of nurses as the first point of contact with patients, while the growth of nurse practitioners and nurse-prescribing, potentially at least, gave nurses a larger role in the management of patient care. There was also evidence that an extended role for nurses as the first point of contact for patients in providing primary care was increasingly accepted by the public and did not compromise quality (Horrocks, Anderson and Salisbury, 2002; Lattimer et al., 1998; Shum et al., 2000). Furthermore, nurses experienced greater opportunities to get involved in the structures of decision-making of primary care – such as PCGs' and PCTs' boards (Audit Commission, 1999c), though their influence remained relatively small (Regen et al., 2001).

Pharmacists

The activities of dentists and opticians in identifying certain diseases at an early stage has already been discussed, and there is further scope for gearing the work of these professions more closely to prevention and early diagnosis, and for greater co-ordination with services for children and the elderly in primary care. Dentistry is further discussed in Exhibit 10.3. But it is perhaps the role of pharmacists that has been most neglected, and where most potential lies. Pharmacists have often complained that their skills are underutilised and that they could play a much bigger role in advising the public on treatments and referring them appropriately to other parts of the health care system (Royal Pharmaceutical Society of Great Britain, 1997).

The Department of Health responded with a new strategy based on two principles: maintaining and improving access, and improving quality (DoH, 2000j, 2002, 2003d). More specifically, the strategy proposed greater availability of drugs without prescription and greater involvement of pharmacists in the management of illness. It also sought to link payment directly to these activities rather than basing it simply on the volume of prescriptions dispensed. Local pharmaceutical pilot schemes were introduced to experiment with new ways of working. These offered services such as medicines management, diagnosis, and assessment and treatment of particular groups of patients (such as people with asthma, for example). They allowed groups of pharmacies to provide a joint community pharmacy service, and permitted PCTs to develop a community pharmacy service, with pharmacists being employed or subcontracted. Meanwhile, negotiations have continued over the new community pharmacy contract, with Government attempting to incentivise quality of services and recognise the wider role of pharmacies in health promotion, promoting self-care, and referring patients to other health care provision. The new contract is also likely to identify specific additional services that pharmacies may provide, including medicine-use review, needle exchange, smoking cessation and care home/intermediate care services.

Exhibit 10.3 NHS Dentistry

Dentistry, though part of the NHS, has always been provided by a combination of the public and private sectors. Most dentists working in primary care are self-employed; few are directly employed by the NHS. Yet few dental practices are wholly 'private', less than 2 per cent do not treat any NHS patients.

For many years, dentistry was an uncontroversial area, apart from occasional concerns about quality of service, triggered by media exposure of poor practice. In the 1980s, however, growing dissatisfaction emerged both in Government and in the profession about the system of remuneration, which was based on fees for specific services set by a national contract. Although there were clear incentives to undertake restorative dental work, prevention went unrewarded. In an attempt to shift the balance towards prevention and continuity of care, a new system was introduced in 1990, with capitation fees for children and payments for registered patients. The plan backfired when the Government underestimated the cost of the new system and, to the fury of the profession, clawed back some of the money by reducing their fees.

Dissatisfaction among dentists with state remuneration, coupled with rising demand for dental treatment and a shortage of dental practitioners (the UK has fewer dentists per head than most comparable nations, around forty per 100,000) led to an expansion of private dental care during the 1990s. In 1992, only 7 per cent of dentists' income came from private practice, rising to over half their income by 2002, by which time over a million people had dental insurance. The market for private dental care grew by an estimated 50 per cent in real terms between 1997 and 2001 alone (Office of Fair Trading, 2003). Meanwhile, the number of adults registered for NHS treatment with dentists fell by 5 million (around 20 per cent) during the 1990s (Hayward, 1999). Complaints about lack of access to NHS dentistry increased, with a third of those seeking to register claiming that they had experienced difficulty (National Consumer Council, 1998) while half of health authorities reported shortages of dental practitioners (British Dental Association, 1999). At the same time, criticism of private dental care grew. The Office of Fair Trading (2003), investigating consumer complaints, called for better information on prices and treatment, improved systems of complaints and redress, improved regulation of professional standards, and reducing unnecessary restrictions on dental businesses in order to increase competition and choice.

The ills of NHS dentistry have been thoroughly diagnosed (see Audit Commission, 2002f; Health Committee, 1993, 2001b; Cm 2625, 1994; DoH, 2000k, 2002l). The central problem is the system of remuneration, which continues to reward treatment rather than prevention and is not linked to the quality of care. Initiatives to deal with the problems of access and quality have been piecemeal. Government has introduced pilot schemes – Personal Dental Service (PDS) pilots – which tested out new ways of service delivery, including greater use of salaried dentists and buying in self-employed dentists to undertake particular

$\longrightarrow$

Exhibit 10.3 continued

→

tasks or sessions of work. Meanwhile, Dental Care Centres, in areas where dentists are in short supply or which have large unregistered populations, were introduced. While these initiatives represent a step forward they remain small-scale, representing less than 5 per cent of the NHS dentistry budget. However, the political pressure to improve NHS dentistry increased following the Prime Minister's pledge that all who wanted an NHS dentist would be able to find one through NHS Direct by October 2001. Interestingly, this commitment did not guarantee that people would receive NHS comprehensive dental care. Later, the DoH suggested placing a duty on PCTs to ensure access to NHS dentistry. PCTs would be responsible for securing high-quality care, promoting oral health and addressing health inequalities in this field. Other proposals included the introduction of oral health assessment – which would go further than the current examination to include preventive work and advice. The Government also endorsed the setting and monitoring of national standards in dentistry. Despite a commitment to experiment with new ways of remuneration and explore ways of linking remuneration to policy objectives, the prospects of immediate reform were not good. Most independent observers agreed that little would change until national contractual arrangements were replaced by the commissioning of services from practices on the basis of population need (see Oliver, 2002).

Note: In Wales, oral health has been given greater priority, with a Welsh Dental Initiative introduced in 1995 to attract dentists to areas where there is a shortage. More recently, the Welsh Assembly has introduced free dental check-ups for people under 25 and over 60, and has frozen the maximum fee for NHS care (which was increased in England). Although there are no PDS schemes in Wales, the Welsh NHS has been active in devising clinical standards in dental care and has embarked on a number of schemes to improve children's oral health, especially in areas of deprivation (Audit Commission, 2002f).

These changes can be seen as an opportunity for pharmacies to become more closely integrated within the primary care system. But they may also represent a threat, particularly to those pharmacies that lack the skills and capacity to change and develop. PCTs may then be seen as the enemy rather than an ally, with pharmacies being squeezed out by their extended role. For the small independent operators, this is combined with the existing threat from the supermarket chains which are driving down prices of products sold in the local chemists, making them less profitable (Lewis, 2001b).

General Practice

GPs, while retaining their dominant role in primary care, have experienced a variety of changes – salaried posts, PMS contracts, delegation of tasks – which, potentially at least, make them more dependent than in the past on other members of the primary health care team. This, coupled with greater intervention by PCTs to promote teamworking and changes in the 'skill mix' of primary care, suggests an era where relationships may be more equitable. Indeed, PCTs, salaried service and practice-based contracts can be seen as posing a significant challenge to the traditional autonomy of GPs (Lewis, 1998; Moon and North,

2000; Audit Commission, 2002h). At the very least, these changes will lead to a restratification of GPs (Sheaff, Smith and Dickson, 2002), which could make it easier for local primary care organisations to 'divide and rule' and bring GPs under managerial control, something they have long resisted (Glendinning, 1999). On the other hand, GPs remain in a powerful position, both individually and collectively within primary care, and continue to exert a strong influence over strategic decision-making, protocol, practice and resources (Peckham and Exworthy, 2003). In the short term at least, their grip on primary care will remain strong.

Much, however, will turn on the introduction of new contracts for GPs, in the form of PMS contracts – which cover an increasingly large area of general practice – and, at the same time, a new national contract, accepted by GPs across the UK in 2003. The new contract is underpinned by three main principles: clear specification of services provided by general practices, a fairer system of funding that reflected the needs of patients, and a closer link between income and quality of service. The main provisions are as follows. First, practice-based contracts will be introduced. This means that individual GP lists will be replaced by practice lists, though patients will still be able to choose to see a particular doctor at the practice. Practices will be accountable to the PCT for resources and on quality issues. Secondly, medical services will be divided into three categories: essential services – which all practices will have to provide (including seeing patients presenting with symptoms); additional services – widely provided but practices will be able to opt out of them (examples include immunisation and child health surveillance); enhanced services (such as minor surgery) which practices can opt in to provide. Thirdly, GPs' 24-hour responsibility for patients will end. From 2004, out-of-hours responsibility will pass to the PCTs. Some practices may continue to provide this service, however, though they cannot be compelled to do so. As already noted, out-of-hours services have been a major issue of contention. Reforms in the mid-1990s led to the creation of co-operatives and primary care centres, which relied more on telephone triage and screening by nurses, and involved a move away from home visits (Hallam and Henthorne, 1998). Overall, patients indicated satisfaction with these services, though there was some dissatisfaction about reduced home visits and long waits in some centres. Although these schemes shifted the balance away from home visits, the heavy out-of-hours workload of GPs continued, with most still providing services at evenings and weekends. Fourthly, there will be changes to practice payments. In future each will receive a 'global sum', a payment per patient according to a national formula, weighted by factors including age, gender, and local death and illness rates. This is expected to go some way to deal with the long-standing problems of inequity in the distribution of general practices. Meanwhile, in a separate development, the Medical Practices Committee, which regulated the location of doctors in an effort to prevent inequities from widening further, was abolished. In addition to the global sum under the national formula, practices will be able to accrue other income by providing enhanced services, such as those mentioned above. A third stream of income can be generated by quality improvements – linked to a new framework of assessment discussed below. Additional payments for career development, seniority of GPs, and for infrastructure, including IT, will also be included in the new contract. Furthermore, to secure sufficient support for the contract among GPs, it was agreed that no practice should be financially worse off under the new regime. Finally a new quality framework will be introduced. Practices will be rewarded for planning and achieving specified service standards in terms of organisational effectiveness, clinical effectiveness and patient experience. The standards will be set by an expert committee and will be based on recognised standards of best practice and evidence. Practices will be reviewed annually by PCTs and periodic visits will also take place. Although there is an element of external scrutiny, practices will provide their own evidence on how they are meeting the standards set.

Accurate predictions about the impact of the new contract are difficult. In theory, PCTs will have more leverage over practices and may be able to reconfigure services more effectively. However, their current capacity to commission services appears to be limited (Audit Commission, 2004b). For the time being at least, the system of quality assessment is in the hands of the practices themselves, which have considerable discretion. It is also possible that the new contract may create greater autonomy for practices, enabling them to offload functions back on to PCTs by opting out of particular services. Much, it seems, will depend on the extent of the Government's relationship with the GPs, the latter's support for reform and their willingness to participate in decision-making and planning. Reports that GPs believe that they lack influence over PCTs (Mooney, 2003), coupled with findings of reduced willingness among GPs to engage with PCTs (BBC News, 2003), therefore suggest problems ahead for the future development of primary care.

Conclusion

Predicting the future of primary care is difficult, largely because the institutions are at an early stage in their own development and face complex challenges. It is clear that in order to achieve their goals, they will have to develop their commissioning roles to a higher level of sophistication. For most observers, this means commissioning around the 'patient's journey' rather than provider organisations, improving the monitoring of performance, and integrating commissioning so that it incorporates needs-assessment, service planning, monitoring and evaluation (NHS Alliance, 2002; Audit Commission, 2004a). It is possible that primary care organisations will evolve into US-style 'managed care' organisations, exerting greater control over the provision of all aspects of care (see Exhibit 5.1). Moreover, other reforms, such as the creation of Foundation Hospitals, greater patient choice and new systems of internal resource allocation, are likely to have a major impact on primary care, and therefore much will depend on how these are actually implemented (Lewis, Dixon and Gillam, 2003b; Walshe, 2003c).

Experts in primary care tend to hedge their bets by identifying a range of scenarios, rather than a single path of future development. For example, Peckham and Exworthy (2003) identify five scenarios: *dynamic conservatism*, where the process of integrating primary care within the NHS continues but diversity is tightly managed; *corporate organisation* – where people get a choice of primary care organisation, which manages care on their behalf; *specialisation*, where secondary care extends into primary care settings, bringing it under the control of specialists; *integration*, where the interface between primary and social care becomes particularly important, with local authorities taking on key roles in relation to primary care; *and public health primary care organisation*, where the PCTs develop as community-oriented bodies, placing great emphasis on partnership working in an effort to promote health.

All these developments may occur within the same institution, with certain features being dominant. The focus on health care, rather than health promotion, is, however, likely to remain strong. There may also be greater diversity between primary care organisations, increasingly likely given devolution and the different arrangements for primary care in different parts of the UK.

_____ *Further Reading* _____

Boaden, N. (1997) *Primary Care: Making the Connections* (Buckingham, Open University Press).

Dowling, B. and Glendenning, C. (2003) *New Primary Care* (Buckingham, Open University Press).

Peckham, S. and Exworthy, M. (2003) *Primary Care in the UK: Policy, Organisation and Management* (Basingstoke, Palgrave).

Starfield, B. (1998) *Primary Care: Balancing Health Needs, Services and Technology* (New York, Oxford University Press).

Health and Social Care

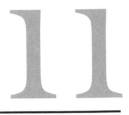

The majority of NHS expenditure is allocated to the care and treatment of elderly people, children, people with mental illness, people with learning disabilities and those with chronic illness. These people, which include the most vulnerable in our society, are also the biggest users of social care. Yet, despite their often pressing and complex needs, it has long been acknowledged that the combination of health and social services for these groups has been poor (Means, Richards and Smith, 2003) which is why they became known as the 'Cinderella services'. This chapter explores how these services have developed in recent years and in particular how government has tried to bring health and social care services together in a more effective way.

Care in the Community?

Debates about the needs of vulnerable and chronically ill people have focused on 'community care'. The community care policy originated from various official documents (Ministry of Health, 1954; Cm 9663, 1956), and ministerial speeches, notably that given by Enoch Powell in 1961, heralding the closure of the large mental hospitals (Barham, 1992). The policy was given further momentum by a series of scandals in the late 1960s and early 1970s in long-stay hospitals (Robb, 1967; Martin, 1984), and critical studies of institutional care (Townsend, 1962; Goffman, 1961; Meacher, 1972; Miller and Gwynne, 1972; Morris, 1969).

The essence of community care is that, rather than being cared for in long-stay hospitals and other large institutions, people should be looked after in their own homes and in non-institutional environments, and with regard to needs and wishes of local people, involving them and their carers more in service planning and provision (Payne, 2000, p. 188). In reality, however, community care was open to a variety of interpretations (Higgins, 1989). Its vagueness – arising from the nebulous nature of 'community' and 'care' (Barnes, 1997) – meant that it could justify many different initiatives, from closing down certain institutions to extending private provision. Although community care policy was essentially about removing people from institutions, it became a particular form of deinstitutionalisation (Jack, 1998). While asylums were closed down and geriatric wards closed, others smaller care institutions flourished – such as private care homes and day centres.

The Shortcomings of Community Care

During the 1960s and 1970s the large institutions remained, and community-based services developed slowly. The policy was revitalised in the 1970s with the publication of White Papers for the mentally ill and mentally handicapped people (Cmnd 4683, 1971; Cmnd 6233, 1975). Joint Consultative Committees and Joint Planning Committees were established at local level to address the problems of inter-agency collaboration (Means, Richards and Smith, 2003; Hudson and Henwood, 2002), supplemented by a programme of joint finance to promote community-based services. However, community care was still plagued by poor collaborative working between different agencies and between the various professionals involved in health and social care (Green, 1986; NAO, 1987; Audit Commission, 1986, 1989, 1992; Social Services Committee, 1985).

During the 1980s, the Thatcher Government realised that community care offered scope to reduce entitlements to free care, promote privatisation and shift the responsibility for care towards families, individuals and voluntary organisations. As one policy document famously stated, 'care in the community must increasingly mean care by the community' (Cmnd 8173, 1981). However, implementation proved problematic. Pressures on hospitals to reduce costs led to earlier discharges, adding to the workload of social care providers and carers, already stretched by demographic trends and the closure of long-stay hospitals. The gap between needs and services was particularly acute in the mental health sector (Groves, 1990; Barham, 1992), while many elderly, sick and disabled people also faced neglect in the community (Jack, 1998, p. 27).

However, the impact on the elderly was alleviated to some extent by changes in social security rules during the early 1980s, which permitted claimants to cover the costs of care in private and voluntary homes. The sector mushroomed, and, by the end of the decade, the public/private sector balance in long-term care had been transformed. In 1979 the independent sector – private and voluntary organisations – had one-third of the market for long-term care. By 1989, its market share had grown to over half, and has since grown further (Player and Pollock, 2001; see figure 11.1).

The Griffiths Report

Although private provision of long-term care was consistent with the Governments' ideological orientation, the rising cost to the tax-payer of this

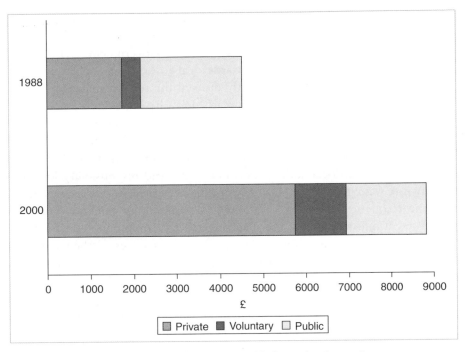

Figure 11.1 Long-term care: Market value by sector
Source of Data: Laing and Buisson (2001), *Laing's Healthcare Market Review 2001/2002*

open-ended commitment to fund long-term care was not. The Prime Minister's advisor, Sir Roy Griffiths, was invited to examine the issue, and he produced a report which outlined three guiding principles for reform: that the right services should be provided early enough, to people who needed them most; that individuals should have more choice and a greater say over services; that people should be cared for wherever possible in their own homes, or as near a domestic environment as possible (DHSS, 1988). Griffiths wanted clearer responsibility for services at all levels: at the top, a minister for community care; at local level, social service departments would identify needs, set priorities, and develop plans for community care; at the individual level, care managers would co-ordinate the assessment of needs and arrange appropriate packages of care.

Griffiths believed that perverse incentives in favour of residential care should be removed by reducing social security payments for people in residential homes to a basic level. The balance (the care element) would then be paid by local authorities on behalf of those requiring residential care. For others, the care element could purchase an alternative package of community services from local authorities, the NHS and the private sector. Griffiths envisaged central government providing substantial resources for community care, allocated through approved local community care plans, and drawn up by councils in consultation with health authorities, voluntary organisations and the commercial sector. He also recommended that central funds should be ring-fenced, so that the funds could not be used for other services.

These recommendations alarmed the Thatcher Government (Wistow and Harrison, 1998), which was hostile towards local government and suspicious of its spending ambitions, and particularly disliked the recommendation to give local authorities a key role. Yet, after a year's delay, having been persuaded that the plans would lead to lower costs, greater private provision and a shift in the responsibility for community care to local councils, the Government accepted most of Griffiths's ideas in its White Paper, *Caring for People* (Cm 849, 1989). Griffiths's idea that local authorities should have lead responsibility for community care was endorsed, as was the principle of individual care management. But the recommendation for a minister for community care was not. The Government refused to grant specific, 'ring-fenced' community care funds for all client groups. Although it was intended that only services for the mentally ill would receive earmarked grants, channelled through health authorities, temporary ring-fencing of community care funding was later introduced.

Caring for People emphasised privatisation more heavily than the Griffiths report. Although Griffiths encouraged independent provision – where it was more economic and efficient than direct provision by the public sector – it did not advocate the widespread replacement of statutory services. The Government stated that maximum use must be made of the independent sector. Council-run homes did not receive the residential allowance – a housing cost element for each resident – which disadvantaged them against commercial and voluntary homes, and provided an incentive for councils to privatise their own homes or place residents in the private sector. The independent sector was encouraged further by the so-called '85 per cent rule', which stipulated that this proportion of new money received from central government had to be allocated to independent sector provision.

Legislation was introduced in the form of the NHS and Community Care Act of 1990 which, as Barnes (1997) observed, was the first time that community care had provided a central focus for welfare legislation. However, most of the community care provisions in the Act were subsequently postponed until April 1993 because of the scale of the changes and Government concerns about the impact of the reforms on local tax bills in a pre-election period.

The Impact of the Griffiths Reforms

Community care was implemented at different speeds and with varying degrees of success in different localities (Wistow et al., 1994). This made an overall assessment difficult, particularly as the Griffiths reforms coincided with other developments in primary and social care (Moon and North, 2000; see also chapter 10). Even so, as evidence accumulated, the impact of the reforms became clearer.

The mixed economy of social care

The Griffiths reforms sought to stimulate a mixed economy in social care (Barnes, 1999) Under the new regime, local authorities became commissioning bodies and were expected to reduce their direct provider role (Bamford, 2001). However, they seemed poorly equipped to commission care and faced problems dealing with market failure, extending choice and maintaining quality of service (Forder, Knapp and Wistow, 1994).

There was evidence that the commissioning process was both bureaucratic and costly (Audit Commission, 1997a; Hawley and Hudson, 1996; Lewis and Glennerster, 1996; Hadley and Clough, 1996). This was exacerbated by poor and adversarial relationships between commissioners and providers (Knapp, Hardy and Forder, 2001). Commissioning tended to reflect not the needs and choices of individuals (Farrell, Robinson and Fletcher, 1999; Audit Commission, 1997a; Clinical Standards Advisory Group, 1998b; Bamford, 2001; Henwood, 2001) but the imperatives of the commissioning process. There was also a tendency to fit existing services to needs, rather than rearrange services to meet assessed need (Hawley and Hudson, 1996). However, given the scale of the changes, much was achieved. There was considerable variation in the experiences of users and carers (Henwood, 1995). Some local authorities clearly offered more choice and were more responsive to users and carers than others (Social Services Inspectorate, 1996; Lewis et al., 1996; Lewis and Glennerster, 1996).

Generally, there was a reluctance to decentralise budgets, which would have brought the processes of commissioning and care management closer together (Knapp, Hardy and Forder, 2001). Most studies commented adversely on the dominance of 'spot contracting' (where services are negotiated and paid for separately rather then being part of a general or block contract – see Bamford, 2001). This inhibited the development of new and more responsive services (Audit Commission, 1996b, 1997a; Lewis et al., 1996). Furthermore, elements of unfair competition were discovered, including 'cherry-picking' by the independent sector, offset to some extent by unwarranted bias in favour of 'in-house services' in some local authorities (Audit Commission, 1997a).

Assessment of the impact of the Griffiths reforms on quality of service proved difficult. Much evidence was anecdotal and based on providers' views rather than those of users or carers. However, the new regime appeared to have an adverse impact on the people providing services, which might have had implications for service users. According to Hadley and Clough (1996), conditions and morale among those working in social care deteriorated in the early 1990s. Social care organisations were beset by greater insecurity, reduced autonomy and more secrecy, leading to a defensive management culture that discouraged innovation and organisational learning.

Although concerns about service quality persisted (Farrell, Robinson and Fletcher, 1999), later studies painted a more optimistic picture, where choice, quality and cost-effectiveness were improving (Knapp, Hardy and Forder, 2001). This was attributed partly to increased emphasis on a more inclusive approach to commissioning that involved users and providers more closely in the planning process. Other factors included new performance management and regulatory systems, discussed later in this chapter. Nonetheless, considerable variations have persisted, with some authorities undertaking their social care role much more effectively than others (Audit Commission, 2002g) and unacceptable variations in services between people living in different areas (Clinical Standards Advisory Group, 1998b). This continues to be reflected in the differences between local authorities in their funding of residential and domiciliary care, which Griffiths had tried to address. In 2001, the proportion of the elderly-services budget spent on residential care by local authorities, which averaged 60 per cent, ranged between 46 per cent and 81 per cent (Audit Commission, 2002g). Overall, though, residential places declined in the 1990s by around 10 per cent, while local authority domiciliary care grew by over 50 per cent, suggesting a significant shift between the two (Knapp, Hardy and Forder, 2001).

Funding and rationing

Despite improvements in commissioning, claims about underfunding persisted. Although large sums were transferred from central government to local authorities in the 1990s, it was claimed that the amounts were insufficient (Laing, 1996; Audit Commission, 1994b, 1996b). This criticism continued after 1997, with reports of severe funding problems in social care, in contrast with the relatively generous increases for the NHS (Player and Pollock, 2001; Henwood, 2001).

To address the gap between needs and funding, local authorities began to prioritise (Audit Commission, 1996b). As they were obliged to publish eligibility criteria in their community care plans, they used these to identify priorities (Lewis and Glennerster, 1996). Although people were increasingly ranked by need (as indicated by factors such as risk and dependency), each authority tended to develop its own system of assessing priorities, defining eligibility, and allocating resources. A more standardised system was later introduced by the Blair Government. However, there was no obligation to provide or commission services to meet the assessed need, a principle tested several times in the courts during the 1990s. Prioritisation meant that those in greatest need received more intensive packages of care. For example, although the average contact hours for home help and care doubled between 1992 and 2001, the numbers receiving help fell by over a quarter (Means, Richards and Smith, 2003, p. 65). Evidence from specific client groups, such as the elderly, indicated that packages of care were targeted at those with higher levels of need (Bauld et al., 2000), while admission to nursing or residential care was also being more appropriately based upon assessment of needs.

Charges were also introduced and extended as local authorities faced increasing financial pressures on them (Baldwin and Lunt, 1996; National Consumer Council, 1995). Although means tests were used, charges affected low-income groups and those with high levels of disability (Scope, 1995; Baldwin and Lunt, 1996). There was a considerable variation in charges between councils and in systems of means testing, which led to geographical inequities (Audit Commission, 2000b; Cm 4192, 1999). The unfairness of charges was criticised (Farrell, Robinson and Fletcher, 1999), and fresh guidance to councils subsequently introduced (DoH and Department for Work and Pensions, 2002). This stated that, when charging for non-residential services, councils must find fairer ways of means testing, should not reduce users' income below a certain level, must provide benefits advice at the same time as assessing means, and must disregard earnings when assessing ability to pay. Furthermore, councils were now required to assess each individual's disability-related expenditure before disability benefits could be taken into account.

Privatisation?

The increased use of charges, and the greater selectivity in the allocation of state-funded social care was in line with the Government's expectation that people would pay more towards the cost of care. Even so, the shift towards private funding should not be exaggerated. Even in long-term care, seven out of ten social care recipients continued to receive state funding by the end of the decade (Laing and Buisson, 2001).

On the supply side, the community care reforms helped to expand further the role of the independent sector. As noted earlier, the majority of residential and nursing homes are now run by commercial and voluntary organisations. However, the growth in the independent residential care sector was partly stimulated by the transfer of local authority homes to voluntary bodies (Bamford, 2001, p. 14). Meanwhile, parts of the independent care sector struggled following the Griffiths reforms (Player and Pollock, 2001). Residential care homes endured a financial squeeze as local authorities sought to reduce costs, and as fewer people entered residential care. As less-dependent people were diverted away from residential care, homes found themselves dealing with a higher proportion of people with complex needs, who were more costly to care for (Fitzhugh, 1995). These problems continued, with the residential and nursing care sector under considerable strain, particularly in the south-east of England (Audit Commission, 2002g).

Efforts to reduce costs in residential and nursing home care, and divert people into domiciliary care, opened other avenues. The independent sector acquired a growing role in the provision of domiciliary services. In England in 1992, only 2 per cent of home-care contact hours funded by local authorities was provided by independent contractors. By 1997 this had risen to 44 per cent

(Wistow and Hardy, 1999), increasing to over half by 2002 (Laing and Buisson, 2001, p. 176). Subsequently, the independent sector looked to benefit from the development of intermediate care schemes, which divert people from hospital and prevent their admission by providing facilities for care and rehabilitation (see Exhibit 11.3).

Interagency collaboration

One of the persistent problems of community care has been poor co-ordination between health authorities and local authorities. During the 1990s, reorganisations, of both the NHS and local government, added to these difficulties (Hiscock and Pearson, 1999). First, the changes created further incentives for organisations to shift costs on to others (Salter, 1994; Clinical Standards Advisory Group, 1998b). In domiciliary care, for example, disputes about which agency should fund or provide care became even more protracted (Social Services Inspectorate, 1996; Henwood, 1995). Moreover, the early discharge of people from hospital increased the financial burden upon social services departments and NHS primary care services. Secondly, the internal market in health care affected collaboration. The extension of fundholding to community health services introduced new priorities at odds with those of the NHS community health trusts and social service departments (Henwood, 1995). This exacerbated historically-poor relationships between GPs and social services staff amid the concerns of doctors that community care would add to their workload (Moon and North, 2000; Kavanagh and Knapp, 1998). Thirdly, the reorganisation process itself disrupted collaborative efforts, even after the new structures had bedded down (Charlesworth, Clarke and Cochrane, 1996; Wistow et al., 1994).

Following Griffiths, efforts to promote joint working were renewed. Health and local authorities were expected to reach agreements on hospital discharge arrangements and continuing care packages. New national guidelines on continuing care were developed to limit inappropriate discharges from hospital. However, monitoring exercises undertaken following the reforms indicated that success in joint working at the individual case level depended greatly on the commitment of local managers and staff (Social Services Inspectorate, 1996). Meanwhile, the individual consequences of poor collaboration were graphically highlighted (Jones, 1998). By the end of the 1990s, the fragmentation of health and social services remained a serious problem, with many receiving poorly co-ordinated services (Audit Commission, 1997a, 1997b; Clinical Standards Advisory Group, 1998b; Farrell, Robinson and Fletcher, 1999).

One of the brighter prospects of the Griffiths reforms was the development of joint commissioning between health and social services. Ideally, this involved health and social services organisations entering into arrangements to plan local services according to needs, and allocating resources accordingly (Rummery and Glendinning, 2000; Hudson, 1995). Other developments, such as the introduction of the Total Purchasing Pilot (TPP) scheme, appeared to encourage joint commissioning, with two out of five schemes engaged in developing continuing and community care services (Moon and North, 2000, pp. 156–7). However, on closer inspection pre-existing strong relationships between health and social care organisations – particularly informal relationships – were the key factors (Lewis and Glennerster, 1996). Furthermore, joint commissioning was less effective in tackling the everyday problems of poor collaboration between professionals at the front line (Rummery and Glendinning, 2000, p. 49). Moreover, the development of joint commissioning was impeded by legal difficulties involved in pooling budgets and establishing joint organisations between local authorities and NHS bodies, though some were removed by subsequent legislation, discussed below.

Exhibit 11.1 NHS Continuing Care and Discharge Arrangements

Eligibility for NHS continuing care, and the appropriateness of discharging vulnerable patients from hospital, became a major political issue during the 1990s (Health Service Commissioner, 1994, 1996a, 1996b). The Major Government responded by setting out general principles for NHS continuing care (DoH, 1995c). Patients requiring continuing care fell into several categories: those needing ongoing and regular clinical supervision because of the complexity, nature or intensity of their needs; those requiring unpredictable interventions; and patients receiving in-patient or hospice care, who were likely to die in the very near future. However, the Government avoided setting national criteria for continuing care. Instead, local health authorities were charged with drawing up local policies and eligibility criteria, and were required to establish panels to review disputed cases. The wider question of funding long-term care was also considered (Cm 3242, 1996). Tax relief was given to those making provision for funding their own care and the capital threshold at which people met the cost of nursing and residential care was raised.

The continuing care guidance was criticised for being unclear and inadequate, and there were renewed calls for national eligibility criteria (Health Committee, 1995b). Many believed that the eligibility criteria restricted access for people with 'intense and specialist needs' (South, 1999). There was evidence that people were still being discharged inappropriately into nursing home care (Jones, 1998; Barnet Health Authority, 1997). Matters came to a head in 1999 when, in a landmark case (North and East Devon Health Authority ex parte Coughlan), the Court of Appeal decided that the closure of an NHS facility and subsequent transfer of disabled patients to local authority care was unlawful. It was adjudged that although local authorities could legally provide nursing care, this had to be ancillary or incidental to the provision of accommodation and of a nature that could be expected from an authority which primarily provided social services. In other words, nursing primarily for health needs must be funded by the NHS. The judgement raised serious questions about other instances where severely disabled patients had been discharged into nursing and residential homes. This, along with the Long Term Care Commission's recommendations, led Government to ask health authorities to review their eligibility criteria, and later to introduce new national guidance (DoH, 2001j). This stated that, for nursing home residents, health authorities and PCTs are responsible for arranging – free of charge – access to GP and primary care services, nursing advice, physiotherapy, occupational therapy, speech therapy,

$\longrightarrow$

Exhibit 11.1 continued

→

dietetics and podiatry, continence and related equipment, specialist nursing and medical equipment normally only available through hospitals, palliative care, and access to hospital care. In the case of residential homes, the range of services was similar (excluding specialist nursing and medical equipment, which would not normally be used in a residential care setting anyway). The scope of review panels and complaints procedures was also extended to other decisions about NHS-arranged or funded continuing health services and free nursing care. Despite the Coughlan judgement and the new guidance, some health authorities apparently made little progress in reviewing their eligibility criteria, meaning that patients continued to be unfairly treated (Health Service Commissioner, England, 2003a).

Other policies had implications for hospital discharges. Intermediate care (see Exhibit 11.3) was heralded as a means of discharging patients into facilities where they could receive short-term care and rehabilitation, free of charge. In addition, a new system of cross-charging social service departments for delayed discharges from hospital was introduced. From 2004, local authorities must reimburse hospitals when patients have been assessed as ready for discharge. Initially this will apply to acute in-patients only. However, the scheme may not work as planned (Health Committee, 2002d; NAO, 2003d; Glasby, 2003), because many of the reasons for delayed discharges lie outside the control of social service departments. Delays in assessments, an important cause of delay, are often due to a shortage of key therapists. Another problem is the shortage of care homes, again not the fault of councils. It has also been suggested that delays in discharge are due mainly to problems in hospitals rather than shortcomings in social services. Reimbursement may also make matters worse. It could distort social care priorities, leading to larger numbers of people being admitted to hospital unnecessarily. Furthermore, it is possible that people could be placed inappropriately in social care settings simply to avoid cross-charges. Above all, it may undermine good relations between the NHS and local government, which are essential for effective collaboration health and social care. Interestingly, in some areas (Warwickshire, for example) trusts have agreed not to impose fines on councils, preferring instead jointly to fund new intermediate care services.

The Blair Government and Social Care

The Blair Government inherited a policy of community care that had become discredited for failing vulnerable people. Consequently, the term 'community care' was used less frequently in official circles, though it did not slip entirely from the vocabulary. Indeed, the new Government's programme impinged on both institutional and community care in several ways, each of which is discussed further in this section: collaborative working between health and social care agencies; long-term care, and in particular how it should be financed; new systems of regulation and performance management for social care.

Collaboration

The Blair Government proclaimed its intention to introduce more effective forms of governance. A key element of this approach was that the public sector was expected to work more coherently. The phrase 'joined-up' government was coined to describe the need for improved co-ordination, collaboration and partnership between public sector agencies (Sullivan and Skelcher, 2002; Balloch and Taylor, 2001). This principle underpinned many new initiatives aimed at addressing the long-standing problems of poor collaboration in health and social care (Glendinning, Powell and Rummery, 2003), while heading off demands for a fully integrated health and social care system (Health Committee, 1999d; Hudson, 1998; Hudson and Henwood, 2002).

The Government's approach was outlined in the White Papers, *The New NHS: Modern, Dependable* (Cm 3807, 1997), *Modernising Social Services* (Cm 4169, 1998) and *Modernising Local Government – In Touch with the People* (Cm 4014, 1998), and a document on partnership working, *Partnership in Action* (DoH, 1998f). Joint guidance on health and social care priorities was issued at national level (DoH, 1998d). Although social care had been prioritised in previous NHS guidance, this was the first time that responsibilities for various health and social care priorities had been detailed. The NHS was expected to lead on waiting times/primary care/cancer/heart disease, and local authorities on children's welfare/inter-agency working/regulation, and a number of responsibilities were shared (health inequalities/mental health/promoting independence). Instead of proposing new statutory health and social service organisations, several initiatives were introduced to improve relationships between local government and the NHS, including the removal of statutory obstacles to joint working. Subsequently, the Health Act 1999 enabled health and local government to pool budgets to commission integrated packages of care, to transfer funds and delegate commissioning functions to each other, and to integrate provision by allowing NHS trusts or PCTs to provide social care, and social service organisations to provide health care.

The Health Act 1999 imposed a duty of co-operation regarding health and welfare on local authorities and NHS bodies. Subsequently, local authorities were given powers to improve the social, economic and environmental well-being of their communities. They were expected to participate in the preparation of health improvement programmes drawn up by health authorities, and were subsequently required to formulate community plans. The requirement to produce health improvement and modernisation plans was later dropped, though local authorities were expected to contribute to NHS local delivery plans (LDPs) which replaced them.

NHS and local authority plans were expected to take account of Joint Investment Plans (JIPs), three-year rolling plans setting out the aims, objectives, responsibilities and resources of health and local government bodies with regard to improving services for particular client groups. JIPs were first mooted by the *Better Service for Vulnerable People* initiative (DoH, 1997a), which paved the way for other policies, such as multidisciplinary assessment and intermediate care for older people (see later). JIPs were initially established for older people and later extended to other client groups, such as people with learning disabilities. Important themes of JIPs were improving service integration, responsiveness to needs, and promoting independence among users. A further initiative complemented this approach to vulnerable people. *Supporting People* (Department of the Environment, Transport and the Regions, 2001), sought to reorient housing-related support services by strengthening local partnerships between local government, the NHS and other agencies. This involved a more systematic approach to mapping and meeting needs. For groups such as the elderly, mentally ill and people with learning disabilities, this raised the prospect of more support for independent living.

Existing mechanisms such as the Joint Consultative Committees (see above) were abolished, while joint finance was absorbed within other budgets. New performance and modernisation funds were established to promote service development, along with earmarked funds for initiatives relating to particular client groups, such as elderly and mentally ill people.

In addition to central directives, financial and legislative changes, the NHS was restructured. PCGs and PCTs were expected to work more closely with providers of social care to improve collaboration. Health Action Zones (HAZ) were introduced to strengthen co-operation. As discussed in Chapter 10, these generated some improvements, no mean achievement given the poor history of interagency relationships. Subsequently, the NHS Plan (Cm 4818, 2000) emphasised integration. The move towards PCTs was heralded as a way of improving joint working. Intermediate care was expanded and Care Trusts introduced to bring health and social care for particular groups, such as elderly and mentally ill people, into one organisation.

The Government, disappointed with the take-up of the 1999 Health Act flexibilities, stated that the use of such powers would become a requirement. Although three out of five local authorities had planned or used these powers by 2000 (Local Government Association, 2000), schemes covered a small minority of patients. However, evaluations of Health Act flexibilities were positive (Hudson et al., 2002). Pooled budgets were popular and many examples of effective joint working were found. Changes were tangible – such as greater co-ordination of processes, protocols and structures, leading to improvements in efficiency and effectiveness. Intangible changes were also apparent – including shifts towards a 'whole system approach' and some dramatic changes in the perspectives of partner organisations, in particular, a strengthened focus on shared achievement rather than a blame culture.

Ironically, the reorganisation that followed the NHS Plan disrupted the improved relationships between local government and the NHS that had resulted from the introduction of PCGs and HAZs. Although it was acknowledged that PCTs were in a good position to redesign health and social care (Audit Commission, 2002g), others believed they placed a low priority on collaboration, largely because of the turbulence of reorganisation and the inconsistency between health authority and local authority boundaries (Hudson, 2003). Plans to create care trusts were heavily criticised for similar reasons. On a more positive note, there was more support for rationalising partnerships between the NHS, local authorities and other organisations at local level through local strategic partnerships. It was argued that LSPs could co-ordinate the various partnerships across the range of health and social care activities, including public health. Their role is discussed further in Chapter 13.

In summary, what has been the impact of the Blair Government on collaboration in health and social care? (see Glasby and Littlechild, 2004). Problems of fragmented and poorly co-ordinated services remain, resulting from constant reorganisation, an overwhelming focus on reducing the demand for acute hospital services, and perverse incentives (Banks, 2002). Furthermore, resource pressures still encourage the shifting of responsibility for care on to other agencies. Cultural differences between the NHS and local government – both organisational and professional – persist. Interestingly, flagship sites for integrated working have faced problems. In Somerset a pioneering effort to integrate mental health services in one organisation did not produce expected benefits in the short term (Peck, Towell and Gulliver, 2001) with staff experiencing increased workloads and more bureaucracy, and users and carers reporting less involvement in care planning. Users also believed that access to services had deteriorated since reorganisation. Meanwhile, in Barking and Dagenham, an initiative bringing health and social care within a single organisational structure collapsed amid recriminations in 2003.

Perhaps central direction can only achieve so much (Hudson, 2002; Hudson and Henwood, 2002). Central government has a key role in establishing a framework conducive to collaboration (Hudson et al., 2002). Inconsistencies in health authority and local government boundaries as well as financial, planning and performance management systems continue to cause problems. But beyond this, it is the cultural barriers between organisations and between professional groups that need to be addressed, in order to produce effective teamworking in a high-trust environment (Hudson et al., 1997; Glendinning, Rummery and Clarke, 1998). Given continuing professional rivalries and entrenched organisational perspectives, this is easier said than done. Policy-makers face a dilemma. Do they wait for new powers and duties to be taken up in an atmosphere of trust and co-operation? Or do they adopt a directive approach which risks alienating those on whom ultimately effective collaborative working depends?

The dilemma is not confined to policy-makers in England. Elsewhere in the UK there are similar requirements for the NHS and local government to work together, and powers to pool budgets and delegate functions. In Wales, efforts were made to bring health and social care more closely together through local health, social care and well-being strategies. These plans are jointly owned by health boards and local authorities. In Scotland, the executive has powers to compel joint working where services are adjudged to be failing. In addition, joint resourcing and management was proposed for particular client groups, initially the elderly. This involves establishing joint management arrangements, identifying the resources to be brought under these arrangements, the setting of joint priorities and performance management frameworks, as well as governance and joint accountability frameworks. In Scotland, there are local partnership agreements between agencies that feed into local plans for health, the community, social care and housing. Meanwhile, in Northern Ireland, where there is a single organisational structure for health and social care, shortcomings have been identified and ways are being sought to make it work more effectively at the local level.

Exhibit 11.2 Care Trusts

The NHS Plan for England proposed new Care Trusts to integrate health and social care within a single organisation (see Glasby and Peck, 2003). Where care trusts are based on PCTs, they take responsibility for commissioning and providing services in primary care, community health and social care. Alternatively, they can be based on NHS trusts, and have a provider role only. This represented a significant policy change. The Blair Government had earlier decided against creating new organisations, placing faith in measures to strengthen collaboration between local government and the NHS. The rationale behind care trusts was that they encourage a consistent approach to service improvement, a common strategy for health and social care at local level, greater flexibility and efficiency, as well as better working arrangements for staff. It was also believed that better communication and multidisciplinary working would arise (DoH, 2001k).

The creation of care trusts was roundly criticised (see Hudson, 2002). It was pointed out that Northern Ireland, where single health and social service boards have existed for many years, faced similar problems as in England (McCoy, 2000). Indeed, it was argued that care trusts could actually undermine relationships between the NHS and local government which had shown recent improvement. Local authorities feared a takeover of social care by the NHS, believing that they would lose control over budgets and priorities, and that, consequently, social care would be attuned less to community well-being and more to the narrower objectives of the NHS. It was also felt that formal integration of social care alongside health might detach it from other local authority responsibilities such as housing, making it more difficult to co-ordinate services affecting the welfare of vulnerable groups.

Local authorities were worried that they would remain accountable for services delegated to the care trust, while their planning and monitoring role remained unclear. They were also anxious about financial issues, particularly the impact of care trusts on their existing budgets. The Government conceded that care trusts could not be imposed by the Department of Health, though it could insist on the use of partnership powers under the Health Act. Local authorities were allowed to nominate representatives to sit on care trust boards.

Nonetheless, the implementation of care trusts was beset with problems. Only five were established in 2002 – two based on PCTs and three on trusts. A further three were established in 2003. Some were responsible for older people's services, others for mental health or learning disability services, while some covered two or more of these areas. Other potential care trusts failed to materialise, discouraged by several factors: difficulties in transferring staff from local government to the NHS owing to differences in terms and conditions; problems of disentangling proposed care trust responsibilities from existing services,

$\longrightarrow$

Exhibit 11.2 continued

$\longrightarrow$

particularly for older people; and boundary problems in the case of PCT-based care trusts – as most PCT/local authority boundaries were not the same (Hudson, 2002). Furthermore, moves to create care trusts broke down owing to local disagreements between the NHS and local government over management structures, financial issues and accountability arrangements.

These problems drained the enthusiasm of the supporters of care trusts (Hudson et al., 2002). The policy was further undermined by reports (Audit Commission, 2002e; Henwood, 2001) cautioning against their widespread creation. Despite these setbacks, the policy retains considerable attraction for Government (Hudson, 2002). Care trusts enable local authority care services to be placed in a centrally run NHS, orienting social care more closely to the Government's health targets – particularly those relating to access to acute hospital care.

Note: In 2003, following the Laming report on the Victoria Climbié case, the Government proposed the creation of children's trusts as a means of co-ordinating services more effectively in this field (see also below).

The Funding and Provision of Long-Term Care

During the 1990s, the Major Government sought to diffuse concerns about the funding and provision of long-term care. But the political pressures remained, with elderly people and their families incensed that their hard-earned assets, including their homes, would be sold in order to pay care home fees, while others paid little or nothing. Such complaints supported a general view that the current system was ungenerous, unfair and inadequate (see Health Committee, 1999a), leading to a renewed interest in methods of funding long-term care (see Wittenberg, Sandhu and Knapp, 2002).

Shortly after taking office, the Blair Government established a Royal Commission on long-term care for the elderly (Cm 4192, 1999; Robinson, 2002a; Deeming and Keen, 2001; Health Committee, 1999d), which identified a 'sense of betrayal, a lack of trust and a genuine sense of hopelessness' in this area. Its favoured solution, supported by all but two of its members, was to separate and redefine the various costs of care. *Living costs and housing costs* would be subject to a means test, with poorer people being exempt from charges. However, *personal costs* – which the commission defined as the additional costs of being looked after as a result of frailty and or disability associated with old age 'that directly involves touching a person's body … and is distinct from treatment/therapy and from indirect care, such as home help or the provision of meals' – would be funded out of general taxation subject to an assessment of need. The Commission subsumed within this latter recommendation that nursing care be exempt from means testing, irrespective of where it was provided. Other ways of pooling risks, such as social insurance and private insurance schemes were regarded as less equitable and efficient compared with general taxation (see Deeming and Keen, 2001; IPPR, 1996; Joseph Rowntree Foundation, 1996).

The Commission maintained that its central recommendation would not place an unreasonable burden on public finances, and involved only a small increase in the share of national expenditure allocated to long-term care. This has been disputed (see Wittenberg, Sandhu and Knapp, 2002). Indeed, two Commission members disagreed with free personal care, arguing that it would add significantly to public expenditure. They did, however, support free registered nursing care. The Blair Government, which took over a year to respond to the Commission's report, backed the minority recommendation and proposed that all registered nursing care in nursing homes be free. This caused controversy, largely because nursing had been narrowly defined. Nurses' organisations, along with groups representing elderly people and those with long-term conditions, argued that in defining nursing as the time spent on supervision, delegation and provision of services by a registered nurse, the Government excluded large areas of personal care from its guarantee of 'free nursing'. The complexity of the assessment process, necessary to implement the policy, was also widely criticised. A further concern was that it would promote the separation of nursing from personal care when people needed a more integrated approach (Heath, 2002).

Free nursing care for people in nursing homes in England was introduced in 2001. This involved transferring the nursing element of funding currently held by local authorities to PCTs. Meanwhile, local authority powers to provide registered nursing care were removed. In England, three bands of payment were introduced to reflect the severity of assessed need. This produced criticism that, for many people, the payments were too low. In Wales and Northern Ireland, a simpler system was adopted with a single, flat-rate payment for nursing costs. The Northern Ireland Assembly and the Welsh Assembly have both endorsed the principle of free personal care, but have no powers currently to introduce it. However, the Scottish Executive followed the Royal Commission's key recommendation and funded personal and nursing care costs from 2002. This raised the prospect of future comparisons with the English system – and may challenge the latter's sustainability (Deeming and Keen, 2001). Members of the Royal Commission later criticised this situation, restating the case for free personal care (Lord Sutherland of Houndwood et al., 2003). They argued that the situation outside Scotland was unfair, and discriminated against patients who had long-term chronic illnesses that needed personal care – such as Alzheimer's Disease. Others also found that the distinction between nursing and personal care was arbitrary and unfair (see Brooks, Regan and Robinson, 2002), and endorsed the Royal Commission's view that the balance between equity and affordability is best struck by making personal care free. The faults of the system south of the border had already become evident. When free nursing care was implemented, some nursing homes simply raised their fees, so that residents were no better off. The Government responded by requiring homes to provide a clear statement of the balance between the charges for nursing and other aspects of care. This, however, is likely to produce further bureaucracy and, by making the relative costs explicit, may lead to further pressures for a more generous system of state funding.

The controversial debate over nursing and personal care overshadowed other important aspects of the long-term care agenda discussed by the Royal Commission, some of which were acted upon by the Blair Government. Other measures taken in response to the Royal Commission's recommendations included disregarding the value of people's homes for three months after admission to residential care. The capital thresholds at which people would have to pay some or all of the residential and personal costs of care was raised to £11,500 and £18,500 (in line with general inflation since 1996 and much less generous than the £60,000 upper limit suggested by the Royal Commission). The Government gave local authorities both powers and funding to defer payment for care costs (so that the family home did not have to be sold), though the Royal Commission actually cautioned against the use of schemes. The Royal Commission made other recommendations regarding joint working between agencies, the regulation of standards and the role of carers, which are mentioned elsewhere in this chapter.

Quality and Standards in Social Care

From the early 1990s onwards, the Department of Health took a closer interest in quality and standards in social care. This was reflected in the monitoring of local authority community care plans. The Social Services Inspectorate (SSI), located within the department, embarked on a programme of national monitoring, which included detailed studies of particular authorities and thematic studies of community care. Meanwhile, the Audit Commission became increasingly involved in monitoring social care as part of its value-for-money role in the NHS and local government. Regulatory systems also came under increasing scrutiny in this period, although the Conservative Government was keen to avoid placing additional 'red tape' on the thriving independent social care market, it eventually conceded that a more comprehensive and integrated system of regulation was needed. The Blair Government continued the trend towards greater central government involvement by outlining plans to strengthen regulation, clarify and raise service standards, and monitor the performance of social services more closely (Cm 4169, 1998).

Regulation

The expansion of social care during the 1980s was not matched by an increase in regulatory capacity (Kerrison and Pollock, 2001), and there were particular concerns about the regulation of care homes (Turrell, Castleden and Freestone, 1998 and, more recently, Fahey et al., 2003). There were no explicit standards to guide the regulatory process and, to make matters worse, the regulatory system was divided – statutory responsibility for residential care homes fell to local authorities, while nursing homes and independent hospitals were regulated by health authorities. The absence of national standards for services encouraged inconsistency, while important areas of care, notably the growing domiciliary care sector, lay outside these regulatory frameworks.

Calls for an integrated and comprehensive system of social care regulation were not new (see, for example, DHSS, 1988; National Institute for Social Work, 1988). Further recommendations from the Government's Better Regulation Task Force (1998) – for a national regulatory body, clear national standards and a more comprehensive system of regulation – bolstered the resolve to create a new regulatory system. The Royal Commission on Long Term Care also endorsed the need for a single body to oversee social care and set national benchmarks (Cm 4192, 1999). Subsequently, the Blair Government introduced regulatory reform in social care in England and Wales, enacted by the Care Standards Act of 2000. A new regulatory framework for Scotland, along similar lines, was introduced by the Regulation of Care (Scotland) Act, 2001.

The Care Standards Act created a new body, the National Care Standards Commission (NCSC), in April 2002. This body acquired a range of regulatory, registration and inspection functions from the NHS and local government, and additional responsibilities for previously unregulated areas of care. Its remit included independent hospitals, and all adult and child care services: care homes, children's homes, domiciliary care agencies, and nurses' agencies. In Scotland and Wales, slightly different arrangements were made. The principal body for social care regulation in Scotland is the Scottish Commission for the Regulation of Care; in Wales, it is the Care Standards Inspectorate for Wales. The Scottish Executive and the National Assembly for Wales are responsible for producing their own guidance and standards within their respective parts of the UK.

The NCSC had barely arrived before the Government decided to bring the regulation of health care providers under a new body, the Commission for Healthcare Audit and Inspection (CHAI). From 2004, CHAI will combine the functions of CHI and the NCSC's regulatory responsibilities for the independent health care sector. Also from 2004, the social care functions of NCSC will be merged with the Social Services Inspectorate (and part of the Audit Commission) to form a new non-departmental public body for social care in England, the Commission for Social Care Inspection (CSCI) in 2004. It should be noted in this context that the Royal Commission on Long Term Care had urged the creation of a national care commission to monitor trends in the provision of care for older people, ensure transparency and accountability in the funding of long-term care, and various other functions, including representing consumers. But it was disappointed with the creation of NCSC and subsequently CSCI on the basis that these were principally regulatory bodies.

In addition, the care standards legislation led to national standards, for both residential and domiciliary care. The old statutory distinction between nursing and residential homes disappeared (though homes providing nursing care must meet additional standards – see Laing and Buisson, 2001, p. 187). In England, guidance was issued, (DoH, 2002o) setting out care home standards in a range of areas: choice of home, health and personal care, daily life and social activities, complaints and protection, environment (including premises and facilities), staffing, and management/administration. Most of the standards came into effect from April 2002. Following lobbying from the independent care sector, the implementation of some standards was delayed, notably requirements that each service user should have a minimum amount of space in his or her private accommodation and that each home should have 80 per cent of places in single rooms, delayed for existing homes until 2007. Care-home owners also lobbied successfully against plans to set fixed staffing ratios (Laing and Buisson, 2001, p. 189). Standards on domiciliary care were also issued to providers in England (DoH, 2003e). It was acknowledged as a difficult area to regulate. Even so, the standards cover a range of areas including user focus, needs-assessment, meeting needs and responsiveness, contracts, confidentiality, privacy and dignity, autonomy and independence, medication, health and safety, protection from theft and abuse, and record-keeping, as well as a range of staffing and organisational issues.

Local care charters were issued that included standards which could be used as a basis for reviewing performance. These documents, which superseded the community care charters of the 1990s, were meant to inform users and carers about what they could expect from local housing, health and social services, and what recourse they had if these expectations were not met. The charters were required to cover six areas: helping users and carers find out about services, understanding and responding to their needs; finding a suitable place to live, helping people to live independently; getting the right health care; and helping carers to care.

The Social care workforce

Notwithstanding the dedication of people working in social care, the overall quality of the social care workforce has long been a concern. This has been underlined by high-profile service failures, coupled with an acknowledgement that the sector has a low proportion of appropriately trained staff, low pay and poor morale. The Blair Government introduced a number of measures with regard to practice standards and the social care workforce (see Cm 4169, 1998; DoH, 2000l).

A Social Care Institute for Excellence was introduced in 2001 to promote high standards of practice based on evidence and experience. It was expected to produce and disseminate guidelines on social care practice and service provision. A General Social Care Council (GSCC) was established in England to regulate standards in social care, with similar bodies being established in Wales and Scotland. The GSCC, which has a lay majority, sets standards for practice and conduct, and is responsible for the registration of qualified care workers, such as social workers. It also regulates social work education. A further organisation, the Training Organisation for Personal Social Services (TOPSS) was established to maintain occupational standards underpinning social care qualifications, identifying training needs, and ensuring that these needs are met. The main vehicle for linking occupational standards with qualifications were Care NVQs (National Vocational Qualifications). Meanwhile, the qualification criteria for new social workers changed with the extension of basic social work training from a two-year diploma to a three-year honours degree course from 2003.

It is impossible to assess the impact of these reforms as they are at such an early stage. However, concerns about social care workforce and training issues has persisted. The King's Fund Care and Support Inquiry, for example, challenged what it saw as the current faith in Care NVQs (Henwood, 2001). It argued for a major overhaul of the assessment and verification of NVQs to ensure that they were sound and reliable indicators of competence. This inquiry also expressed concern about the impact of financial pressures on training and staff development, and recommended new incentives to encourage employers and employees to develop skills. Finally, it called for efforts to improve the image and status of social care work, and to improve recruitment and retention – including improved pay and conditions.

Monitoring and performance management

The Blair Government changed the way in which social care was monitored. In England, a new performance assessment framework was introduced, based on performance indicators (see Humphrey, 2003). This was later accompanied by a star rating system, similar to that used in the NHS in England. Councils that performed well on the star rating system (achieving three stars) were promised greater autonomy and a 'lighter touch' from central government. The worst performers (no stars) could expect closer scrutiny and more intervention. The first star ratings for social services departments were published in 2002, and were based on key performance indicators and qualitative data generated by service inspections and reviews undertaken by SSI and the Audit Commission (Cutler and Waine, 2003).

Another element in an increasingly centralised performance management system is 'Best Value'. The Blair Government introduced a statutory duty of Best Value on local authorities in 2000, to replace the competitive tendering regime imposed by the previous Government. This forced local authorities to scrutinise the cost-effectiveness of their services and how economies and improvements could be achieved. This was integrated into the performance management regime in the form of joint Best Value inspections, undertaken by SSI and the Audit Commission. This provided further information about the performance of local services, and created pressures to conform with central government policies (see Maile and Hoggett, 2001; Geddes and Martin, 2000).

These new systems of performance management have been criticised on several grounds. First, it is argued that the performance indicators used are crude and based on poor-quality information (Humphrey, 2003). The star ratings have attracted particularly strong criticism on these grounds. Reliance on a small number of quantitative measures can be misleading, while qualitative data – based on reviews which are themselves open to subjective and inconsistent assessment – can be inaccurate (Cutler and Waine, 2003). Secondly, the system is geared towards shifting the blame for failure to the local level, while increasing central control, which is bad for accountability (Humphrey, 2003; Cutler and Waine, 2003). Thirdly, despite the rhetoric which places equal emphasis on economy and improved quality, it is clear that, in practice, cost is the crucial factor (Humphrey, 2003). Indeed, the Best Value regime has been criticised for placing too much emphasis on cost reduction over quality improvement (Henwood, 2001).

Fair access

As already explained, a raft of measures addressed the problems of fair access to health care (Chapter 8). In social care, the public/private mix, both in the supply of and payment for services is greater than in the NHS, making equity more problematic. It is also an area where the reservoir of unmet need is believed to be even greater than in health care, implying greater selectivity and targeting of services. Rather than setting access targets, the Government's initiative – Fair Access to Care Services (FACS) – introduced guidance about how councils should establish and operate criteria on eligibility for services (DoH, 2001t). The guidance did not require them to adopt identical criteria on eligibility, as this would have stimulated demands for equal treatment from users. Instead, the guidance set out a common framework which councils must adopt when establishing their own eligibility criteria. The framework was based on the impact of services on the risk to independence: critical (e.g. life-threatening); substantial (e.g. abuse or neglect has or will occur); moderate (e.g. inability to carry out several personal care routines); and low (e.g. inability to carry out one or two personal routines). Councils were told that when devising and using their eligibility criteria, and in determining eligibility for individuals, they must prioritise those with greatest immediate and longer-term needs. The framework stressed that assessment procedures should be co-ordinated and integrated across local agencies and should not discriminate against individuals unfairly. It emphasised the importance of care plans to record assessed needs and risks, outcomes, contingency plans, service provided, contributions and charges, and dates for review. Finally, the importance of risk assessment and prevention was highlighted.

While the framework pressed councils to adopt a more explicit and systematic approach to eligibility, it did not deal with the problem of variations in access between different areas, nor did it explicitly address inequities arising from socio-economic or ethnic status. Indeed, variations in access to social care still depended largely on the amount of public funding for social care services, and the willingness and ability of people to pay for private care services.

Policies for Specific Care Groups

In addition to its policies on health and social care, the Blair Government introduced strategies and service frameworks for specific care groups, such as the elderly, people with mental illness, people with learning disabilities, and children. It also developed policies for the users of social care and their carers (see also Exhibit 12.1).

Elderly People

The National Service Framework (NSF) for older people was introduced in England in 2001 (DoH, 2001e), with other parts of the UK adopting similar strategies. The NSF outlined a ten-year programme and identified eight service standards:

- *Age discrimination*: health and social care services provided on the basis of need, not age.

- *Person-centred care*: integrating health and social care and enabling older people to make choices.

- *Intermediate care services*: (see Exhibit 11.3).

- *General hospital care for older people*: delivered through appropriate specialist care and skilled staff.

- *Stroke prevention*: the NHS working in partnership with other relevant agencies.

- *Falls*: the NHS working in partnership with councils to prevent falls and fractures in older people, and providing effective treatment and rehabilitation, as well as prevention advice through a specialised falls service.

- *Older people with mental health problems*: to have access to integrated mental health services.

- *The promotion of active, healthy life in older people*: promoted through a coordinated programme involving councils, led by the NHS.

The NSF set key interventions and milestones. These included: audits of age-related access policies by October 2001; a single assessment process by April 2002 and a single community equipment service by April 2004; the appointment of joint intermediate care co-ordinators in each health authority by July 2001; all general hospitals to have identified an 'old-age' specialist multidisciplinary team and lead nursing responsibilities for elderly people by 2002; all general hospitals to introduce a specialised stroke service by 2004 and all hospitals caring for stroke patients to follow Royal College of Physicians clinical guidelines; all health and social care systems to have an integrated falls service by 2005, and by 2004 to have agreed protocols on the management and care of mental health problems in the elderly (as well as service plans that included the development of an integrated mental health service for older people). In addition, local plans were expected to include a programme to promote healthy ageing and to prevent disease by April 2003, with local health systems improving the health and wellbeing of elderly people in several areas, including flu-immunisation, smoking cessation and blood pressure management, by April 2004. A commitment was also made to improve the management of medicines, including medicine reviews for elderly people and new systems to extend pharmacists' role in helping and advising them.

The NSF for Older People raised the profile of services for older people and emphasised the importance for this particular group of joint working between different agencies and professions (see Glasby and Littlechild, 2004). This was further enhanced by the appointment of a national clinical director for older people's services, complemented by local 'champions' and teams to lead and co-ordinate implementation. According to the Department of Health (DoH, 2003f), early improvements included a review of written policies in the NHS to ensure they did not discriminate against older people. Such action has not, however, provided a guarantee against age discrimination (see Roberts, Robinson and Seymour, 2002). Progress was also made in intermediate care (see Exhibit 11.3). There was also a fall of 1500 in the number of patients experiencing delayed discharge. Those receiving intensive home care services reportedly increased from 72,300 to 77,400 between 2001 and 2002. Other achievements reported included an increase in the proportion of hospitals with stroke units and in the uptake of flu-vaccination among the over-65s.

Exhibit 11.3 Intermediate Care

When people with complex health and social needs are cared for outside hospital, they need a co-ordinated network of good-quality health and social care services to support them. Although this has long been acknowledged, concerted efforts to develop such a network are relatively recent. The imperative to improve cost-effectiveness and throughput in the hospital sector, coupled with the introduction of national service frameworks for elderly and mentally ill people, have focused attention on practical ways of reducing pressure on

⟶

Exhibit 11.3 continued

$\longrightarrow$

hospital services, hence the official backing for intermediate care, defined by the Department of Health (DoH, 2002m, p. 3) as 'a range of integrated services to provide faster recovery from illness, prevent unnecessary acute hospital admission, support timely discharge and maximise independent living'.

The NHS Plan outlined several commitments, including an additional 5000 intermediate care beds by 2003/4, 1700 'places' in non-residential homes, and an expansion in rapid response and admission prevention to a further 70,000 people. By 2003, an additional 3300 intermediate care places had been created, according to the Department of Health (DoH, 2003f). The main focus of intermediate care was on the elderly, though it is of relevance to other groups, including people with mental illness and physical disabilities. Intermediate care schemes vary considerably (Vaughan and Lathlean, 1999), though their principal aim is comprehensive assessment of health and social care needs and appropriate care and rehabilitation services. They are based on local partnerships between different agencies – social services, the NHS and the independent sector – and involve different professional groups.

In England, intermediate care was further clarified as services that meet all the following criteria:

- are targeted at people facing unnecessarily prolonged hospital stays or inappropriate admission to acute in-patient care, long-term residential care, or continuing NHS in-patient care
- are provided on the basis of a comprehensive assessment, resulting in a structured individual care plan that involves active therapy, treatment or opportunity for recovery
- have a planned outcome of maximising independence and enabling patients to resume living at home
- are time-limited, normally no longer than six weeks (and frequently as little as one to two weeks, or less)
- involve cross-professional working, with a single assessment framework, single professional records and shared protocols

Although the development of intermediate care services is generally viewed positively, there have been criticisms, including insufficient funding (Moore, 2002). Although the NHS Plan announced that £900 million would be allocated to the development of such services, less than a third was allocated to the NHS. Of the remainder, most was allocated to local authorities, but was not earmarked for specific use on intermediate care. Some believe that intermediate care is a form of privatisation that will accelerate the numbers cared for in the independent sector, either in nursing homes or by using private agencies to support domiciliary care. Some fear that intermediate care will reduce entitlements to free NHS care (Pollock, 2000), even though the Government stated that intermediate care (defined as lasting no longer than six weeks) would be free.

Impact of intermediate care on the workload of primary health and social care professions has also been a concern, though the evidence is unclear (Wilson and Parker, 2003). Some schemes increase workload, while others may reduce it. Doubts exist about the quality of care provided. Quicker discharge and delayed admission may have an adverse effect, particularly on frail, elderly people. There is a danger that they may be inappropriately admitted to nursing and residential homes and may have difficulty accessing the health services they need (Janzon et al., 2000). Even so, there have been positive evaluations of the efficacy of some services (such as Hospital at Home schemes – see Wilson et al., 1999; Jones et al., 1999; Shepperd et al., 1998a, 1998b), while others have been negative on both efficacy and cost grounds (Steiner et al., 2001).

Even so, problems became apparent. In some areas, joint assessment proved problematic, with confusion over objectives, roles and responsibilities. Indeed, the deadline for single assessment was revised to 2004. Despite implementation problems, benefits to users seem to have accrued, including the identification of unmet needs and access to financial help (Drennan et al., 2003). Moreover, the requirement to produce a single assessment process appears to have stimulated local debates about interprofessional and interagency relationships, and how best to improve services for older people (Audit Commission, 2002e).

Change has been slow. The Social Services Inspectorate (2002) found that councils generally worked well with health agencies and that services continued to improve, but criticised the rate of change at an operational level. Complaints about inconsistency and unreliability of domiciliary services were found. This report identified problems with commissioning and assessment processes, and noted that care plans were too often service-led. Serious shortfalls in monitoring and reviewing and in care packages were found, leaving many vulnerable people at risk in community settings. The SSI was also consistent with other reports (Brown, Tucker and Domokos, 2003; Audit Commission, 2002e) that improvements in information systems and technology were needed to improve care management and communication between health and social care agencies.

Mental Health

Mental health, so long a neglected area of health and social policy, was propelled up the political agenda during the 1990s (Rogers and Pilgrim, 2001). This resulted from several high-profile service failures, a number of which raised fears about public safety. The Conservative Government responded with a plan to improve services and control patients discharged into the community (Peck and Parker, 1998). Mental Health had become an official priority in the early 1990s. The Blair Government enhanced this by providing additional funding and clarified policy objectives (DoH, 1998g). These were to provide *safe* services that protected the public, *sound* services that ensured patients and carers had full access to services, and *supportive* services that worked in partnership with patients, users, carers, families and communities. In addition, a review of mental health legislation was announced. New targets for reducing suicide and undetermined injury were also introduced (Cm 4386, 1999).

An NSF for mental health was introduced in England (DoH, 1999b), and again other parts of the UK developed their own approach. The English NSF outlined service standards and models for adults up to 65 (children and the elderly were covered by other NSFs). The mental health framework covered mental health promotion, primary care, access to services, effectiveness of services, carers and suicide prevention. For each area, standards and objectives were outlined, along with details of how progress would be monitored. For example, standard two stated that 'any service user who contacts their primary health care team with a common mental health problem should have their mental health needs identified and assessed' and 'be offered effective treatments, including referral to specialist services for further assessment, treatment and care if they require it' (DoH, 1999b, p. 128).

The NSF was criticised for several reasons (see Rogers and Pilgrim, 2001, pp. 214–15): the document appeared to be an amalgam of academic and political discourse, and, as a result, lacked consistency; it legitimised the status quo and did not challenge current service arrangements; it used evidence and selectively and emphasised technological over social interventions. However, it was regarded more positively for including hitherto neglected issues such as mental health promotion and carers' needs. Moreover, the publication of the document itself underlined the importance of mental health policy as a Government priority, sending out a strong message to the NHS.

Mental health was subsequently highlighted as a core priority in the NHS Plan, and additional service targets were set (Cm 4818, 2000). A National Director for Mental Health was appointed and subsequently a National Institute for Mental Health in England established to bring together research, development and implementation of policy. In addition, the Government proposed integrated service providers in the form of care trusts. However, mental health user groups, and many professionals, were concerned that policy continued to be dominated by concerns about public safety, and, indeed, protested vigorously against proposals to reform mental health legislation on these grounds. There was also dissatisfaction about the funding of mental health services and access to effective drugs. Furthermore, it has been suggested that the objectives of NSF may be jeopardised by staff shortages in key areas (Health Committee, 2000b). However, some advances have been made: in primary care – increased provision of outreach services, early intervention teams, and home treatment services; in inpatient care – more secure beds and staffed beds available 24 hours a day. However, it has been acknowledged, even by the National Director for Mental Health, that change has been slow (Smith, 2003; see also CHI, 2003d). Over half of mental health trusts had difficulty implementing National Service Framework action plans (Audit Commission, 2003b). It appears that funds were less generous than planned and possibly diverted for other uses (Lewis, Eaton and Carlisle, 2002; Sainsbury Centre for Mental Health, 2003). Other criticisms include overemphasis on national targets for mental health over local priorities, neglect of users' needs (Carlisle, 2002; Moore, 2003d), and the low priority given to acute in-patient mental health care (Carlisle, 2003c). Finally, although collaborative working in mental health has generally improved, problems remain, with examples of poor relationships between agencies and professionals in mental health in some areas (Rosen and Jenkins, 2003).

Carers

There are an estimated 6.8 million carers aged 16 or over in Britain, 20 per cent of whom provide more than 50 hours of care a week (Maher and Green, 2002). Many carers are young (Aldridge and Becker, 2003; Becker, Dearden, and Aldridge, 2001) – 150,000 carers are under 18 – and many are elderly, with 16 per cent of people aged 65 or over having caring responsibilities. Carers themselves suffer from poor health. Over half of those caring for 20 hours a week or more reported a long-standing illness. The health of elderly carers is very poor, with around half reporting long-term illnesses that limit their activities. Almost 40 per cent of carers say their health has been affected by caring. In addition, they face many other social and economic problems, such as isolation and deprivation. Less than half those caring for over 20 hours per week are in paid employment, and many report financial problems (Child Poverty Action Group and Carers UK, 2001).

It has been estimated that carers save the economy around £57 million a year (Carers UK, 2002). But they too have important needs, and it is only recently that these have been acknowledged. Several important policy developments have occurred, beginning with the Carers (Recognition and Services) Act 1995, which gave 'regular and substantial' carers an entitlement to have their needs assessed and taken into account by local authorities. However, the legislation, while raising the profile of carers, was largely symbolic. Local authorities were reluctant to undertake separate assessments and could not be compelled to meet assessed needs (Carers National Association, 1997). Moreover, there was limited understanding and knowledge of the legislation among both managers and carers (Seddon and Robinson, 2001).

Recognising the limitations of the legislation, and influenced by an increasingly effective carers' lobby, the Blair Government introduced a national carers' strategy in 1999 (Her Majesty's Government, 1999). This had three strategic aims: *better information for carers* – including a new charter on long-term care, discussed earlier; *more support* – including the involvement of carers in planning and providing services; and *care for carers* – including a right to have their health needs met, new powers for councils to provide services to carers, and regular breaks for carers, including a new special grant for this purpose. The strategy promised additional funding (£140 million) for carers' breaks and other financial changes, including reductions in council tax, access to pensions for carers, and the possibility of increased allowances for carers in the future. Help with finding work was promised for carers of working age, and additional support was promised for young carers.

The strategy promised further legislation. Subsequently, the Carers and Disabled Children Act (2000) gave carers a right to an assessment in their own right, independent of any assessment of the person for whom they were caring.

It also empowered local authorities to provide services direct to carers following assessment, and to make direct payments to carers for services that met their assessed needs, extending a scheme introduced earlier for service users. Direct payments, discussed more fully in Chapter 12 in the context of patient and user involvement, allow individuals to purchase their own care and support. The Act also enabled local authorities to operate a voucher system for carers needing short-term breaks. In addition, local authorities were permitted to charge for services to carers, providing they did this in a reasonable way.

Despite the fanfare surrounding its introduction, the strategy initially had a limited impact (Lloyd, 2000). One survey found positive changes alongside continuing problems (Carers UK, 2003). Direct payments were viewed positively, though some carers experienced problems with managing payments. Some people appeared to be getting more help with respite care. For those carers with health problems, most assessments covered their health. However, most respondents claimed they were not getting necessary help, though in some cases this was because the person cared for was refusing assistance from other people. Only a third had actually received a carer's assessment. Of these, problems experienced included a failure to assess the need for carers' breaks. Just under two-fifths experienced an increase in services (though not all assessments call for an increase). Another report had earlier found that the Carers' Special Grant was helping to promote and realise breaks for carers, though local implementation was variable (Banks and Roberts, 2001). It also reported that the new grant was stimulating a range of services for carers and bringing carers' issues into mainstream service planning.

Learning Disabilities

Learning disabilities, which affect around 2 per cent of the population, have been defined as 'a lifelong condition which reduces a person's ability to understand new or complex information, to learn new skills and to cope with life independently' (King's Fund, 1999, p. 1). This has been a neglected area, indicated by the 30-year gap between the two key policy documents: *Better Services for the Mentally Handicapped* (Cmnd 4683, 1971) and *Valuing People: A New Strategy for Learning Disability for the 21st Century* (Cmnd 5806, 2001).

As in other areas of social care, the key policy objective has been to move away from large institutional provision. Most people with learning difficulties now live in hostels, flats and shared houses, or with their families. Support is community-based, and includes social care provided in day centres. However, there is evidence that people with learning disabilities continue to face social isolation, lack of access to health care, and problems with housing, employment and the benefits system (King's Fund, 1999).

The main themes of current policy are that more must be done to support the independence of people with learning disabilities and their integration in society. Services must be person-centred and involve users and carers in service planning and review. Government reforms promised more information for carers, a new advocacy network and additional funding for advocacy groups. An expansion of direct payment schemes among people with learning disabilities was also endorsed. Another important theme was collaboration. As with other groups, such as the elderly and mentally ill people, health and local authorities are expected to draw up joint investment plans to improve services for people with learning difficulties. In addition, local authorities with social service responsibilities are expected to establish partnership boards in this field (including representatives from health agencies and the voluntary sector). New funds were announced to support service developments and research. Finally, there was a commitment to improve housing and employment opportunities for people with learning disabilities. With regard to housing, improved provision of advice and information by housing authorities was promised, alongside new systems of allocating housing-related support announced in *Supporting People* (Department of the Environment, Transport and the Regions, 2001). With regard to unemployment, new targets for increasing the numbers of people with learning disability in work were introduced, alongside changes to the Government's support programme for disabled workers.

Scotland and Wales have their own programmes for people with learning disabilities (Scottish Executive, 2000b; National Assembly for Wales, 2001b). These have similar objectives as in England, namely to increase independent living, to improve collaboration between agencies, to improve the responsiveness of services to individual needs, and to promote better integration in society.

Children and Young People

Since 1997 children and young people have been at the centre of many policy initiatives. These include policies aimed at tackling social exclusion and poverty, policies on the family, and policies affecting the health of children and young people, such as those on smoking, drugs and food, and sexual health. In addition, various schemes were introduced to improve services for children, including programmes such as the National Childcare Strategy (Harker, 1998), and *Sure Start*, which aimed to improve access to child care, health, early education and support for children aged under four and their families in disadvantaged areas.

These various initiatives did little to address the variable quality of health services for children. In children and adolescent mental health services, for example, the Audit Commission (1999b) found a wide variation in expenditure on services between different areas that was unrelated to needs. During the late 1990s the Bristol case exposed the variable standards of children's cardiac surgery. To improve the overall standards of children's health care, the Government proposed a national service framework. In England, the NSF focused on six areas: acute and hospital services; maternity services and babies; children in special circumstances; mental health; children with disabilities and long term illness; healthy children and young people. The standard for hospital services, published in 2003 (DoH, 2003g), covered the design and delivery of hospital services around the needs of children and families; the quality and safety of hospital services; and the suitability of hospital services for the care of children. Wales has developed a children's NSF along similar lines to England, while Scotland has a separate strategy for children's health which emphasises the need for a combined children's health service; integrated services across health, local authority and other service providers; the appointment of child commissioners in NHS boards; and local child health strategies and implementation plans.

Meanwhile, long-standing concerns about social care for children, culminated in the Victoria Climbié inquiry (Cm 5730, 2003). The inquiry, which investigated the abuse and murder of a little girl by her aunt and partner, followed other similar investigations by uncovering evidence of poor co-ordination between services. It also found a failure to pass on information, weak accountability, poor management, lack of staff capacity, inadequate training, and staff shortages. Efforts to improve services had already been undertaken in England, most recently by the *Quality Protects* initiative introduced in 1998. This included interagency guidance to safeguard children, and a new framework for assessing the needs of children and their families. With regard to residential care, also plagued by high-profile scandals (Utting, 1997), standards were brought within the remit of the National Care Standards Commission

In response to the Climbié inquiry, the Government proposed a reform programme (Cm 5860, 2003). Local authority children's services, education and social services would be brought under a single director and a lead council member held responsible for all children's services. At national level, an independent children's commissioner would be appointed, a post already established in Wales. Scotland also decided to introduce an independent commissioner for children and young people (Scottish Executive, 2000c). Ministerial responsibility for children, young people and families was consolidated into a single post within the Department for Education and Skills, though health and social care responsibilities for children remained with the Department of Health. To promote effective joint working at local level, new duties were proposed for agencies such as the police, health, education and social care bodies to safeguard children and promote their wellbeing. Councils, primary care trusts and other bodies were to be given powers to create children's trusts, to bring together child health, education and welfare functions (see Hudson, 2003), an idea similar to care trusts. It was envisaged that professionals, such as teachers, social workers and health professionals, would be brought together in multidisciplinary teams based in schools and community-based children's centres. Common training for professionals involved in child care was also proposed, alongside a workforce strategy to encourage recruitment and retention of child-care workers. Although this initiative is at an early stage, there are concerns that reorganisation could lead to even more upheaval and disruption of services.

Conclusion

At national level there has been much activity in terms of new policies and reforms in health and social care. These have been general – concerning health and social care policy across all client groups – as well as specific to the needs of particular groups such as the elderly, mentally ill people, children, and people with learning disabilities. At local level, efforts are being made to integrate services more effectively and promote independent living among service users. But much remains to be done. There is a long history of both policy activity at national level and local initiatives coming to little. A great deal depends on central government maintaining its emphasis on these areas and providing the necessary framework, including resources. Also of great importance is the willingness and ability of local health and social care agencies to work together effectively in response to the needs of service users and their carers. As this chapter has indicated there is still much to do to bring about the kind of seamless service that central government, and service users and carers, desire.

_____ *Further Reading* _____

Bamford, T. (2001) *Commissioning and Purchasing* (London, Routledge).

Glasby, J. and Littlechild, R. (2004) (2nd edn) *The Health and Social Care Divide – The Experiences of Older People* (Bristol, Policy Press).

Glasby, J. and Peck, E. (2003) *Care Trusts: Partnership Working in Action* (Abingdon, Radcliffe Medical).

Hudson, B. (ed.) (2000) *The Changing Role of Social Care* (London, Jessica Kingsley).

Lewis, J. and Glennerster, H. (1996) *Implementing the New Community Care* (Buckingham, Open University Press).

Means, R., Richards, S. and Smith, R. (2003) *Community Care: Policy and Practice*, 3rd edn (Basingstoke, Palgrave Macmillan).

Patient and Public Involvement

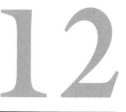

During the 1990s, concerns about a 'democratic deficit' in the NHS centred on the inadequacy of existing mechanisms to involve patients and the public in decision-making (Cooper et al., 1995). A series of health scandals – notably the Bristol case – led to calls for stronger accountability to patients. Indeed the Bristol inquiry recommended that the involvement of the public in the NHS must be embedded in its structures, and that perspectives of patients and the public must be taken into account in decisions about the provision of health care. Meanwhile, patients appeared less deferential towards professionals and more willing to complain and seek redress. It was also believed that they were becoming more like consumers, seeking out information and wishing to exercise greater choice in health care. This chapter examines the reaction to these trends by exploring the development of policies on patient and public involvement, complaints and advocacy, and patient choice.

Watchdogs, Advocates and Complaints

Community Health Councils

From the inception of the NHS, lay representatives have been appointed to health authorities and boards. However, these are regarded as fairly weak mechanisms of representation and accountability. While lay representatives can introduce a 'public perspective', they are appointed under ministerial authority and not perceived as independent. To strengthen the voice of the community in the NHS, Community Health Councils (CHCs) were established in 1974 in England and Wales (Klein and Lewis, 1976). Similar bodies were created in Scotland and Northern Ireland. As well as their representative function, CHCs undertook other roles: monitoring local services, informing the public about services, and assisting with complaints. In addition, health service organisations had to consult them when considering substantial changes in services.

Exhibit 12.1 User and Carer Involvement in Social Care

User and carer involvement has been promoted in social care as well as health care. Pressures to strengthen the role of users arose from several sources (see Bamford, 2001): first, the emphasis placed on the social model of disability, which highlights disabled people's rights and choices, independent living, and the need to challenge prejudice, discrimination and paternalism in the provision of services and in society (Oliver, 1990); secondly, the rise of organisations representing disabled people, people with mental illness and learning disabilities and other marginalised groups, such as the elderly; thirdly, the managerial agenda, which placed greater emphasis on service outcomes, and user-satisfaction measures.

These trends encouraged the involvement of carers. The social model of disability champions carers by highlighting their need for support (Bamford, 2001). Carers have become extremely well organised and lobbied effectively for recognition (see Chapter 11). Although they are also seen as proxy users when service users are severely incapacitated, it must be recognised that carers' and users' views are not identical and there are tensions between them (see Rogers and Pilgrim, 2001, with regard to mental health).

The views of users and carers can be surveyed. They can be consulted about services individually or in groups. Representatives of user or carer organisations can be included on advisory or decision-making fora. It is generally acknowledged that users' and carers' views are stronger when expressed collectively and can be influential (Barnes et al., 1999). However, it is also acknowledged that user/carer group representatives can be isolated when in a minority on committees (Bamford, 2001), and their representativeness may be called into question. Moreover, user (and carer) organisations can be undermined by unstable funding regimes and limited human resources (Barnes et al., 1999). The fact that such groups include chronically ill people can affect the continuity of representation (see also Rhodes and Small, 2001). Groups can be manipulated by managers and professionals, who may adopt a selective approach to user/carer involvement, accepting groups when it suits them and ignoring them when not (Barnes et al., 1999).

Users and carers can be involved directly in the management or commissioning of services (Bamford, 2001). Services can be delegated to voluntary organisations run by users and/or carers, though there are tensions between the roles of service provider and citizen advocacy. Another approach is to delegate the payments for care services to the individual service user or carer. Such schemes, known as direct payment schemes, have been encouraged in recent years. In 1996 the Community Care Direct Payments Act enabled local councils to transfer resources direct to disabled people once their needs had been assessed. This has been described as 'a real transfer of power from professionals to users' (Bamford, 2001, p. 43). Even so, as the scheme is not mandatory, implementation has been slow and only a few thousand people benefited from such schemes in the first five years. More could be done to encourage the take-up of direct payment (Bamford, 2001; Henwood, 2001), including better and more widely available information that is geared to the needs of users, as well as better support and advice for those wishing to use direct payment schemes. Measures to improve take-up have included a national information campaign, the extension of direct payments to adults over 65 (following a recommendation from the Royal Commission on Long Term care – see Chapter 11; and to carers (following the Carers and Disabled Children Act 2000).

CHCs' activities were limited by small budgets relative to the demands placed upon them (Moon and Lupton, 1995). Their independence was threatened, particularly when challenging unpopular decisions (Hogg, 1986; Hunter, 1995). Occasionally, their very existence was in doubt. Governments – both Conservative and Labour – questioned the wisdom of funding organisations that publicised problems and exposed flaws in their policies. The CHCs' national body – the Association of Community Health Councils of England and Wales (ACHCEW) – was a particular irritant, exposing long waiting times and other shortcomings in services.

The development of health service commissioning during the 1990s offered new opportunities for CHCs to become involved in priority-setting, identifying needs, monitoring compliance with contracts, and quality assurance. But they were wary, believing they could become incorporated in these processes and lose independence. But failure to engage actually led them to be further marginalised (Pickard, 1997). Meanwhile, the development of new methods of gauging public views on health care, such as citizens' juries, focus groups and surveys, compounded this marginalisation.

The effectiveness of CHCs was called into question, though much of this was unfair. They were under-resourced. Their legal powers were restricted, particularly with regard to primary care. They had poor access to information and could be excluded from key meetings. While some CHCs were ineffective, they were not in the majority. In general they provided a valuable service for local people needing advice and assistance – particularly with complaints – and were a rallying point for those unhappy with the NHS.

Politically, CHCs were weak, and both their supporters and detractors acknowledged that a review of their function was overdue. A review did take place in the mid-1990s, but was shelved (Insight Management Consulting, 1996). However, in 2000, the Blair Government decided to replace CHCs in England with a new statutory system of patient and public involvement. CHCs and ACHCEW mounted a rearguard action, which delayed parts of the intended legislation until after the 2001 general election. Subsequently, some compromises were reached, but CHCs did not survive. The new statutory framework in England that replaced them is discussed later in this chapter. Notably, CHCs survived in Wales, and indeed were promised stronger powers.

The Health Service Commissioner

The health service commissioner, also known as the 'health ombudsman', investigates complaints about the NHS from the public regarding hardship, injustice, maladministration and service failure, including failure to provide a service. Currently, the English and Welsh health ombudsman posts are held by the same person. This person also acts as the parliamentary ombudsman and Welsh administration ombudsman, investigating complaints about government departments and public bodies. In Scotland, the health commissioner role is undertaken by the Scottish public services ombudsman, who examines complaints about all Government departments, public bodies and local government organisations. Northern Ireland also has an ombudsman to consider complaints about certain public bodies, including the NHS.

The health ombudsmen are independent of both Government and the NHS. However, their powers of investigation are limited (Giddings, 1993). They may not examine cases that are likely to come before a tribunal or the courts, and can only act when the earlier stages of the NHS complaints procedure – discussed below – have been exhausted. Indeed, most of complaints made to the ombudsman for England are rejected because they are premature or lie outside her jurisdiction (Health Service Commissioner, England, 2003b). Another problem is the lack of jurisdiction over local government issues. Unlike Scotland, there is a separate system of local ombudsmen in England and Wales. However, there is increasing co-operation here between health and local government ombudsmen on cases involving both health and social care. Private health care mostly lies outside the remit of the health ombudsmen, though care of NHS patients in private hospitals is covered (private medical care in NHS hospitals is not). Prior to 1996, when a new complaints procedure was established, ombudsmen could not examine clinical complaints, nor cases relating to family practitioner services. But now all aspects of the NHS except personnel issues are included within their remit.

Although ombudsmen can recommend compensation and redress, they cannot force a health service organisation to act. The only weapon currently available is bad publicity, which, given the level of media interest in the ombudsmen's reports, can elicit a response. The ombudsmen may exert further pressure by revisiting cases where there has been inaction. Furthermore, in England, the ombudsman's work is scrutinised by the House of Commons' Select Committee on Public Administration, which can cross-examine those who have ignored earlier recommendations.

Complaints Procedures

The Health ombudsmen are at the pinnacle of the NHS complaints system, and only a small proportion of complaints reach them. In 2002–3 the NHS in England received over 90,000 written complaints about hospital and community services and over 40,000 about family health services, but fewer than 4,000 complaints were received by the health ombudsman for England, of which fewer than two hundred were accepted for investigation. Even if a complaint falls within the remit, further investigation will only take place if added value is likely. Investigations focus on cases where the earlier stages of the complaints process have failed and where more can be achieved for the complainant. It is to these earlier stages that we now turn.

The present system owes much to an inquiry by the Wilson committee, established in the 1990s following criticism from professional groups and consumer organisations about the deficiencies of the existing system (DoH, 1994c). In 1996, the committee's recommendations led to the introduction of a three-stage national complaints system covering all types of complaint (clinical and non-clinical matters), replacing the complex array of procedures that previously existed (DoH, 1995d).

Stage one of the new procedure was called *local resolution*. Its underlying principles were that complaints should be resolved closest to the level at which the problem had occurred, and in a way that was flexible, fair and conciliatory. So, with regard to family health services, the individual practice became responsible for local resolution. In the case of health authorities, trusts and subsequently PCTs, initial responsibility for complaints was given to front-line staff and their managers, with complaints managers and chief executives becoming more closely involved in the more serious and complex cases. The chief executive of the organisation was required to give a written reply to each written complaint, though, as health ombudsman reports have shown, this does not always happen in practice.

Approximately 3 per cent of complainants took matters to the next stage – known as *independent review*. Dissatisfied complainants could request that the organisation with overall responsibility for the service consider establishing an independent review panel to examine the complaint. The procedure as introduced in 1996 was as follows. A non-executive member of the health authority, trust or PCT would be designated as a convenor for each case and would be expected to consult with an independent lay person, drawn from a list of suitable candidates. If satisfied that the complaint was not associated with any impending legal action, and that there was potential for the issue to be resolved by independent review, a review panel would be established. Alternatively, the case could be sent back to the local resolution stage, or other avenues, such as conciliation between the parties, might be attempted.

If an independent review was to proceed, an independent lay person (usually the person consulted by the convenor) would chair the panel. The convenor would also serve on the panel, along with other nominees and lay representatives, the exact composition depending on whether the organisation establishing the review was a health authority, trust or PCT. Where complaints involved clinical judgement, it was required that appropriately qualified assessors be appointed to advise the panel.

The independent review panel took evidence from the various parties (such as the complainant and the professionals involved) and produced a report, a copy of which was sent to the complainant and the relevant chief executive. The latter was required to write to the complainant setting out what action if any would be taken. Targets were set for the completion of reviews. For example, health authority and trust complaints should be completed within 120 days.

It proved difficult to meet these targets, largely because of the shortage of independent reviewers and clinical assessors, and the difficulty of arranging mutually convenient times for meetings.

If complainants remained dissatisfied, either because of a refusal to grant an independent review, or because they disagreed with its conclusions and recommendations, they could ask the health ombudsman to investigate the complaint. The ombudsmen can also respond to complaints by staff about unjust treatment in the investigation of a complaint. They may comment on the overall workings of the NHS complaints procedure as well. For example, the English ombudsman has been very critical and has argued that the procedure is too complicated and time-consuming, that independent review panels are not perceived as independent, and that there is a reluctance to give financial redress. Consequently, the ombudsman recommended stricter time limits on local resolution, 'fast-tracking' of cases where local resolution had been effective, and a code of practice on redress (Health Service Commissioner for England, 2002).

Others, too, voiced discontent. A report from the Scottish Association of Health Councils (1998), was sceptical about the independence of the convenors in the independent review procedure. The Health Committee (1999c) recommended that the role of convenors be abolished, enabling patients and carers to appeal directly to an independent review panel. The committee also wanted a system that could fast-track complaints alleging serious shortcomings in performance. Wallace and Mulcahy (1999) also criticised the role of convenors and recommended fast-tracking of cases that had implications for patient safety. They called for explicit guidance on the rules and conduct of panels, procedures for monitoring the implementation of panel recommendations, better support for complainants, and regional complaints centres to handle independent reviews.

In 1999 the Blair Government initiated a review of the complaints procedure. An evaluation of the current system (System Three Social Research/York Health Economics Consortium, 2001) found high levels of dissatisfaction among complainants with both local resolution and independent review. Only a small minority believed their complaint had been handled well. The main causes of dissatisfaction included poor attitudes of staff, poor communication, lack of support and information, and a lack of independence of the review process, particularly regarding the role of convenor. In contrast, most staff who had been complained against were broadly satisfied with the process. Among those operating the complaints process, the main concerns were a perceived lack of independence, the time and cost involved in operating the system, the difficulty of completing reviews on time, and the need to improve the link between complaints and action. The evaluation report made a number of recommendations, including a uniform procedure for primary care and hospital services, clear guidance on the application of the complaints procedure, a stronger link between clinical governance and complaints, clearer lines of responsibility for the performance of complaints systems, and standardised financial and administrative support. The report also recommended improvements in independent review, including the development of consistent criteria for convening review panels, new ways of convening panels, regional bodies (or a new independent national authority) to hold panels to account, wider powers for panels to summon witnesses, and steps to ensure implementation of remedial action.

Following a long delay, new proposals for England emerged (DoH, 2003h). The new Commission for Healthcare Audit and Inspection (CHAI) was given responsibility for the independent scrutiny of complaints, while the health ombudsman's role at the top of the system would remain. It made sense to involve CHAI as it was already responsible for clinical governance, raising the prospect of a closer link between complaints and service improvement. The new system also held the possibility of referring complex or urgent cases more quickly to the heath ombudsman. Another possible advantage was a closer link with complaints about social care, under the remit of another new body, the Commission for Social Care Inspection, with which CHAI was expected to work closely. Less optimistically, CHAI and CSCI faced crowded agenda and it was unclear where complaints would be in their order of priorities. Moreover, CHAI was a national body, at some distance from where complaints arose. It would also come to this area with no previous experience of complaints handling (Health Service Commissioner for England, 2003b).

Other parts of the UK responded differently. In Wales (NHS Wales, 2003), a new independent review secretariat accountable to the Welsh Assembly was established. Independent lay reviewers and clinical assessors are appointed by this secretariat. Local health boards and trusts are expected to establish procedures for the overview and management of complaints and required to produce action plans following reports from independent panels. In addition, local health boards are expected to help family practitioner services establish effective complaints procedures, facilitate local resolution, and follow up independent review panel reports about services. CHCs, which survived in Wales, were given a greater role in providing independent advocacy to those wishing to complain. At the time of writing, the policy on complaints in Scotland has not been finalised, though it is likely that new responsibilities will be placed on local NHS bodies to guarantee patient feedback and effective local resolution of complaints. In addition, support and information services for people wishing to raise concerns and make complaints will probably be strengthened. It is also likely that, as in England and in Wales, the responsibility for independent review will be taken away from local health bodies, and given either to a new national complaints authority or transferred direct to the Scottish ombudsman (see Scottish Executive, 2003b).

New Patient Advice and Advocacy Services

Meanwhile, in England, a new service to advise and inform patients was introduced. The NHS Plan announced the creation of a Patient Advocacy and

Liaison Service (PALS) in every trust by 2002. The aim of PALS was to establish an identifiable person if people had a problem or needed information. The scheme built on local projects, such as in Brighton, where the introduction of a patient advocacy service was believed to have reduced complaints and promoted changes in training, care delivery and facilities (Dunman, 2001).

PALS services were introduced in a number of trusts and PCTs during 2001. Following concerns about confusion with independent advocacy services, discussed later in this chapter, their name was changed to Patient *Advice* and Liaison Services. PALS core functions were as follows (DoH, 2002p; 2003i): to be identifiable and accessible to patients, carers, friends and families; to provide on-the-spot help and agree immediate to speedy resolution of problems; to provide relevant information or support; to act as a gateway to independent advice and advocacy support; to act as a catalyst for improving services, linking closely with clinical governance systems; to support staff in developing a culture more responsive to patients and their families; to promote a seamless service, with PCT PALS leading on issues cutting across primary, secondary and social care.

Evaluations of PALS were mainly anecdotal, citing good practice – usually improvements in services that had followed contacts with patients or relatives. Few evaluations collected data systematically. An exception was the evaluation of the PALS pathfinder at George Eliot Hospital NHS Trust by Baggott and Buchanan (2002). This study found that the service was well received by stakeholders, such as patients groups and staff; almost all queries were resolved within ten working days; and official complaints had fallen by 9 per cent since the implementation of the scheme. The service appeared to reduce staff defensiveness when dealing with patients' concerns, though it was too early to say whether cultural change was taking place. It was also recognised that PALS had a role to play in triggering specific improvements, alongside other mechanisms such as complaints and clinical governance processes. Meanwhile, a review of PALS in London (NHSE London Regional Office, SILKAP Consultants, 2001) found that they had been positively received by staff and users, and that they helped to create a more open and responsive culture. It identified ways of improving PALS, including better training for PALS staff, more explicit structural links within the trust to provide feedback on services, closer links with the trusts' public involvement activities, efforts to improve cultural-awareness skills and translation services, and improvements in local relationships with other PALS, PCTs and hospitals. Research by Kirkcaldy, Robinson and Perkins (2003) into PALS in the north-west of England found that these services facilitated quick resolution of concerns, but a more consistent service needed to be developed across different sites. This study also found that some PALS were more accessible to some users than others (see also Heaton and Sloper, 2003).

Another study was highly critical of the new service (Hill and Marks, 2003), based on 100 telephone inquiries to trusts. In three cases, the trusts declared that they had no PALS service, despite having details of the service posted on their websites. Only half the calls made were answered in person by PALS staff, though over a quarter were connected to an answering service and may have been followed up later. The study judged that of the 51 calls answered in person by the PALS service, only 28 gave a credible response. Furthermore, only 72 per cent of responses provided information about independent advocacy. These findings indicated wider problems of implementation as highlighted by the Health Committee (2003b). A particular problem was that PALS services often relied on a small number of officers and volunteers, with a large workload and limited resources. In addition, there was a tendency in some trusts to offload other patient-information, liaison and feedback functions on the PALS service, so that its essential role of handling patient queries was swamped by other tasks. A further problem in some trusts was confusion arising from unclear and overlapping responsibilities among others who handled complaints, concerns and demands for information – including receptionists, complaints officers and nursing staff.

The Government acknowledged that PALS would not provide independent advocacy. In the Health and Social Care Act 2001, it introduced a statutory duty on the Secretary of State for Health to make arrangements to provide independent complaints advocacy services (ICAS). ICAS provide independent support for those wishing to complain about services, rather similar to a function previously undertaken by CHCs. This support will vary according to the individual, as some people need more assistance than others when negotiating complaints procedures. PCT patient and public involvement forums, discussed further below, will be responsible for commissioning ICAS from 2004. In the interim, ICAS were commissioned directly by the Department of Health (Cole, 2003). The decision to introduce ICAS before PCT Patient and Public Involvement Forums had been established was criticised (Health Committee, 2003b). It is also unclear how ICAS will work with PALS and existing advocacy services catering for specific client groups such as mental health service users and people with learning disabilities. In Wales, ICAS is now the responsibility of CHCs, while in Scotland it has been proposed that health boards will have the responsibility for commissioning ICAS, subject to the approval of a new national body (see below).

Patient's Charters, Choice and Consumerism

Internal Markets

The Conservative Governments of the 1980s and 1990s conceptualised patients as consumers. From this perspective, it was argued that health services had little incentive to improve performance or to respond to the needs and preferences of patients. Indeed, consumer models of health stressed the weakness of the latter (Arrow, 1963). Patients lacked information about the quality of health care and the competence of providers, they were dependent on the expertise of professionals, they were often vulnerable, and found it difficult (and in some situations impossible) to make choices about health care. Even if they could, they had few alternative providers to choose from.

The internal market, introduced by the Conservatives in the early 1990s, emphasised the importance of market forces in satisfying the needs and preferences of patients. Indeed one of the key aims of *Working for Patients* was 'to give patients, wherever they live in the UK, better health care and greater choice of the services available' (Cm 555, 1989, p. 3), while one of the key changes heralded was 'to make the Health Services more responsive to the needs of patients, as much power and responsibility as possible will be delegated to the local level' (p. 4). But the scope for patient choice remained limited in practice and competition was weak. Patients' preferences were indirectly articulated by purchasers of health care – GP fundholders and District Health Authorities. Moreover, patients and users did not act like conventional consumers of commodities, even when they did have scope for choice – such as the choice of GP for example (see Leavey, Wilkin and Metcalfe, 1989; Salisbury, 1989; Shackley and Ryan, 1994; Lupton, Donaldson and Lloyd, 1991; Thomas, Nicholl and Coleman, 1995). Private patients were able to exercise greater choice between various packages of care and providers, but even they exhibited little sign of consumerism (Calnan, Cant and Gabe, 1993). Indeed, in both the private and the public sectors, professionals and providers remained powerful relative to service users.

The Patient's Charter

Recognising the difficulties of achieving change through market forces, the Major Government introduced the *Citizen's Charter* to promote a more consumerist ethos within public service organisations (Cm 1599, 1992; Deakin, 1994), while a separate initiative – *the Patient's Charter* – was introduced into the NHS (DoH, 1991). The original charter set out national rights and service standards that patients could expect from the NHS with regard to access to services, in particular waiting times; personal consideration and respect; information; and the making of complaints. The charter was later revised (DoH, 1996a), and specific charters introduced for various groups, including children and young people, pregnant women and mentally ill people. In addition to these national charters, the Department of Health encouraged local health and social care organisations to introduce their own charters.

Although there was support for an explicit statement of rights and standards in principle, the *Patient's Charter* attracted criticism. Most of the proclaimed 'rights' were not new, such as the rights to receive emergency treatment or be registered with a GP. Many were vague, such as the right to detailed information about local health services. The rights were not enshrined and there was no way of guaranteeing them in practice. Even so, some rights were new and subjected to close scrutiny by Government, such as the right to guaranteed admission within a specified time limit – initially two years, reduced to 18 months. In the later version of the charter it was alleged that people were waiting longer than the official limits. There was no independent assessment of these statistics, and consequently great scope for manipulation (see Chapter 8). Some of the standards were vague, such as 'you can expect to be cared for in an environment that is clean and safe' (DoH, 1996a, p. 15) while others were deliberately worded to avoid an imperative. For example, patients could 'expect' to receive a written explanation of the hospital's food policy, and patients admitted to mixed sex wards 'should' have access to separate washing and toilet facilities.

Other standards related to the cancellation of operations, a named qualified nurse, midwife or health visitor for each patient, and discharge from hospital. These three areas were later identified by Bruster et al. (1994) as not meeting the *Patient's Charter* standards. Others included privacy, dignity, religious and cultural beliefs, informing relatives and friends of progress, clear explanation of proposed treatment, access to health records, signposting of premises, choice about participating in medical education and training, and guaranteed admission within two years. This research was based on patients' reported experiences rather than Government statistics. A later study (Farrell, Levenson, and Snape, 1998) found that few patients were aware of the contents of the *Patient's Charter* and that it tended to conceal rather than highlight problems that needed action. Many of the targets of the *Patient's Charter* were criticised as short-term. On a more positive note, however, it was credited with raising awareness of the needs of patients and promoting a cultural change towards a user perspective.

The *Patient's Charter* did little to empower health service users. The Blair Government initiated a review (Dyke, 1998), which recommended a more localised approach. It argued for a new charter package, rather than a single document, comprising: a clear set of values at national level along with a few key minimum service standards; local charters, expressing how these principles would be achieved, including service and process standards that would be effectively monitored; and disease-specific guides for health service users, aimed at helping them understand relevant clinical performance standards and become more active partners in their care. However, a new document '*Your Guide to the NHS*' (DoH, 2001l) was later introduced. This restated the core principles of the NHS, set out in the NHS Plan: the provision of a universal service for all, based on clinical need not ability to pay; the provision of a comprehensive range of services; shaping services around the needs and preferences of individual patients, their families and carers; responding to different needs of different populations; working continuously to improve quality services and minimise errors; supporting and valuing staff; devoting public funds solely to services for

NHS patients; working with others to provide a seamless service; keeping people healthy and working to reduce health inequalities; and respecting the confidentiality of patients and providing open access to information about services, treatment and performance. The guide emphasised that people should take responsibility for their own health and use services responsibly, including following advice on healthy lifestyles. The guide also outlined some of the key performance targets set out in the NHS Plan and elsewhere. In Wales, a new *Patient's Charter* was also developed along similar lines. A Health and Social Care Guide was published (Welsh Assembly Government, 2002a), setting out what people could expect from health and social care services now and in the future. The document also gave details on how people could get more information about health services. As well as setting out the principles on which care and treatments should be based, the document also set out responsibilities of patients. Meanwhile in Scotland, a new statement of rights and responsibilities for health service users was drafted with the assistance of consumer organisations. A final version is expected in 2004.

Elements of the *Patient's Charter* approach survived. Many of the Labour Governments' targets followed on from indicators introduced by the *Patient's Charter*. In addition, other commitments referred to in the *Patient's Charter*, on hospital discharges, cancelled operations and mixed sex wards, for example, were extended. Hospital discharge arrangements were revised and new commitments on cancelled operations included in the NHS Plan of 2000. With regard to mixed sex wards, the Blair Government continued its predecessor's drive to eliminate them – though this had still not been achieved at the time of writing (Moore, 2003c).

New Imperatives

The Blair Government did not abandon the consumerist approach of its predecessor (Crinson, 1998), but extended it. It introduced new services heralded as being more responsive to patients' needs and preferences, such as NHS Direct, Walk-in Centres, and the increased use of booking systems in primary care (see Chapter 10). It began to emphasise the importance of making the NHS more 'patient-centred', in part a response to the Bristol case and other scandals. Coupled with this was another imperative. The Government interpreted public dissatisfaction with aspects of the NHS as a rationale for a more consumerist approach. Certainly people were unhappy with waiting times for treatment, for example. But there was nothing new in this, and overall dissatisfaction with the NHS was actually higher in 1991 than in 2000 (Mulligan and Appleby, 2001; Appleby and Rosete, 2003). There was evidence that the NHS could respond more effectively to the health care needs and preferences of its users. The Wanless report (2002) stated that patients wanted more involvement in decisions, more information, better explanation of tests and treatments, and more opportunities to discuss anxieties and concerns. It also acknowledged research findings that, in future, patients would expect more from the NHS, and that it would have to respond to demands for quicker, more flexible access to services, improved relationships with health care professionals, more participation in care, and high-quality and timely information (Kendall, 2001). Interestingly, Wanless did not find any evidence that choice was a current key priority for the public, but asserted that this would become more important in the future. One should beware of generalisations in this area. For example, it is acknowledged that some people have different attitudes to information and choice (Kendall, 2001) in health care. The variation in attitudes of patients was captured in research drawn on by the Wanless report (Henke, Murray and Nelson, 2002). Six different types of patients were identified: *dependers*, who depend on contact with health services for reassurance, and *anxious seekers*, motivated by fear of ill health, are both high users of services. *Stoics*, who mostly avoid health care, and *avoiders*, who are in denial until major symptoms appear, are medium users. Meanwhile the low users are the *proactives*, who have an active role in relation to their own health and have strong personal control and motivation, and *receivers*, who are trusting and passive.

The NHS Plan made several commitments to extend choice, including more information about health and health services, through NHS Direct and other sources; more information about individual care (with patients receiving copies of letters between clinicians regarding their care); and an extension of hospital booking schemes, giving patients more choice over appointment dates and times. Furthermore, NHS trusts and PCTs would be expected to survey patients' and carers' views about their services, with all NHS organisations and care homes being required to publish a patient prospectus – an annual report on views received by patients and resulting action taken. This was also expected to contain details of local services and performance ratings.

The use of consumer surveys had been encouraged since the early 1980s. The Griffiths report gave a major impetus to this approach (Allsop, 1992), as did the internal market in health care, which led health authorities to commission surveys about local priorities. The Blair Government introduced large-scale, national patient surveys. The first in 1997 collected the views about general practice, followed by surveys on coronary heart disease and cancer services. These surveys are now part of the remit of the Commission for Healthcare Audit and Inspection (CHAI) and are used to evaluate the quality of services from the patient's perspective.

Surveys of patient's views can be useful, but must have clear objectives about the scope and nature of feedback required (Draper, Cohen and Buchan, 2001). They can provide information about the quality and performance of services (Straw et al., 2000). However, they also can produce inconsistent results

(Cohen, Forbes and Garroway, 1996), may fail to pick up on the intensity of opinion on an issue, and are regarded as a relatively weak instrument for promoting change (Avis, 1997). Moreover, they are seen as clearly part of the 'market research model' (Beresford, 1988) of consumerism, and may be regarded as a narrow and flawed instrument for measuring views and preferences. Even if properly conducted, they can be manipulated. Indeed, like market research in the business world, surveys can be used to present a false image of a service, for example by reporting levels of satisfaction, rather than dissatisfaction. On the other hand, negative findings can be exaggerated and used to justify interventions. Moreover, surveys are costly to commission and take up staff time that could be spent on patient care.

Extending Choice

The Blair Government decided that NHS patients should have more choice about care and treatment. It stated that by 2005 all patients would be able to choose where they are treated, whether this be local NHS hospitals, the new diagnostic and treatment centres, private hospitals, or even hospitals abroad (DoH, 2001u). Subsequently, patients waiting over six months for heart operations were offered the choice of an alternative provider, later applied to other elective specialties, such as eye and orthopaedic surgery. Later, the Government announced that patient choice would be extended into areas such as children's health services, older people's services, long-term conditions, emergency care, mental health, maternity services and primary care (Cm 6079, 2003). Planned actions included: giving patients more opportunity to record their views about treatment in a form accessible to clinical teams; access to alternative providers, including the private sector, in primary care; greater choice over when and where to get medicines; more choice for patients at point of referral for surgery; and greater choice in other areas of care, beginning with maternity services and terminal care.

The impetus towards greater patient choice came from several sources. Initially, a number of European Court judgements increased the scope for patients facing 'undue delay' to seek treatment in other EU countries where they could access 'indispensable treatment' (see Price and Pollock, 2002; Kanavos and McKee, 2000). Subsequent cases reinforced and strengthened this principle (Laurance, 2003). Also, patient choice was seen by Government as a way of meeting key NHS performance targets. By allowing greater patient choice, it was believed that more people would be treated by private providers at home and overseas, thereby maximising use of this capacity. In cardiac surgery, for example, waiting times over six months fell dramatically following the involvement of the patient-choice scheme – although the exact contribution of the scheme was unclear. Finally, the Government argued that extending patient choice would be popular. There was some evidence to support this. An opinion survey undertaken on behalf of the BMA found that over four out of ten patients would be willing to travel outside the UK for treatment and over half stated that other organisations, including the private sector, should be involved in providing services to NHS patients (BMA, 2002).

However, increased patient choice has drawbacks (see Appleby, Harrison and Devlin, 2003). There are concerns about the impact on other priorities. Equity may be undermined by greater choice – some people may be more willing or able to make choices than others. Moreover, if NHS providers lose income as a result of increased competition from private providers, their financial problems may adversely affect patient services. Efficiency could also be affected. The creation of additional capacity to respond more flexibly to choice will be expensive and not necessarily cost-effective (see Carlisle, 2003b). Also, there are the additional costs of responding to patients' choices, finding out individual preferences, and arranging services accordingly. Moreover, there is no guarantee that choice will improve the quality of treatment. Indeed, it is possible that it may have an adverse effect if patients are not fully informed about quality of care or if regulatory systems fail to guarantee minimum standards are being met. Arguably, as the supply side of health care market becomes more fragmented and includes more organisations from outside the NHS, it will become more difficult to ensure effective regulation of health care and the provision of high-quality consumer information.

Consumerism

Many of the initiatives to improve the welfare of NHS patients and service users have been based on a narrow consumer model of health. This may be regarded as a useful approach, particularly if, as some suggest, patients are becoming more informed and confident about making choices (Sloan, 2001). It may reflect what some have called 'the commodification of health care' in modern society (see Henderson and Petersen, 2002). However, there has been much criticism of what some have called the 'supermarket model' of consumerism (Winkler, 1987). Critics argue that, even though there may be greater assertiveness of patients and availability of information about health, a consumerist approach is inappropriate (see Hogg, 1999). Consumerism has market connotations, yet service users in health and social care do not necessarily act as rational purchasers and remain at a considerable disadvantage compared with professionals and service managers (Twigg, 2000; Barnes, 1997; Shackley and Ryan, 1994). Indeed, with regard to services that involve compulsory treatment or in situations where people are unable to express their wishes, the term 'consumer' seems bizarre. For example, in relation to mental health, Rogers and Pilgrim (2001, p. 113) have argued that 'no logical case can be made for calling detained patients consumers or customers'. Others have attacked the moral basis of consumerism in health care and have argued that consumerism tends to misrepresent the NHS and the position of users within it (Sorell, 1997). Some have responded to this by taking a broader view of consumerism. According to Williamson (1992), for example, consumerism should be viewed in terms of interests rather than in a narrow market sense. This allows for the inclusion of political factors and relationships, and a focus on participation of patients and users in care, standard-setting and planning. Others have adopted a similar approach (Allsop, Baggott and Jones, 2002). Nonetheless, consumerism is disliked by those who continue to see it as a loaded term. They argue for a broader conceptualisation of health care users which explicitly recognises other dimensions of participation in health care, such as democratic accountability, partnership in decision-making, scrutiny of service providers, and even direct control of services by users, in the context of improved rights for individuals as citizens rather than simply consumers of health services (see Winkler, 1987; Barnes, 1997). The remainder of this chapter explores these aspects in further detail.

Patients' Rights

People can have specific rights in relation to health care, though it has long been acknowledged that these rights are limited (Hogg, 1999). Recently, however, there have been important changes affecting rights to care and treatment, access to information, confidentiality, and consent. These occurred for several reasons. First, at the international level, there were moves to establish stronger protection both of human rights generally and of patients' rights. Secondly, domestic policies on freedom of information, confidentiality and data protection – also shaped by European obligations – affected patients' rights. Thirdly, evidence of specific instances of poor or harmful practice led to reforms. Fourthly, pressure from citizen advocacy organisations, health consumer groups and the media added to the impetus for change. Finally, the Government's own emphasis on consumerism in health care encouraged demands for stronger rights in areas such as information and complaints.

Rights with Regard to Care and Treatment

Over the past decade, international efforts have been made to strengthen the position of service users within the health care system. Institutions such as the WHO Regional Office for Europe (1994) and the Council of Europe (Council of Europe, Committee of Ministers 2000) have issued declarations stating the importance of patients' rights and patient participation in health care decision-making. Although only a few European states have actually introduced patients' rights legislation, such as Holland for example, they have been under pressure to take action to adopt certain principles in their domestic policies. These include the clarification of patients' rights with regard to participation in health care and the availability of health care information.

More specifically, rights to care and treatment in the UK have been made more explicit by the Human Rights Act 1998, which enshrined the European Convention on Human Rights into domestic law. Although it did not give individuals an absolute right to care and treatment, the Act was expected to strengthen claims regarding access to services or the quality of care received (Hewson, 2000; Loveland, 1999). Indeed, the NHS, as a public body, has a statutory duty to comply with the Act. Several of the rights set out under the Act may provide a basis for legal action, including the right to life, prohibition of inhuman and degrading treatment, respect for a private and family life, right to information, right to found a family, and right not to be discriminated against on grounds of race and gender. Following its implementation in 2000, the Act did not have a major immediate impact (Sunkin, 2001), though a number of community care and mental health cases were based on human rights arguments – a continuation of previous practice. Its full impact, however, can only be assessed in the longer term, as more and more cases are brought and legal precedents are established.

Access to Information and Confidentiality

Patients, and their nominated representatives, have rights of access to information held on their personal records. Changes in the law in the 1980s and 1990s included the Data Protection Act 1984, which gave access to computer-based health records, and the 1990 Access to Health Records Act which extended these rights to manual records. However, in practice, patients were often deterred from accessing records by unhelpful staff, illegible, handwritten notes, and excessive administrative charges (see Association of Community Health Councils for England and Wales, 1998). Barriers also included legitimate grounds for refusing access, namely where serious harm to the patient or others was likely, or where information would be disclosed about a third party.

Future access to health information will also be governed by the Freedom of Information Act of 2000, to be fully implemented in 2005. This Act introduced a general right of individuals to recorded information held by public authorities, including the NHS. It will supersede an existing code of openness in the NHS introduced in the mid-1990s, currently policed by the health ombudsman. Under the new regime, penalties will be imposed on public authorities which destroy or alter data, fail to maintain accurate records, or which unfairly refuse access to information. In addition, a new tribunal is to be established to enforce rights to information. The Freedom of Information Act requires authorities to establish publication schemes, which will be approved by an Information Commissioner. It should be noted that there are several grounds for preventing information from entering the public domain, including commercial interests, health and safety issues, and national security. Authorities must also balance the need to disclose information with the need to maintain confidentiality.

With regard to confidentiality, data protection laws have forced Government to introduce new guidelines. In the mid-1990s the circumstances in which information collected by the NHS could be passed on to others was clarified. Subsequently, a system was established to oversee access to patient-identifiable information, as recommended by the Caldicott report (DoH, 1997b). 'Caldicott Guardians' were established in health authorities, PCTs and trusts to ensure good practice. NHS organisations were expected to develop local protocols for anonymising of data and the disclosure of such information, to restrict access to such information, and improve organisational performance with regard to staff training and compliance with guidance. In addition, the 1998 Data Protection Act required health bodies to secure informed consent for data in addition to its use in care and treatment. It also strengthened legal provisions governing the transfer of data to third parties, and clarified responsibilities for the control and security of data. The new Act covered all records, including manual records, and set maximum fees for access (£50 for manual records; £10 for computer records). Furthermore, in 2000 a National Confidentiality and Security Advisory Body was established to advise and promote best practice on patient-confidentiality.

These moves failed to allay public concerns. Indeed, new rules enabling ministers to sanction access to confidential information without patients' consent, permitted by the Health and Social Care Act 2001, were strongly opposed. The Government argued that the measure was necessary but transitional, to enable researchers to access vital information without having to obtain permission from each patient. Access could also be granted to public health bodies and other organisations where this supported 'essential NHS activity'. As a safeguard, and to placate opposition, the Government established an advisory group to consider requests for such confidential information.

Developments in information technology raise important issues about access and confidentiality. Only time will tell whether electronic records, accessible by multiple parties, will be more secure than traditional manual or computer-based records. Greater patient access to electronic records has been proposed, through 'smartcards' for example, the technical feasibility of which is being evaluated. Patients have also been promised greater control over health records and opportunities for contributing information about how they want to be treated (Cm 6079, 2003). Meanwhile, delicate issues remain about how much information patients should see about themselves, particularly with regard to the safeguards on harm and the protection of third parties mentioned in the Data Protection legislation.

Consent

During the late 1990s, issues of consent achieved a high public profile. There was a public outcry in cases where parents found that their children's organs had been retained by hospitals without permission. Such practices came to light during the Bristol inquiry and attention later centred on Alder Hey Children's Hospital, Liverpool, where it was found that pathologists had acted illegally and unethically (The Royal Liverpool Children's Inquiry, 2001). Consequently a national census of organ retention was undertaken, which revealed that over 50,000 organs had been retained by English hospitals across the country between 1970 and 1999, many without fully informed consent (DoH, Department for Education and Employment, Home Office, 2001a). Further investigations revealed that the law was ambiguous, and requirements for consent poorly understood (DoH, Department for Education and Employment, Home Office, 2001b). The Government proposed changes in the law, requiring positive consent for retained organs, making it easier to establish whether a criminal offence had been committed, and imposing penalties for breaches of the law (DoH and Welsh Assembly Government, 2002). In the meantime, interim guidance on the use of human organs and tissue was issued (DoH and Welsh Assembly Government, 2003). A code of practice on communication with families about post-mortems, along with new standard consent forms for organ retention, were also introduced (DoH, 2003j). In addition, an independent commission was established to oversee the return of organs and tissues. Changes to the coroner's system and death certification were proposed, issues also taken up by the Shipman inquiry.

Issues of consent have arisen elsewhere. The operation in 2000 to separate the Siamese twins known as 'Mary' and 'Jody' was controversial, not only because it led to the certain death of the first child, but also because the parents' refusal to consent to the operation was overruled by the courts. Other controversies included the case of a 15-year-old girl whose refusal of a heart transplant was similarly overruled (Dyer and Boseley, 1999). Adults can also be treated against their will. In the past, the courts have ruled against women unwilling to undergo Caesarean operations. However, the Court of Appeal has since ruled that, in future, no woman having the capacity to decide for herself can be forced to have an operation. This principle applies to any case – male or female – involving questions of capacity to decide on invasive treatment. Even in the mental health field – where issues of capacity are more complex–powers to compel treatment have been challenged (see Chapter 11). Professionals and the Government recognise that patient consent can no longer be taken for granted. Indeed, the Department of Health, the General Medical Council and other professional bodies have introduced guidance in recent years, clarifying legal requirements and setting out good practice (see DoH, 2001m, 2001n; GMC, 1998)

Patient and Public Involvement

Patient and public involvement can occur at different levels: in policy issues, in service planning, and in relation to individual treatment. The latter aspect is considered further in Exhibit 12.2. The remainder of this section explores the role of patients and the public in health policy and service planning.

Encouraging Patient and Public Involvement in the 1990s

The Conservative Government's internal market reforms provided a stimulus for those purchasing health care to find out more about people's preferences and needs (Lupton, Donaldson and Lloyd, 1998). In addition, the Department of Health urged purchasers to listen to local communities when setting priorities (NHSME, 1992). This later developed into a commitment in the NHS priorities and planning guidance given for 1996/7, where it was stated that there should be greater voice and influence given to NHS service users and carers in their own care, the development and definition of local service standards, and NHS policy at local and national level (NHSE, 1995).

During the 1990s, NHS organisations began to experiment with various means of gauging patient and public opinion, including surveys, as well as new methods of engaging with the public, patients and their representatives. Citizens' Juries were established to advise on issues such as hospital closures, local priorities and alternative ways of providing services (Stewart, Kendall and Coote, 1996; Smith and Wales, 1999: Elizabeth, Davies and Hanley, 1998; McIver, 1998). They involve the appointment of a panel of around 20 to 25 people drawn from the local community to consider a particular set of options relating to a decision. This body takes evidence from various expert witnesses, and, following a period of deliberation, issues a verdict. Citizens' juries have a number of advantages and disadvantages (see Pickard, 1998). They can generate public debate and, in some cases, wider support for a particular option. They may improve public understanding of an issue and thereby help to overcome public opposition to a particular proposal. By bringing different values to bear on an issue, they may encourage innovative solutions. However, as they are disbanded after completing their task, they represent a very limited and temporary form of accountability. They also have limited independence. Even where the authorities that establish them do not seek directly to interfere in their work, the juries are still dependent on their information, resources and expertise. It is also very difficult for juries to set their own agenda, as the key questions are usually determined in advance. Their decisions are not binding on the organisation that establishes them, so their recommendations could be rejected. Another shortcoming is that although efforts are made to ensure citizens' juries reflect the broad composition of the general population, they cannot really claim to represent the community. They are not linked to the community by any representative mechanism such as nomination or election, so their representativeness is purely symbolic.

Exhibit 12.2 Patients, Partnership and Care

It would wrong to see the impetus for greater involvement of patients in health care decision-making as coming entirely from service users. Indeed, professionals increasingly recognise that patients and service users have a role to play in their own care. The philosophy of partnership, where patients and professionals (and others, such as carers) play a part in health care decision-making has attracted stronger support in recent years and has, to some extent, challenged the traditionally paternalistic approach of the health professions. This has occurred for a number of reasons (Coulter, 2002; Williamson, 1992, 2000): a recognition that patient-involvement can improve outcomes, that it can build stronger and more trusting relationships between professional and service users, that it can help construct realistic and achievable standards of care that satisfy both parties, and that it can reduce the burden on professionals by promoting self-care.

But, in practice, there is still much disagreement about the appropriate extent of patient involvement. From a narrow professional perspective, involvement should be undertaken only where improved outcomes are forthcoming, for example where it leads to improved communication between professionals and patients, better diagnosis and compliance with treatment regimes. Many professionals remain wary of empowering patients in ways that could undermine their dominant position in the provision of health care. Few professionals are comfortable with the idea of being controlled by users, though the majority recognise that most patients cannot be regarded simply as passive recipients of care.

Indeed, patients can be regarded as experts in their own right. They possess information, knowledge and expertise about their condition which professionals do not possess. In 2001, the Expert Patients Initiative was launched by the Department of Health (DoH, 2001q). This built on the experience of self-management programmes for people with chronic diseases such as arthritis. The aim was to promote patient expertise in various ways: integrating user-led self-management into NHS national service frameworks and NHS services; expanding practical support for user-led self-management programmes; promoting professional awareness of the benefits of self-management. Although these have been widely regarded as positive steps towards improving the quality of life and self-esteem of people with chronic illness, critics argue that they do not significantly challenge professional assumptions about people with chronic illness, nor do they necessarily lead to greater empowerment of such patients (see Wilson, 2001; Thorne et al., 2000).

There is only patchy evidence about the impact of shared decision-making between patients and professionals on health outcomes (see Coulter, 1997; Stewart and Brown, 2001). Moreover, the benefits of shared decision-making in one area, such as cancer, (Gattellari, Butow and Tattersall, 2001) may not arise in others. It should also be noted that not all patients wish to take control of their care (see Degner et al., 1997 with regard to breast cancer patients), while others unable to do so because they are mentally incapacitated or unconscious. But it is still important that patients' concerns, wishes and values be incorporated into health care decisions (Guadagnoli and Ward, 1998).

Partnership with patients has gone beyond their participation in decision-making. Patients, and in some cases carers, have been incorporated into processes of standard-setting and

$\longrightarrow$

> **Exhibit 12.2 continued**
>
> ⟶
>
> audit at several levels. Patients and their representatives have been included on committees established by professional and regulatory bodies such as the Royal Colleges and the Commission for Healthcare Audit and Inspection. They have also been appointed to panels monitoring the quality of care in relation to specific services such as stroke care or cancer treatment. In addition, patient-satisfaction surveys have been used to evaluate the quality of care provided.

While citizens' juries are a 'one-off', user panels are ongoing and can be used to sound out opinion over a longer period. User panels have their origins in patient-participation groups set up by GPs in the 1970s (Pritchard, 1981; Brown, 1999). These groups were quite diverse, but usually restricted their discussions to feedback on practice organisation, the provision of voluntary and self-help services, and, in some cases, the development of new services. During the 1990s, there was growing interest in establishing bodies to provide a patient-perspective on the quality of services (see Exhibit 12.2) and on planning and commissioning issues. Health authorities, trusts, some GP fundholders and, later, primary care groups began to establish user panels with this wider brief. In some cases (see, for example, Bowie, Richardson and Sykes, 1995) these bodies considered priorities. However, like citizens' juries, user panels only had advisory status, and similarly could be ignored.

At the local level, the development of public involvement was haphazard. Some health authorities were very positive about encouraging user involvement and proactive in encouraging other NHS organisations to establish means of engaging with patients and the public. Some produced good practice guides that were drawn on by others when establishing their own arrangements (see, for example, Barker, Bullen and De Ville, 1997; Chan, 2000; Nottingham Health Authority, 1999). Nonetheless, there was much cynicism about efforts to involve patients and the public. Citizens' juries, user panels and other consultation fora were seen as ways in which decision-makers could be informed, and their decisions legitimised rather than shaped (Davis and Daly, 1999; Milewa, Valentine and Calnan, 1998; Milewa, 1997; Harrison and Mort, 1998). There were worries about the representativeness of the people who sat on such bodies (see Hogg and Williamson, 2001). It was argued that public and user involvement was not systematic, but 'bolted on' to an NHS dominated by professional and managerial interests (see Hogg, 1999). Effective involvement required fundamental changes in policy and practice, alongside a more democratic structure of decision-making (Popay and Williams, 1994).

There was also a lack of consistency, owing in part to the lack of a clear national policy on patient and public involvement. The Department of Health tried to address this by introducing a patient-partnership strategy (DoH,

1996b) which set out several key aims: to promote users' involvement in their own care, to encourage informed choice, to make the NHS more responsive to the needs and preferences of users, and to support the effective involvement of users. This initiative was continued by the Blair Government, which, in its 1997 White Paper on the NHS, set out as one of its key principles 'to rebuild public confidence in the NHS as a public service, accountable to patients, open to the public and shaped by their views' (Cm 3807, 1997, p. 11). Health authorities were expected to involve the public in service planning and priority-setting, Health Action Zones were required to work with the public and service users in developing their activities, while primary care groups and trusts had a specific brief to develop arrangements for public involvement (see Chapter 10). This was followed by a joint publication by the Department of Health and other bodies (NHSE/IHSM/NHS Confederation, 1998) offering advice and guidance to NHS organisations on how to consult the public, and a revised patient-partnership-strategy document (DoH, 1999f).

Primary care was seen as a key area for promoting patient and public involvement at the local level. Yet research has shown that primary care organisations faced several obstacles in attempting to involve patients and the public and often struggled to develop effective ways of involving local communities (Alborz, Wilkin and Smith, 2002; Regen et al., 2001). These organisations had limited skills and support for this function, meagre resources, including time, and also some negative attitudes among both board members and the public (Rowe and Shepherd, 2002). In addition, others found an emphasis on short-term initiatives and a failure to commit to identifiable changes in policy or practice (Gillam and Brooks, 2001). Indeed, there was little evidence that PCG/Ts saw patient and public involvement as a means of responding to local preferences. Rather, their activities were rationalised in terms of improving quality and responsiveness from a professional perspective (Milewa et al., 2002). On a more positive note, there was evidence of good practice, with some organisations actively seeking to engage with users, through local community groups, for example (see Anderson et al., 2002; Regen et al., 2001). There was some indication that efforts to involve patients and the public could provide a means for giving them a greater say, though this depended greatly on the overall commitment of the organisation to user-involvement and its willingness to link this activity to existing programmes of change (Anderson et al., 2002). Much also depended on the priority given to users' views in relation to other factors such as professional judgement, planning and operational constraints, and limited resources (Milewa et al., 2002).

At the national level, ministers and civil servants began to involve health consumer groups more closely in the policy process. For example, groups representing patients, users and carers were appointed to the bodies which drew up national service frameworks, advisory committees of NICE (Quennell, 2001), and, later, the Modernisation Action Teams that fed into the NHS Plan of

2000. Subsequently, Chapter 10 of the NHS Plan (Cm 4818, 2000) introduced a wide range of initiatives for public and patient involvement. A commitment was made to increase lay and citizen representation on professional and regulatory bodies and on key government committees. Indeed, a third of the members of the newly-created NHS modernisation board, which oversees the implementation of the NHS Plan, consisted of patient and citizen representatives. The Government also promised a new system of patient and public involvement for England, replacing CHCs with local advisory bodies and patients forums, alongside the new PALS services already discussed. Greater scrutiny of NHS decisions by local authorities was also proposed, with new committees established for this purpose.

As already noted, these proposals caused controversy and were modified. CHCs survived for longer than originally envisaged, as the new framework was delayed. PALS were renamed as patient advice and liaison services and new independent complaints advocacy services (ICAS) were endorsed. The original plans for local advisory bodies and patient forums were replaced by a more complex structure overseen by a new, national patients' organisation (see DoH, 2001o, 2001p).

The New Statutory Framework for England

The features of the new system were as follows. First, the introduction of a statutory duty in the Health and Social Care Act of 2001 on strategic health authorities, PCTs and NHS trusts to make arrangements for service users to be involved in and consulted upon the planning and provision of services, proposals for changes in service provision, and decisions affecting the operation of services. This duty was supported by guidance in 2003, setting out how health bodies could ensure that this was fulfilled (DoH, 2003k). As well as establishing duties to ensure independent complaints and advocacy services (ICAS), the 2001 Act introduced a requirement for local authorities to establish overview and scrutiny committees (OSCs) for health services. In 2003, OSCs were formally established in local authorities with social services responsibilities, though some councils had earlier established similar bodies. NHS organisations must provide information to OSCs about services, and decisions that affect services, and their senior officers must attend meetings to answer questions. The NHS must also consult OSCs on any substantial changes in services, and the latter can refer such changes to the Secretary of State for Health. Some believe that this form of accountability is too limited. One option might be to enable local authorities to take over public and community health functions and the commissioning of health services (Morley and Campbell, 2003). Others include democratising primary care trusts, partnership bodies and public involvement forums.

The National Health Service Reform and Healthcare Professions Act 2002 provided the legislative framework for national and local bodies for patient and public involvement. At local level, patient forums were created in each PCT and trust in England to monitor and review services; obtain the views of patients and carers and report these to the trust; provide advice, reports and recommendations about services to the trust; give information and advice to patients and carers; and assist them and their families in prescribed circumstances. Patient forums were also given powers to refer concerns to OSCs, Strategic Health Authorities, the national patients' body (CPPIH – see below) and others. PCT patient forums were given additional responsibilities, including the arrangement of ICAS, making information available about complaints, representing public views about health, and monitoring, promoting and advising upon public involvement. In order to enable them to carry out their function, patients' forums were given specific powers to enter and inspect premises, and to request relevant information to enable them to monitor services. It was decided that in each trust a member of the patient forum would serve as a non-executive director. Confusingly, patient forums were later renamed Patient and Public Involvement Forums (PPIFs), despite the fact that the original legislation referred to patient forums.

A statutory Commission for Patient and Public Involvement in Health (CPPIH) was established, with the following functions: advising ministers on public involvement and consultation, and on the provision of ICAS; representing the views of PPIFs and voluntary organisations; advising and assisting PPIFs and co-ordinating their activities; advising and assisting providers of ICAS; setting and monitoring standards of PPIFs and ICAS; appointing the members of PPIFs; reporting matters of patient welfare or safety to regulatory bodies; and generally promoting public involvement in health. The CPPIH was also responsible for providing administrative support to the PPIFs, though it actually contracted this function out to a number of voluntary sector organisations. These 'local network providers' were also expected to help PPIFs to recruit members, and to communicate with each other, with other agencies and with CPPIH.

With the demise of CHCs and the emergence of these new institutions, the landscape of patient and public involvement begins to look very different. In many ways, the new framework is radical. It has a stronger statutory framework and is more comprehensive than that which it replaced. It is far too early to assess its impact, though there has already been criticism of both the policy and the implementation of the changes (see Cole, 2003; Health Committee, 2003b; Banks, 2001).

One of the main criticisms is fragmentation; the patient or citizen is faced with a bewildering array of institutions whose roles are poorly understood, even by experts. Indeed, the area is now full of confusing acronyms – PALS, ICAS, PPIFs, CPPIH – adding to public incomprehension. Even ministers appeared confused about the various responsibilities of these bodies (see Health

Committee, 2003b, para. 26). The CHCs were by no means perfect, but they hosted various functions 'under one roof' – assistance with complaints, advocacy, consultation, and scrutiny. Now that these have been scattered among different institutions, it appears that the new system is less rather than more coherent.

The dismantling of CHCs may have affected the capacity of local patient and public involvement systems. As experienced staff have departed, crucial expertise has ebbed away. In some cases, individuals have reappeared in new roles as PALS officers or in patient forums. But others have gone elsewhere and have thus been lost. The new system may also lack expertise as a result of the contracting process used to establish the CPPIH local network providers that support PPIFs. Some contracts were awarded to organisations without local knowledge, or with little or no knowledge of the NHS (Muir, 2003).

There was criticism of the amount of resources allocated to the new system. Claims that it would be more expensive to run than the chronically under-resourced CHCs were superseded by fears about inadequate funding. The Association of Community Health Councils for England and Wales (2002) calculated that new PPIFs would require almost twice the staff currently employed by CHCs to provide a 'fit for purpose' service and around a 50 per cent increase to provide a basic service, but that the necessary funding was not forthcoming. There were delays in setting up the new system. The process of establishing PPIFs took so long that CHCs were given a stay of execution until the end of 2003. The appointment of PPIF members proved difficult, with around 10,000 people needed to fill these vacancies (Health Committee, 2003b). Moreover, as already noted, the delays meant that the ICAS had to be established by different means. The DoH had to take over their commissioning role from PPIFs as an interim measure.

Further criticism focused upon the lack of consistency between the new statutory framework and other initiatives. In particular, the proposed foundation trusts, required to involve service users in their governance arrangements, appeared to supersede the system of patient and public involvement heralded in the NHS Plan. Initially it was stated that foundation trusts would not have to appoint PPIFs. The new system of patient and public involvement would scarcely have been implemented before being partially dismantled, as trusts acquired foundation status. The Health Committee (2003b, para. 34), which had earlier raised doubts about the arrangements for public involvement in foundation trusts, expressed its amazement that the connections between 'these two divergent and conflicting policies on patient and public involvement' had not been drawn out before the new system had been implemented. Ministers later conceded that foundation trusts must have PPIFs.

Even so, the changes in patient and public involvement initiated by the NHS Plan were criticised for their lack of consistency with other initiatives to promote public involvement and citizen participation (Banks, 2001). Although wide-ranging, the reforms did little to bring together good practice from other areas such as social care (see Exhibit 12.1) and regeneration. Also, by creating an additional system of public involvement, this risked adding to the 'consultation fatigue' experienced by local communities. Subsequently, the DoH (2003l) urged closer links between health, local government and the voluntary sector on these issues and highlighted the role of local strategic partnerships (see Chapter 13) in promoting greater coherence in public involvement activities.

Representing Patients

In recent years the number of voluntary groups representing patients, users and carers has increased (Wood, 2000). These include groups focused around a particular condition (such as the Parkinson's Disease Society or the British Cardiac Patients Association), groups representing a particular section of the population (Age Concern; Action for Sick Children); or alliances of groups covering several conditions (Long Term Medical Conditions Alliance; Neurological Alliance), and groups protesting about a particular issue or service (such as the Bristol Heart Children's Action Group, and PITY II which supports people affected by the organ-retention issue – see above). Moreover, many groups now combine their traditional role of providing advice, information, self-help and mutual support (Kelleher, 1994) with a more active lobbying role. In some areas, such as mental health and maternity services, there is a long history of political activity (see Rogers and Pilgrim, 2001; Hogg, 1999; Durward and Evans, 1990).

Groups representing patients, users and carers – health consumer groups – have become more active at national level, seeking to influence policy on a range of issues (Allsop, Baggott and Jones, 2002). They have been incorporated into the policy process, and have been included on various boards and committees. Groups have been influential in many ways: getting issues on to the agenda (for example, highlighting the poor standards of care of elderly people in hospital), shaping decisions (for example, extending breast cancer screening to older women), and the implementation of policy (for example, the creation of specialist stroke units in hospitals) (see Baggott, Allsop and Jones, 2004). Even so, it is acknowledged that they remain less powerful than the more established interests such as the medical profession and the drugs industry (Hogg, 1999; Salter, 2003). This is largely because they are disadvantaged in terms of political resources. Even so, their ability to speak on behalf of patients, users and carers, and their expertise are increasingly recognised by policy-makers and other interest groups (Baggott, Allsop and Jones, 2004).

Patient, user and carer groups also operate at the local level (see Wood, 2000). Some local groups are branches of national organisations, while others are free-standing. In some cases, national organisations have grown out of local initiatives, as in the case of the British Cardiac Patients' Association, which began as a local self-help group. Local groups are consulted by health authorities and PCTs (Milewa et al., 2002). They are acknowledged as speaking on behalf of local patients, users and carers, adding legitimacy to the decisions taken by health service organisations. Dialogue with these groups is seen as one way in which the NHS can fulfil its statutory duty to consult and involve service users (DoH, 2003l).

However, the role of health consumer groups has been challenged. Like many other voluntary organisations, they are often run by highly committed individuals, and there is a danger that they may not accurately represent the views of ordinary service users. In particular, there are fears that the representation of users depends too much on 'the usual suspects', a small number of people who have the time, skills and expertise to participate in consultation processes. Although it is true that the numbers of people involved is relatively small, and the same people tend to be appointed to advisory committees at national level, this does not mean that they cannot represent a wider constituency of users. Indeed, many groups actively seek the views of patients, users and carers, and this is used as evidence by their representatives. Moreover, Government claims to be wary of groups that cannot support their arguments with evidence (see Baggott, Allsop and Jones, 2004).

Another, related problem is that there are considerable inequalities between health consumer groups. They vary in terms of the resources at their disposal, and their political leverage. These inequalities are not necessarily related to the intensity of the needs these groups claim to represent. Some constituencies are well-organised and/or well-connected. These include the elderly, the mentally ill, long-term conditions, maternity services, and carers. Others – people with rare conditions, ethnic minorities, the users of acute services – are less well-organised. Indeed, it is possible that for some conditions no group exists and therefore their interests may not be articulated to decision-makers and service providers. In view of this, it is important that efforts be made to consult and involve patients, users and carers who are 'hard to reach' (Tritter et al., 2003), and perhaps to facilitate organisation where barriers exist.

Public Involvement in Wales and Scotland

In Wales, a series of policy documents since the late 1990s have emphasised the importance of public and patient involvement (Welsh Office, 1998; National Assembly for Wales, 2001a). NHS bodies in Wales are required to consult and involve the public. Local health boards (and formerly local health groups) and trusts were required to undertake base-line assessments of their public and patient involvement activities. In addition, they must produce annual involvement plans, and an annual prospectus, including patients' views. The activity of NHS bodies with regard to public and patient involvement is monitored through the performance assessment framework for Wales. In addition, the Welsh Assembly has promoted good practice in public and patient involvement (National Assembly for Wales, Office for Public Management, 2001; Welsh Assembly Government, 2003a). CHCs, as noted earlier, were not abolished in Wales. Indeed, the Welsh Assembly proposed measures to strengthen their role, including new statutory powers to provide independent advocacy and to review health services. In addition, extended rights to consultation on service changes and additional powers of entry to and inspection of NHS facilities were promised. Proposals to change the composition of CHCs and to introduce a new Welsh national body for CHCs were also announced.

In Scotland, too, there has been a greater emphasis on patient and public involvement in recent years (Scottish Executive, 2001; Scottish Executive, 2003c). The main aims of this policy have been to improve capacity, communications, patient information, involvement and responsiveness. Health Boards and trusts are required to respond to the needs and wishes of patients and their efforts are monitored through the Scottish performance assessment framework. Meanwhile, changes have been proposed to the system of Scottish health councils, bodies similar to community health councils. It has been proposed that these should be replaced by a new system that is founded on three key functions: *assessment* of health board activities in promoting patient and public involvement; *feedback* of patients' and carers' views; and *development* of good practice in patient and public involvement. The proposals involve the replacement of the local Scottish health councils with a single national body to be known as the Scottish Health Council. This will be responsible for infrastructure, staff support, training, and spreading good practice, and is to be based in local offices operating with a small staff. In addition, it is likely that local advisory committees will be established in each NHS board area to ensure that the national body is aware of local issues and concerns.

Conclusion

Traditionally, patients, service users and carers have been the passive actors in the health care system (Alford, 1975). Changes have been made which in theory strengthen their position, putting them at the centre of the NHS. Even so, these interests remain at a political disadvantage compared with traditionally powerful interests such as the medical profession and the drugs industry. They are also open to manipulation by Government, which sees patients, users and carers as allies in its reform programme. There is a tendency for Government to wish to minimise criticism and accentuate praise from this quarter. It will be interesting to see how the new statutory framework maintains its independence in the face of these pressures.

It is clear that patient and public involvement must be linked more closely to citizen engagement. The NHS needs to work alongside other public authorities to design public involvement systems that are cost-effective and that do not place an undue burden on patients, users and carers. Not all people want to get involved. Some may be 'too ill to talk' (Rhodes and Small, 2001). But some way of discovering their preferences and values is necessary. A more consistent approach to public involvement is also required to extend public participation into health promotion as well as health care. Engaging with the public on these matters is likely to be crucial in order to improve individual health (Wanless, 2002, 2004) while producing public health policies that are coherent, effective, and accepted by the people.

Further Reading

Anderson, W., Florin, D., Gillam, S. and Mountford, L. (2002) _Every Voice Counts: Primary Care Organisations and Public Involvement_ (London, King's Fund).

Baggott, R., Allsop, J. and Jones, K. (2004) _Speaking for Patients and Carers: Health Consumer Groups and the Policy Process_ (London, Palgrave).

Barnes, M., Harrison, S., Mort, M. and Shardlow, P. (1999) _Unequal Partners: User Groups and Community Care_ (Bristol, Policy Press).

Gillam, S. and Brooks, F. (2001) _New Beginnings: Towards Patient and Public Involvement in Primary Health Care_ (London, King's Fund).

Hogg, C. (1999) _Patients, Power and Politics. Health Policy from a User Perspective_ (London, Sage).

Rhodes, P. and Small, N. (2001) _Too Ill to Talk? User Involvement and Palliative Care_ (London, Routledge).

Wood, B. (2000) _Patient Power?: The Politics of Patients' Associations in Britain and America_ (Buckingham, Open University Press).

Public Health

13

What is Public Health?

According to Smith and Jacobson (1988, p. 3), public health 'involves the promotion of health, the prevention of disease, the treatment of illness, the care of those who are disabled, and the continuous development of the technical and social means for the pursuit of these objectives'. Public health has many different aspects (see Griffiths and Hunter, 1999; Baggott, 2000; Hunter, 2003) and there is disagreement about the relative importance of these aspects, for example about the appropriate balance between the treatment of disease and the promotion of health. Nonetheless, there is agreement that public health is primarily concerned with the efforts of the community to improve health, rather than the treatment of disease manifested in the individual.

Action to promote the health of the whole community dates back to the earliest civilisations (Rosen, 1993). The Ancient Greeks recognised the links between location, environment, lifestyles, nutrition and the health of the community. The Romans, too, were aware of these factors, and sought to improve public health through large-scale engineering works such as water supply systems and sewers. Centuries later, the Victorians established a legislative and administrative framework that led to improvements in health through better housing, sanitation and a cleaner environment, while laying the foundations of the modern welfare state. For most of the twentieth century, however, health policy was mainly concerned with the provision of health care, rather than with the promotion of good health. This reflected to some extent the dominance of the orthodox biomedical approach (see Chapter 2), the low status of public health doctors compared with other medical practitioners, the power and resources of the hospital sector, and the fragmentation of Government responsibilities affecting health, which made it difficult to co-ordinate action.

In recent decades there has been a revival of interest in public health. It is now realised that many of the challenges facing the health system, outlined in Chapter 1, require something more than an expansion and improvement of health services. Governments around the world have responded by developing strategies aimed at improving the health of their populations.

The Challenge of Public Health

Many significant causes of mortality and morbidity discussed in Chapter 1 can be prevented at the community level to some extent. Governments have pursued strategies aimed at preventing health problems and identifying illness at a stage where treatment is more likely to be effective. Essentially, these strategies have three main elements (Jacobson, Smith and Whitehead, 1991):

1 *Education*: to persuade individuals to adopt healthy lifestyles and reject or moderate habits harmful to health – such as smoking and heavy drinking. Education strategies may also be aimed at groups and private institutions in an attempt to encourage collective action to prevent ill health, for example alcohol-awareness programmes in the workplace.
2 *Clinical prevention*: this includes services to monitor health and detect illness at an early stage, for example the provision of screening facilities to detect the early signs of breast and cervical cancer. Also included in this category are other preventive interventions, for example immunisation against diseases such as mumps, measles and rubella (German measles).
3 *Intervention at the social and environmental level*: this involves adopting policies to tackle the root causes of ill health in society. The state has considerable legislative and financial powers to promote health. It can ban or restrict activities harmful to health, or impose penal taxation upon such activities. It has the capacity to co-ordinate national and local policies to ensure that health objectives are not compromised, and may regulate powerful vested interests, such as the alcohol, tobacco and food industries, whose activities can undermine public health. Individual states may also come together to agree strategies to deal with threats to health at the international level (see below), including activities of multinational corporations. Furthermore, the state arbitrates between individuals' rights and liberties. Some individuals in a liberal society may choose to indulge in health-damaging behaviour even when fully informed. These rights, however, impinge on others. The issue of smoking restrictions in public places exemplifies how the state must balance the conflicting rights of its citizens.

Public Health Policies in the UK

The Postwar Period

The creation of the postwar welfare state was itself a major public health effort aimed at the root causes of disease – one of Beveridge's 'five evils'. The creation of the NHS in particular was a key public health intervention: it represented an attempt to improve the population's health by providing comprehensive health services – including preventive services – free at point of delivery (though charges for prescriptions and appliances were subsequently introduced). In addition to these major reforms, other significant measures were introduced over the years to improve public health, for example the 1956 Clean Air Act, which tackled the problem of urban smog – a major cause of respiratory problems in industrial areas. But such specific measures were few and far between. The NHS remained a 'sickness service' and was dominated by the hospital service and in turn by the doctors who practised there – the consultants – who were concerned mainly with treating disease manifested in individual patients, rather than with promoting preventive action at the community level.

In the mid-1970s, policy-makers in many countries began to turn their attention to public health strategies. This was a period of severe economic crisis, which led to a squeeze on publicly-funded health services at a time when demand for these services was perceived to be increasing. Improving public health by preventing illness was seen as a more cost-effective option – though it has since been recognised that higher costs may be incurred by a preventive strategy as people live longer (Normand, 1991), though the benefits in terms of a healthier population may well be greater in the long run. The UK Government identified key areas for future action: inequalities in health status, heart disease, road accidents, smoking-related diseases, alcoholism and mental illness, drugs, diet, and sexually transmitted diseases (DHSS, 1976c). A subsequent White Paper (Cmnd 7047, 1977) fell far short of the coherent public health strategy some expected. Interventionist measures were avoided, for fear of upsetting commercial interests and the public, whom politicians believed would resent attempts to regulate lifestyles. Aside from an increase in health education spending, Government was reluctant to provide extra resources to encourage prevention, and to divert resources from high-technology medicine.

The Thatcher and Major Governments

The Conservative Governments of the 1980s and 1990s were ideologically opposed to public health interventions because of strong associations with collectivism and the 'nanny state' However, they began to adopt such policies, for various reasons. First, they faced a series of public health crises which forced them to adopt a more coherent approach to public health. In the 1980s, a wave of problems, including food poisoning outbreaks, other infectious diseases such as Legionnaire's Disease, not to mention HIV/AIDS, attracted public attention and revealed the weakness of existing arrangements. An inquiry into public health, though confined to public health functions rather than wider policy matters, nonetheless found shortcomings. The Acheson report (Cm 289, 1988) led to an attempt to strengthen local public health leadership, with

Directors of Public Health (DsPH) being appointed by health authorities to advise on and develop policy on prevention and health promotion, to co-ordinate control of communicable disease, and to give medical advice on priorities and planning. Among the DsPHs' tasks was the production of an annual report on the state of public health.

Secondly, the Conservative Governments were concerned that the public did not trust them on matters of health and health care. They identified policies that were popular with the public and which might reassure them that the NHS was safe in their hands. Hence, screening programmes for breast and cervical cancer were introduced at a time when public suspicion of the Government's motives in this field were high. The Government also introduced a new remuneration package for GPs which emphasised health promotion activities such as immunisation, screening and health checks, activities that would be highly visible to patients. Similarly, mass publicity campaigns on smoking, heart disease prevention and drugs, though ostensibly aimed at getting people to change lifestyles also portrayed the Government as concerned about the people's health. These campaigns also emphasised a key element of the Conservatives' philosophy – individual responsibility. Ministers would argue that they were putting across the facts – about smoking and health, for example – though it was down to the individual to change his or her lifestyle accordingly.

Thirdly, the Conservative Governments' attempts to get more value for money out of public services led to efforts to relate the healthcare system more closely to policy objectives and performance measures. Initially this took the form of targets such as the reduction of waiting lists and times. But Government then began to focus on targets for reducing levels of disease. At the same time, reforms of the NHS introduced a purchaser – provider split and an internal market which in theory encouraged health authorities (and the GP fundholders) to assess need and fund activities (health care and other interventions) to improve health as well as health service standards. In practice this did not happen as envisaged, and the focus on treatment services continued to dominate the agenda.

These various strands combined to produce a much greater emphasis on public health. Under the Thatcher Government, proposals for a national plan for health improvement were resisted largely on ideological grounds. However, the Major Government developed this idea, culminating in the *Health of the Nation* strategy (Cm 1986, 1992), which set out a range of disease targets in several areas: coronary heart disease and stroke, cancer, mental health, accidents, HIV/AIDS and sexual health. Risk factor targets were also set, including a reduction in the proportion of the population smoking and a reduction in obesity levels. The strategy was to be implemented through improved co-ordination at all levels of Government, including alliances at the local level (consisting of business, the voluntary sector, local government and the NHS).

The *Health of the Nation* strategy was an important landmark. But its impact on public health was limited by several factors. There was a lack of resources, and consequently little incentive to improve health promotion activities. Indeed the health promotion agenda continued to be regarded as much less important than treatment service issues, with waiting lists dominating government priorities. This was reinforced by the internal market reforms and performance management systems, which emphasised the importance of treatment services.

Critics also argued that the targets had been selected because they were largely achievable within the timeframe on the basis of current trends (Mooney and Healey, 1991). Despite these accusations, some of the targets proved elusive; levels of obesity, smoking among schoolchildren, and women's alcohol consumption all deteriorated. Yet the Major Government refused to countenance policies that might have been more effective, such as more interventionist policies on diet or exercise, or a ban on tobacco advertising, for fear of offending powerful industrial lobbies.

The targets were also criticised for being too disease-oriented and for reflecting medical rather than social aspects of health. The Thatcher Government ignored the recommendations of the Black report (Berridge and Blume, 2003; DHSS, 1980; Townsend, Davidson and Whitehead, 1992) which highlighted the link between socio-economic inequalities and ill health and called for policies to improve the material conditions of the poor. Inequalities in health widened further during the 1980s (Blane, Smith and Bartley, 1990; Whitehead 1987). These developments mirrored income inequalities (Joseph Rowntree Foundation, 1996) which persisted throughout the 1990s. The share of the poorest fifth of the income distribution fell from 9.4 (1979) to 7.9 per cent (1995).

The welfare state continued to redistribute income between socio-economic groups, despite policies to reduce entitlements to benefits and to limit the level of benefits. Even when this is taken into account, inequalities in income continued to grow in the period 1984–90 (Larkin, 2001) Government policies accentuated inequality by prioritising wealth creation and enterprise over full employment and redistribution. Meanwhile, privatisation, deregulation (of low wages and working people's rights in particular) and tax cuts benefited the well-off and disadvantaged the poor. This compounded economic and social pressures, promoting greater economic and social inequalities including the decline in full-time, long-term employment, the growth of low-paid casual work, the rise of dual-income families and the rise of single parenting. These economic and social trends were characterised by Hutton (1996) as the 40-30-30 society: 40 per cent of the population having secure employment and a good material standard of living; 30 per cent having insecure and casual employment; 30 per cent marginalised, unemployed and living in poverty.

The Thatcher and Major Governments were reluctant to acknowledge the existence of health inequalities, but even when they did, they blamed statistical factors (see Chapter 1), selection (inequalities due to those who were ill being unable to hold down jobs) or behaviour (the poor and manual classes indulged in unhealthy activities by choice). In the Major years, ministers acknowledged that 'health variations' (a less contentious phrase) could be a significant barrier to improving the health of the population. But crucial issues of socio-economic disadvantage continued to be ignored.

By focusing on disease targets, and by separating the issue of health inequalities from wider social and economic inequalities, the Conservative Governments in effect conceptualised public health as an issue for the NHS alone, rather than a cross-sectoral issue in which all policies – economic and social – could play a part. This restricted Government policy and inhibited partnerships between the health sector and those who could contribute to improved public health, including regeneration agencies and local government. The Conservative Governments were also accused of ignoring wider environmental causes of ill health, such as pollution. However, under pressure from the Green lobby and the EU, and in the light of broader international concern about global warming, the Thatcher and Major Governments did introduce new legislation and regulatory processes. Moreover, the Major Government proposed that environmental health should be added to the *Health of the Nation* strategy, but this was overtaken by the change of Government in 1997.

The Blair Government and Our Healthier Nation

Senior Labour Party politicians also endorsed the idea of a national health strategy while in opposition during the 1990s, but placed greater emphasis on social, economic and environmental factors. On taking office, the Blair Government signalled the importance of public health by creating the post of Minister for Public Health. This was widely welcomed though some observers were unhappy that it was not a Cabinet-level post.

The Blair Government's public health strategy was set out in a much-delayed Green Paper of 1998 entitled *Our Healthier Nation* (Cm 3852, 1998). Following a long period of consultation, a White Paper was published (Cm 4386, 1999) entitled *Saving Lives*. Separate public health policy statements were set out for Wales and Scotland, as well as Northern Ireland.

One of the main themes of the revised English health strategy was a 'new contract' between the state and the individual, involving Government, local communities and individuals in partnership to improve health. This was portrayed as a 'third way' between a 'nanny state' and a 'victim-blaming' approach, which the new Government identified as features of previous public health policies. The Blair Government also proposed simplifying and reducing the number of national targets. The new targets were as follows:

- reduce the death rate from heart disease and stroke and related illnesses among people under 75 years old by at least two-fifths.

- reduce the death rate from accidents by at least a fifth and reduce the rate of serious injury by at least a tenth.

- reduce the death rate from cancer amongst people aged under 75 years by at least a fifth.

- reduce the death rate from suicide and undetermined injury by at least a fifth.

Exhibit 13.1 Public Health in Wales and Scotland

Wales became the first part of the UK to launch a public health strategy (Welsh Office NHS Directorate, 1989) which set out ten priority areas for achieving sustained improvements in health status or 'health gain': cancer, maternal and child health, mental handicap, mental distress and illness, injuries, emotional health, respiratory illness, cardiovascular diseases, healthy environments, and physical disability/discomfort. Although this ambitious plan had only a marginal impact (NAO (National Audit Office), 1996), it represented a clear attempt to shift the emphasis towards the improvement of health.

The change of Government in 1997, followed by plans for devolution and a new Welsh Assembly, presented further opportunities to develop a distinctive approach. A revised health strategy for Wales (Cm 3922, 1998) and a subsequent strategic framework (National Assembly for Wales, 1998) were introduced. The Welsh strategy appeared to focus more upon the economic and social context of health than the English strategy. It confirmed a number of health-gain targets (Welsh Office, 1997) including back pain, arthritis, dental heath, the consumption of fruit and vegetables, alcohol consumption, smoking, and breast, cervical and lung cancer. Subsequently, the Welsh Assembly set out proposals to improve health, which placed greater emphasis on social, environmental and economic roots of ill health, alongside plans to reorient health services to improve health as well as provide high-quality treatment (National Assembly for Wales, 2001a; Welsh Assembly Government, 2002b). Compared with the English NHS Plan, this placed much more emphasis on public health and health promotion. This continued with the introduction of health, social care and well-being strategies (Welsh Assembly Government, 2003b), which seek to bring about a stronger public health focus across health boards and local authorities, and other organisations. In addition, Wales adopted an action plan to promote healthy and active lifestyles and a food and well-being strategy to reduce diet-related ill health (Welsh Assembly Government, 2003c; Food Standards Agency/Welsh Assembly Government, 2003). It should also be noted that Wales has its own public health service which provides public protection and communicable-disease surveillance, and expertise on public health issues. Each local health board has a public health director drawn from the national public health service.

In Scotland, there is even more scope for divergence, given the greater self-governing powers vested in the Scottish Parliament. The Scottish strategy was initially outlined in a consultative document (Cm 3854, 1998) then subsequently in a White Paper, *Towards a Healthier Scotland* (Cm 4269, 1999). The Scottish approach differed from that in England in a number of ways. First, targets for dental health, smoking, alcohol and teenage pregnancy featured alongside coronary heart disease and cancer in the headline targets set by the strategy. Secondary targets were also set, relating to diet, smoking, alcohol, physical activity, strokes and dental health. Mental health was mentioned as a priority in the White Paper, though no target was set (in contrast to the English strategy). Accidents were identified as an important area for intervention and a commitment was made to develop a new target here. As in Wales, the Scottish strategy indicated a stronger commitment to dealing with

→

Exhibit 13.1 continued

$\longrightarrow$

social, economic and environmental factors, and an explicit commitment was made to monitor inequalities within the target areas. In addition, four demonstration projects at a cost of
£15 million were announced in the Scottish White Paper relating to sexual health, coronary
heart disease prevention, cancer prevention, and pre-school children's health. Subsequent
developments in Scotland included a diet action plan to improve lifestyles, the creation of a
public health institute to focus upon and co-ordinate efforts to improve health (subsequently
merged with the Health Education Board for Scotland to create NHS Health Scotland), new
initiatives to strengthen the public health role of nurses, and the appointment of public health
practitioner posts in local health care co-operatives and joint health improvement posts in
local authorities. Furthermore, the Scottish NHS Plan placed a high priority on health promotion (Scottish Executive, 2000a). Subsequently, the Scottish Executive (2003b, 2003d)
restated the importance of public health. This strategy aimed to put health improvement at
the top of the agenda, integrated within all Government programmes. This involved, among
other things, a new Health Improvement Director within the Scottish Executive, stronger co-
ordination between Scottish Government departments and agencies, co-ordination of
health promotion information campaigns, concentration of national expertise about public
health in one body – NHS Scotland – to support implementation of the national strategy,
integration of health improvement in public sector planning, and the development of learning networks to spread good practice. Also, new integrated programmes were announced
for children and young people, teenagers, the workplace and communities, physical activity, healthy eating, smoking, alcohol, mental health and well-being, homelessness and sexual health. Further structural change has also been introduced to strengthen health
improvement at the local level. Community health partnerships will be expected to promote
health improvement and to work with other agencies to achieve this (see Chapter 10).

The revised public health strategy for England incorporated a greater awareness
of social, economic and environmental factors compared with *the Health of the
Nation*. On taking office, the Blair Government established an inquiry into
health inequalities, chaired by former Chief Medical Officer, Donald Acheson
(who had previously undertaken the inquiry into the public health function in
the late 1980s). This second Acheson inquiry concluded that health inequalities were a key problem and proposed action in several policy areas to reduce
them. Its 39 recommendations included evaluating all policies for their impact
on health inequalities, policies for improving the material well-being and health
of elderly people, reducing income inequalities, improving nutrition, improving
the quality of housing, and reducing poverty in families with children
(Independent Inquiry into Inequalities in Health, 1998). The relevance of
health inequalities, a taboo subject under the previous Government, was
reflected in the two goals stated in *Saving Lives*: 'to improve the health of the
population as a whole by increasing the length of people's lives and the number of years people spend free from illness; and to improve the health of the
worst-off in society and to narrow the health gap' (Cm 4386, 1999, p. 5).
Specific policies, such as Health Action Zones and Healthy Living Centres,
were advanced as a means of promoting health in specific areas where needs

were greatest and had considerable potential to reduce health inequalities (see Chapter 10). National Service Frameworks – see Exhibit 7.4 – also addressed prevention and inequality issues. However, some were disappointed that the Acheson recommendations were not more enthusiastically endorsed by the Blair Government. They doubted its commitment to deal with the legacy of socio-economic inequalities from the two previous decades, particularly in the light of manifesto commitments not to raise income-tax rates. Even though New Labour's budgets redistributed towards the poorer sections of the community, economic inequality continued to widen in the late 1990s (Larkin, 2001). Indeed, in 2000/1 the bottom tenth of the income distribution had a quarter of the weekly disposable income of the top tenth. This figure had remained stable since the mid-1990s. However, in the late 1970s the bottom tenth had over a third of the income of the top tenth (Office for National Statistics, 2003).

However, there was a renewed emphasis on reducing poverty in this period, including a long-term commitment to end child poverty, and a series of changes to welfare and regeneration programmes focusing upon low-income families and deprived communities. The Joseph Rowntree Foundation (2003) reported that poverty in Britain had been reduced overall. However, 22 per cent of people still lived below the poverty line. Others also found that although child poverty had been reduced, it would remain much higher than in the late 1970s (Sutherland and Piachaud, 2001).

The importance of reducing health inequalities was also highlighted, both in the White Paper on public health and in Department of Health guidance (DoH, 1998d). Although the English strategy did not set national targets for reducing health inequalities at this stage, targets were later announced in the NHS Plan and introduced in 2001. These targets, to be achieved by 2010, were: (1) a reduction in the gap in infant mortality between manual groups and the national average by at least 10 per cent, and (2) at least a 10 per cent reduction in the gap between the bottom fifth of health authorities (later altered to local authority areas) with the lowest life expectancy rates at birth and the population average. The agenda was taken forward by a cross-cutting review of health inequalities across Government (Treasury/DoH, 2002). This backed a range of interventions, later developed into a strategy (DoH, 2003b), which set out a range of actions focusing on supporting families, mothers and children, engaging communities and individuals, preventing illness and providing effective treatment and care, and addressing the underlying determinants of health and long-term causes of health inequalities. Specific commitments included targets for improving social housing, eradicating fuel poverty, encouraging more children to walk and cycle, reducing child poverty, improving diet, nutrition and exercise, and reducing smoking and drug abuse. The strategy also promised an expansion of *Sure Start*, child care and support centres for children, improved mental health services for children, and improvements in the social

and health context of school life. However, most of the proposals were a continuation of, and in some cases a repackaging of, existing initiatives. There was
much cynicism about how and to what extent these various programmes would
be co-ordinated and achieved. Even so, new performance targets were set,
which might provide a stronger impetus to local organisations. Moreover, it was
expected that there would be greater co-ordination at regional and local level.
With regard to the latter, local strategic partnerships – involving local councils,
health bodies and others, such as the voluntary sector – were expected to play
a co-ordinating role.

The minister of public health was given the role of improving co-ordination
of policy across Government departments. A Cabinet committee of ministers
drawn from 12 departments was created to develop health policy across
Government (notably the Major Government had established a similar ministerial subcommittee but this had not been very active). In addition, the
Government expressed an intention to gear other policies – in fields such as welfare, housing, crime, education, transport and the environment – to public
health objectives. Health impact assessment – the calculation of the health consequences of policies, programmes and projects (see Scott-Samuel, 1996) – was
endorsed for key government policies, echoing more forcefully the earlier commitment to take into account health implications when formulating policies.
The Blair Government also sought to incorporate health considerations within
broader policies to regenerate communities and prevent social exclusion such as
the Neighbourhood Renewal Strategy. In addition, specific programmes – such
as *Sure Start*, which aims to improve the health and well-being of pre-school
children in deprived areas through the provision of additional, improved and
integrated services – addressed some of the socio-economic roots of ill health
in these areas. In a further move, it was announced that public health directors
would be located in Government Offices of the Regions, responsible for co-
ordinating Government policy at the regional level. Others, however, suggested
that public health powers should be exercised by democratised regional assemblies (see Morley and Campbell, 2003).

The Blair Government initially appeared keen to take on some of the corporate interests whose products were associated with ill health. A White Paper on
Smoking was introduced (Cm 4177, 1998) – with an expansion in assistance for
smokers trying to quit. The Blair Government announced its intention to ban
tobacco advertising. In the latter case it was frustrated by legal challenges,
though its credibility was challenged by allegations – strenuously denied – that
the Government had tried to exempt Formula One motor racing tobacco sponsorship in return for party political donations. Eventually, tobacco advertising
was banned in 2003, though the Government frustrated anti-tobacco campaigners by refusing to legislate to ban smoking in public places. Road safety
policy was limited by a combination of the power of the roads lobby, which
strongly resisted tougher speed limits, and opposition from the motoring public.

Proposals to reduce the alcohol limit for drink-driving, though attracting some public support, were defeated by the combined efforts of the roads lobby, and the drinks and leisure industries. Efforts to curb the impact of motoring on pollution and global warming – through policies such as higher petrol taxes – were successfully opposed by business interests, especially the farming and road haulage sectors. In particular, the fuel protest of 2000, which demonstrated strong public support for the farmers' and lorry drivers' campaign on fuel taxation, deterred Government at national and local level from adopting transport policies which might reduce pollution and improve environmental health.

A proposal to change the law to make it easier to secure convictions for corporate killing was delayed. Furthermore, an alcohol policy document promised in 1998 took six further years to develop and was heavily influenced by the drinks industry (Cabinet office, Prime Minister's Strategy Unit, 2004). The Government was concerned about adverse public response to policies restricting alcohol. Indeed, it actually relaxed the licensing laws, believing this to be a populist measure. Although it created a tougher food regulator – the Food Standards Agency – the Blair Government was as reluctant as its predecessors to take on the food industry on nutrition issues, despite the rising levels of obesity noted in Chapter 1. It did adopt a more pro-active sport and physical activity strategy, though concern was expressed that the policy did little to encourage exercise amongst those who were inactive. New schemes to provide free fruit and vegetables for children and low-income families, and its national campaign on diet, aimed at encouraging people to consume at least five portions of fruit and vegetables per day, were welcomed. But critics believed that greater regulation would be needed in order to deal with the marketing practices of the food industry (see Hastings et al., 2003).

The Blair Government addressed lifestyle issues in the area of sexually transmitted disease and teenage pregnancies. It set a target of reducing teenage pregnancy by half by 2010, and expanded education programmes in this area. This accompanied a sexual health strategy which aimed to reduce specific diseases such as AIDS/HIV and gonorrhoea by 25 per cent. The strategy included a new public education programme and screening for chlamydia, as well as national standards for sexual health services and improved access to such services (DoH, 2001s). However, the Health Committee (2003c) among others believed that more needed to be done to address these problems.

A great deal of emphasis was placed on reducing drug abuse. The approach was very high-profile. It emphasised both prevention and improved collaboration at local level to combat drug abuse, alongside other related social problems such as deprivation, poor education and crime (Cm 3945, 1998). The strategy was later revised, focusing more on heroin and cocaine, though the Government was cautious about easing controls on 'soft drugs'. Pressure to decriminalise cannabis, for example, was resisted, though the Government did allow research into the medical use of cannabis. It also changed the classification of cannabis (from a class B to a class C drug), following recommendations from a number of sources including the Independent Inquiry into the Misuse of Drugs Act 1971 (2000) established by the Police Foundation.

The Blair Government replaced the Health Education Authority (HEA) with a Health Development Agency, to maintain and disseminate an evidence base for health improvement, to advise on standards for public health and health promotion, and to commission and carry out health promotion campaigns. There was some unease about this, as the HEA (and its predecessor body, the Health Education Council) had challenged Government on health promotion issues in the past. Furthermore, each region would have a public health observatory, linked with universities, to monitor health and highlight areas for action and to evaluate progress by local agencies to improve health and reduce inequalities. Proposals were also set out to improve training in public health, to strengthen the public health roles of nurses, midwives and health visitors and to create a new post of Specialist in Public Health, open to professionals outside medicine. In a further development as part of the NHS Plan of 2000, a 'healthy communities collaborative' was proposed to disseminate best practice in the field of health promotion. Meanwhile, the system of control, advice and surveillance of hazards (such as infectious disease, chemical hazards, poisons) was reformed with the creation of a new Health Protection Agency for England and Wales to bring together the expertise of various organisations such as the Public Health Laboratory Service and the National Poisons Information Service.

Local Strategies

In the past, local health strategies have been influenced by international initiatives, such as the *WHO Healthy Cities* project, which focused on improving the health of the poor and disadvantaged, on the need to reorient medical services and health systems away from hospital and towards primary care, and on public involvement and partnerships between public, private and voluntary sectors (Ashton, 1992; Duhl, 1986). Participants in the initiative were expected to adopt specific interventions based on the WHO's *Health for All* principles, to monitor and evaluate these interventions, and to share experiences. Cities that were not officially part of the programme began to adopt similar strategies based on *Health For All* and *Healthy Cities* and, as a result, hundreds of cities in the European region have accepted to some degree the concepts and principles of these policies (Tsouros and Draper, 1992). While international initiatives provided an important stimulus for local health strategies, other factors were also influential in their emergence and development. During the 1980s many local authorities in cities such as Liverpool, Manchester and Sheffield became increasingly concerned about the health of their communities and began to devise strategies (see Harrow, 1991). This was a reaction to deteriorating urban conditions such as deprivation and industrial decline, and was stimulated to some extent by local dissatisfaction about national policies on unemployment, welfare and urban regeneration. The development of local health strategies during the 1990s was further stimulated by a concern for the environment. In 1992 the Rio summit set out an international programme of sustainable development in the form of Agenda 21, which encouraged local authorities to draw up their own local Agenda 21 (LA21) plan in consultation with their communities. Although LA21 was primarily concerned with the environment, the decision-making processes it sought to encourage had potentially wide implications for all sectors, including public health. In particular, it encouraged joint working on environmental and socio-economic causes of ill health.

Central government also began to encourage the development of local strategies during the 1990s. Health authorities were given the task of identifying health needs at the local level and commissioning services to meet them. The first Acheson Report prompted clarification of public health responsibilities at the local level. Subsequently, the *Health of the Nation* strategy provided central guidance for local strategies, and in particular encouraged the formation of 'healthy alliances' between the NHS and local agencies and organisations such as local government, the voluntary sector and employers. These promoted local strategies with regard to specific health problems such as heart disease and child accident prevention (DoH, 1998h, pp. 101, 121–34). Some alliances appeared to work well, particularly where good relationships already existed between local authorities and health authorities, where activities took place against the background of high-profile national campaigns such as AIDS awareness, heart disease prevention, road accident prevention and anti-smoking campaigns, and where funding was available (see Trevett, 1997; Levenson, Joule and Russell, 1997).

But many healthy alliances were less effective (Nocon, 1993; Ewles, 1993; DoH, 1998h). Fragmentation of responsibilities was problematic, particularly where a large number of authorities and organisations were involved. In some cases this situation was exacerbated by fundamental disagreements between organisations – often of a long-standing nature – regarding their respective roles. There was also concern that most healthy alliances were not central to the processes of commissioning and contracting, and that this undermined their effectiveness. Finally, a lack of resources for joint initiatives inhibited collaboration in some areas. Not all authorities earmarked resources for the development of alliances and even where budgets were allocated the sums tended to be small.

The Blair Government reiterated the importance of improved co-ordination at the local level on health matters. At local level, it sought to advance public health by identifying a number of settings in which health promotion initiatives could develop: schools, workplaces and neighbourhoods. Once again, this built on its predecessor's approach, which identified similar settings as a focus for such initiatives. To place greater emphasis on this activity, the Government announced health improvement programmes (later renamed Health Improvement and Modernisation Plans, which have also been superseded by local delivery plans – see Exhibit 7.3) – led by health authorities and agreed with other stakeholders such as local authorities and voluntary organisations. Both health and local authorities were expected to work more closely together on health-related issues alongside other relevant organisations such as voluntary organisations and business. This was underlined in the Health Act of 1999, which required NHS bodies and local authorities to co-operate on health and welfare matters and placed a statutory duty on local authorities to participate in such plans. However, as Hunter (2003) has noted, their impact in promoting the public health agenda was both variable and limited. In this context the primary care groups and primary care trusts were given an explicit brief to promote health improvement and to work with other agencies. While health improvement was not a key priority initially for PCGs and PCTs, it became more important (see Chapter 10). In some areas, improvements in partnership working were observed. Gillam, Abbott and Banks-Smith (2001), for example, reported significant links between PCG/Ts and agencies responsible for regeneration, housing and education. Other factors are undoubtedly at work here, including other policy initiatives to 'join-up' Government at the local level, including, for example, the Government's strategies for regeneration, neighbourhood renewal and crime prevention as well as other NHS initiatives such as Health Action Zones and National Service Frameworks. Local statutory agencies and voluntary organisations work together on a range of issues, many of which have a public health dimension. There are numerous examples of good practice, many of which focus on improving the health of specific population groups such as children, young people, elderly people and deprived communities. Examples include joint action on housing improvement and related illness, accident prevention, sexual health, smoking cessation and physical activity/exercise (Gillam, Abbott and Banks-Smith, 2001; *Health Service Journal*, 2003).

The creation of PCTs was seen as a further opportunity to improve joint working on public health. PCTs' performance is assessed on the basis of indicators of health improvement, as well as improved services, giving them an incentive to promote health and work with others to this end. However, the organisational upheaval involved in the move to PCTs was seen as undermining their health improvement work (Chapter 10). Another issue related to the reorganisation of responsibilities following the NHS Plan. PCTs were given the key role in delivering public health and reducing health inequalities. There were fears that PCTs were ill-equipped for this. Indeed, problems were experienced in recruiting staff with specialist knowledge. Another concern was that public health expertise would become fragmented. In response to this, the Government proposed the establishment of public health networks to supply specialist expertise for local public health organisations (see Singleton and Aird, 2002).

In 2000 local authorities were given powers to promote or improve the economic, social and environmental wellbeing of their area. They also have a community leadership role which involves a duty to produce a community plan. Increasingly, health and local authorities are working together to draw up common plans for health improvement. Interestingly, in Wales local councils and local health boards must draw up a common health, social care and well-being plan. Meanwhile, central government has encouraged local performance agreements, where local authorities work more closely with other agencies to identify common targets and ways of improving their performance towards these targets. As a means of bringing agencies together more effectively, and to address the confusion caused by 'partnership fatigue' – the growth in joint activities across a range of issues and services – central government promoted local strategic partnerships. These are overarching arrangements whereby different agencies can co-ordinate their joint working efforts (such as regeneration partnerships, health and social service partnerships, HAZs, Crime and Disorder Partnerships, and Education Action Zones). Progress has so far been limited, though in some areas considerable efforts have been made to streamline partnerships and focus more on health improvement (Hunter, 2003, p. 135; Hamer and Easton, 2002).

International Strategies

Finally, local and national health strategies must be seen in a broader, global context. As already indicated in this chapter, public health plans have been stimulated and shaped by initiatives at the international level. For example, the World Health Organisation (WHO) has long played a significant role in promoting public health strategies, while, more recently, European Union institutions have increased their involvement in this field. In this section, the role of these supranational institutions is further explored.

The World Health Organisation and Other International Bodies

The WHO *Health for All* programme has exerted an enormous influence on the development of public health strategies at national and local level. Its principles, endorsed at international conferences such as Alma Ata (1978), Ottawa (1986), Adelaide (1988), Sundsvall (1991) and Jakarta (1997), and promulgated in various documents published by WHO from the late 1970s onwards (WHO, 1978, 1981, 1986, 1998c), are as follows:

- Health is a fundamental human right and a social goal. Health is defined in a positive sense, in line with the classic WHO definition (see p. 1).

- There should be an equitable distribution of health resources, both within and between countries.

■ Health is shaped by many factors, social, economic, lifestyle and environmental, and policy makers must construct 'holistic' and 'intersectoral' policies that take account of other sectors of decision-making which impinge upon health. Governments should adopt 'healthy public policies' which strongly reflect health priorities, co-ordinate the actions of Government agencies, and are based on assessments of their health impact (Milio, 1986).

■ Health policies must be pre-emptive and precautionary, the aim being to prevent the problems from arising at the earliest possible stage.

■ Health improvements require a community-wide response. This involves partnership between agencies drawn from all relevant sectors and at all levels. Health promotion must include and involve the community, responding to its concerns, while at the same time promoting healthy lifestyles and supportive environments.

■ Health services must be reoriented towards primary health care and geared to promoting health rather than simply treating illness.

■ Clear performance targets and review mechanisms must be adopted in order to guide health strategies and achieve their objectives.

The original *Health for All* strategy, which set global targets for the year 2000 (WHO, 1981), have since been revised for the 21st century (see WHO, 1998c). In addition, European countries are guided by the WHO European Regional Office's own *Health for All* targets, published in 1985 (WHO Regional Office for Europe, 1985), updated in 1991 (WHO Regional Office for Europe, 1993) and revised in 1998 (WHO Regional Office of Europe, 1998). Specific, detailed targets accompany these main targets. For example, Target 12 includes three specific targets to be attained by 2015: that the proportion of non-smokers should be at least over 80 per cent (and close to 100 per cent in under-15-year-olds); that per capita alcohol consumption should not exceed 6 litres per annum (and should be close to zero in under-15-year-olds); and that the prevalence of illicit psychoactive drug use should be reduced by at least a quarter and mortality by half.

Exhibit 13.2 WHO European Region Targets for the 21st Century

1 By the year 2020, the present gap in health status between member states of the European Region should be reduced by at least one third.

2 By the year 2020, the health gap between socio-economic groups within countries should be reduced by at least one-fourth in all member states, by substantially improving the level of health of disadvantaged groups.

3 By the year 2020, all newborn babies, infants and preschool children in the Region should have better health, ensuring a healthy start in life.

$\longrightarrow$

Exhibit 13.2 continued

→

4 By the year 2020, young people in the Region should be healthier and better able to fulfil their roles in society.

5 By the year 2020, people over 65 years should have the opportunity of enjoying their full health potential and playing an active social role.

6 By the year 2020, people's psychosocial well-being should be improved, and better, comprehensive services should be available to and accessible by people with mental health problems.

7 By the year 2020, the adverse health effects of communicable diseases should be substantially diminished through systematically applied programmes to eradicate, eliminate or control infectious diseases of public health importance.

8 By the year 2020, morbidity, disability and premature mortality due to major chronic diseases should be reduced to the lowest feasible levels throughout the Region.

9 By the year 2020, there should be a significant and sustainable decrease in injuries, disability and death arising from accidents and violence in the Region.

10 By the year 2015, people in the Region should live in a safer physical environment, with exposure to contaminants hazardous to health at levels not exceeding internationally agreed standards.

11 By the year 2015, people across society should have adopted healthier patterns of living.

12 By the year 2015, the adverse health effects from the consumption of addictive substances such as tobacco, alcohol and psychoactive drugs should have been significantly reduced in all member states.

13 By the year 2015, people in the Region should have greater opportunities to live in healthy physical and social environments at home, at school and in the local community.

14 By the year 2020, all sectors should have recognised and accepted their responsibility for health.

15 By the year 2010, people in the Region should have much better access to family- and community-oriented primary health care, supported by a flexible and responsive hospital system.

16 By the year 2010, member states should ensure that the management of the health sector, from population-based health programmes to individual patient care at the clinical level, is oriented towards health outcomes.

17 By the year 2010, member states should have sustainable financing and resource-allocation mechanisms for health care systems based on the principles of equal access, cost-effectiveness, solidarity and optimum quality

18 By the year 2010, all member states should have ensured that health professionals and professionals in other sectors have acquired appropriate knowledge, attitudes and skills to protect and promote health.

19 By the year 2005, all member states should have health research, information and communication systems that better support the acquisition, effective utilisation, and dissemination of knowledge to support *Health for All*.

20 By the year 2005, implementation of policies for *Health for All* should engage individuals, groups and organisations throughout the public and private sectors, and civil society, in alliances and partnerships for health.

21 By the year 2010, all member states should have and be implementing policies for *Health for All* at country, regional and local levels, supported by appropriate institutional infrastructures, managerial processes and innovative leadership.

Source: WHO Regional Office for Europe (1998) *Health 21: The Health Policy Framework for the WHO European Region*

The WHO has done much to focus attention on the key factors that influence health and illness, and has introduced many initiatives to encourage its HFA principles (such as *Healthy Cities*, for example). It is not, however, without its critics, who have focused on its bureaucratic nature and its lack of resources and political leverage, and poor leadership in recent decades (see Beaglehole and Bonita, 1997, p. 227–9). Other international institutions – such as the World Bank and the International Monetary Fund – have, to some extent, taken on the leadership role in the health field, particularly with regard to developing countries (see Walt, 1994). Responding to this, the WHO has tried to reassert itself in recent years, focusing more on the fundamental aspects of health promotion and disease prevention.

The international level is important because so many potential threats to public health are global in nature. One thinks of the spread of infectious diseases resulting from increased mobility, the threats to health posed by environmental factors and climate change, the international traffic in illegal drugs, the impact of international trade in health, and the impact of economic inequalities on the health of the world's population (see Chapter 1), not to mention the effects of war and terrorism. A variety of international bodies have the capacity to improve public health worldwide by tackling these underlying causes of illness and disease. Examples include the UN bodies on narcotic drugs and the environment; the institutions responsible for promoting economic development, such as the UN Development Programme; aid institutions, such as UNICEF; and the institutions of world trade, such as the World Trade Organisation. A major difficulty is getting these institutions and their member states to develop coherent strategies, upon which all can agree, to secure improvements in public health at the global level, in a way that is accountable to the world's population as a whole (see Kickbusch, 2000). A further problem is the domination of many international institutions by the wealthier countries and their reluctance to challenge multinational corporations.

The European Union

The involvement of the EU (and, prior to its creation, the European Community) in health matters has increased since the early 1990s. Hitherto, aside from isolated initiatives in occupational health and safety, cancer prevention, food standards, HIV/AIDS, and drug abuse, public health was viewed as a matter for member Governments. One reason was that the original Treaty of Rome contained no health provisions. However, Community action was permitted under the Single European Act of 1987, which stated that harmonisation of trade must be based on regulations offering a high level of health protection. This had implications for policy in a number of areas, including food hygiene and health and safety at work. Subsequently, the Maastricht

Treaty of 1992 created a new community responsibility for public health. The legitimate areas for community action were the prevention of disease through research, information and education. The European Union has since developed a framework for action on public health. On the basis of this, a network for the control and surveillance of communicable diseases was established. In addition, the Council of Health Ministers in 1995 agreed plans to initiate programmes in several areas: cancer prevention, HIV/AIDS and other communicable diseases, drug addiction, and health monitoring. Subsequently, approval was given for programmes in three further areas: pollution-related disease, injury prevention and rare diseases. The emphasis on the provision of funds, research and information rather than on regulation remained, though a tougher regulatory approach did emerge in some areas, notably on smoking and on food safety, the latter being prompted by the BSE crisis and concerns about GM food.

Subsequently, the Amsterdam Treaty of 1997 increased the powers of the EU with regard to health. It stated that 'a high level of human health protection shall be ensured in the definition and implementation of community policies and activities' (European Union, 1997, p. 39). Community action was extended to include measures 'directed towards improving public health' as well as 'preventing human illness and diseases'. In addition, greater co-operation was agreed in a number of areas including health monitoring and epidemiological surveillance of infectious disease.

A further development has been the decision to adopt a new public health programme in the EU. This programme has three aspects: (1) improving health information and knowledge for the development of public health (2) enhancing the capability of responding rapidly to threats to health (3) addressing health determinants. This new programme intends to draw together established EU and national networks and expertise to implement public health interventions. It does not seek to undertake functions which fall within the competence of existing states but seeks to add value to these activities by supporting structures and programmes which strengthen existing institutions and organisations and by promoting an improved EU response to health threats such as infectious diseases, pollution and contamination. Indeed, a new EU institution – the Centre for Disease Prevention and Control – will soon be established. The EU programme aims to contribute to the definition of minimum quality standards applicable to health. It also sets out to make proactive use of other EU policies – such as structural funds and social policy – to influence health determinants. More generally the new programme aims to integrate health concerns into all EU policies and to ensure that all sectors of the EU policy process deliver a high level of human health protection.

Conclusion

Health strategies operate at a number of levels: national, international and local. They do not operate in isolation, but interact with each other. Hence, local and national strategies have been influenced by international developments, while national and international developments are in turn shaped by local experiences. Strategies are undoubtedly a useful guide for action. The very fact that they exist is an important development in itself, indicating a shift in emphasis from the provision of health care services to promoting public health. But the extent of this should not be exaggerated. Health strategies have been criticised on a number of grounds, including design flaws, implementation failure, unwillingness to tackle vested interests, problems of co-ordination, a refusal fully to address the social, economic and environmental causes of ill health, and for being inadequately resourced. Strategy alone is meaningless without the will to achieve objectives. Goals and targets can only set direction; they cannot guarantee success.

Nonetheless, public health has risen up the political agenda in the last decade. From time to time ministers have its restated importance, as in 2002 when the then Secretary of State for Health, Alan Milburn, called for a re-emphasis on prevention (Hunter, 2003, p. 2). The focus on health inequalities and, more recently, the desire to promote a more sustainable health care system through public health measures, has also been significant. Indeed, a further report by Derek Wanless (2004) – see also Chapter 7 – argued that public health objectives, roles and functions should be clarified and strengthened in order to promote the maintenance of good health. The Government responded by declaring its intention to publish a further White Paper on public health later in the year. Increasingly, those responsible for planning within the NHS will have to take into account the public health perspective and will be expected to liaise with other agencies whose work is relevant to public health, such as local government and the voluntary sector. At the same time, managers and professionals working within the NHS will be increasingly expected to be more aware of the public health dimension of their work and, especially in the primary care sector, to work effectively with those employed by these other agencies.

That being said, public health has a long way to go. As Wanless noted, the evidence and information base for public health intervention is poor. There is a shortage of expertise and capacity in public health. Its practitioners are still relatively weak within the NHS and still lack the clout of professionals involved in hospital-based treatment. The political and organisational obstacles to joint working on public health remain quite strong. Despite the calls for more 'joined-up' government from the centre, it is here, ironically, where narrow organisational interests remain most firmly entrenched. And one cannot ignore the powerful commercial interests that can bring enormous pressure to bear when they feel threatened by public health policies. Finally, despite the undoubted importance of good health, the key to a politician's survival in the field of health care depends foremost on issues of access and the quality of treatment services. The promotion of good health, though a desirable long-term objective, is a matter for the statesman rather than today's breed of careerist politician. This bias is reinforced by the performance management system within the NHS, especially in England which concentrates mainly on health care provision. Until these incentives are properly addressed, and local managers and professionals are rewarded for their efforts in maintaining, protecting and improving health and well-being, the architects of public health strategies will struggle to achieve their aims.

Further Reading

Baggott, R. (2000) *Public Health, Policy and Politics* (Basingstoke, Palgrave Macmillan).

Garrett, L. (1995) *The Coming Plague: Newly Emerging Diseases in a World out of Balance* (Harmondsworth, Penguin).

Hunter, D. (2003) *Public Health Policy* (Oxford, Polity Press).

Jones, L., Sidell, M. and Douglas, J. (2002) *The Challenge of Promoting Health*, 2nd edn (Basingstoke, Palgrave Macmillan).

Orme, J., Powell, J., Taylor, P., Harrison, T. and Greg, M. (2003) *Public Health for the 21st Century: New Perspectives on Policy, Participation and Practice* (Buckingham, Open University Press).

Rosen, G. (1993) *A History of Public Health*, expanded edn (New York, Johns Hopkins University Press).

Wanless, D. (2004) *Securing Good Health for the Whole Population* (London, HM Treasury).

Conclusion

14

Britain is not alone in seeking to reform its health care system (see, for example, European Observatory on Health Care Systems, 2002; Freeman, 2000; Saltman, Figueras and Sakellarides, 1998). Other countries face similar problems and challenges arising from threats to public health, health inequalities, demographic pressures, the cost of health care, technological innovations, and concerns about the quality of health services. There are, of course, differences in emphasis. In the USA, for example, the exclusion of a large proportion of the population – over 40 million citizens are uninsured – is a major issue. While, in the UK, the main concerns have been the speed of access to care and the equity of access to new treatments. Such national variations are reflected in opinion surveys which reveal common concerns about the quality of care, but different priorities (see Blendon et al., 2003).

Each health care system generates its own particular configuration of issues. Moreover, as Tuohy (1999) has observed, each has its own logic and dynamics which enable differences to persist. Even where reform principles are similar across countries, policies on which they are based are inevitably shaped by the political context. Indeed, Jacobs (1999) found that the design and implementation of reforms varied considerably across countries. Both Tuohy and Jacobs highlighted the importance of pre-reform conditions and structures, and political circumstances and institutions in maintaining differences between health care systems (Wilsford, 1994; Greener, 2004). Nonetheless, one cannot deny that there are pressures in the direction of convergence. Common economic, social, political and technological factors faced by health care systems often generate similar policy ideas (Moran, 1999; Ruggie, 1996; Reinhardt, 1996). States often draw on the experience of others and seek to adapt policies to their own circumstances. Indeed, it is widely acknowledged by convergence theorists and their critics alike that common themes of reform are found across industrialised nations. These include: the shifting of responsibilities for health care risks – by the introduction of various forms of managed care and decentralised budget holding; the increasing use of quasi-markets in the delivery of health care; a heavier reliance on the independent sector; greater selectivity and targeting of health care resources; specification of standards and increased regulation of health care provision; an increased emphasis on evidence-based interventions; an acknowledgement of the importance of primary care and community-based services; and a greater recognition of the wider socio-economic and environmental factors in illness.

Britain's Health Reforms

Over the past three decades, the pace of health care reform in Britain has increased markedly. Back in the 1990s, it seemed like a permanent revolution in health care was taking place (Baggott, 1994). No sooner had one set of reforms been introduced, than another was formulated. There were several reasons why this occurred. Central government was under pressure to improve the NHS and to secure quick results. But some policies were not fully implemented, or were frustrated by countervailing actions of managers and professionals at local level, while others had unforeseen consequences which raised further problems that needed to be addressed. Since 1997, if anything, the zeal of central government for health reform has increased. The pace of reform, according to one study, has been 'relentless, almost hyperactive' (Appleby and Coote, 2002, p. 5). There was a torrent of new initiatives, some of which marked important and unexpected shifts in policy. For example, in the Blair Government's 1997 White Paper on the NHS there was no mention of the private sector, but within three years a concordat was agreed, paving the way for it to play a larger role in the provision of NHS care. In April 2002 the National Care Standards Commission began its work. Yet, in the same month, the Government issued new proposals to transfer its functions to two new bodies, the Commission for Healthcare Audit and Inspection and the Commission for Social Care Inspection. Another example occurred when a new statutory system of patient and public involvement was introduced in 2003. As this was being implemented, an entirely different model of public involvement associated with the introduction of foundation trusts was being enacted.

The impact of the constant upheaval of these reforms should not be underestimated. The scale of organisational change is disruptive, undermining capacity and internal and external relationships. The enforced creation of PCTs, for example, was criticised on these grounds. Constant reorganisation and policy changes can also lead to cynicism about reform and general fatigue among those who actually provide services (Greener and Powell, 2003). No wonder then that the restructuring of the NHS following the NHS Plan was labelled by some as 'a redisorganisation' (Smith, Walshe and Hunter, 2001). In addition, the Blair Government has created many new bodies at national level, all of which have had to develop an identity, build capacity, mark out their territory, and build relationships with other national bodies and the NHS at local level. Again the impact on the NHS has been confusing, with a plethora of bodies issuing guidance and monitoring activity. Finally, the multiplicity of policies, and their associated plans and targets, has added to the confusion.

Rather than repeat in detail the policy developments from the 1980s to the present day, it is more appropriate to summarise the broad themes of policy, and the shifts and continuities they exhibit. It is helpful to divide the period into 5 stages;

1 *Early Thatcherism*: radical ideas about privatising parts of the NHS gave way to a more pragmatic approach. Only services at the margins of the NHS were subjected to privatisation and market testing at this stage. Meanwhile, business-style management methods were introduced to try and improve efficiency and greater accountability to central government. Tight control was exerted over the NHS budget and there was a perennial quest for efficiency savings.

2 *Late Thatcherism*: a return to more radical ideas that saw market principles introduced into the NHS. The internal market was one of the last significant pieces of legislation initiated by the Thatcher Government. There was a small gesture towards the private health sector in the form of tax relief for elderly people. In primary care, there was greater emphasis on financial incentives for specific service developments. Tight control of the NHS budget continued.

3 *The Major Years*: an attempt was made to balance markets with national standards and accountability requirements. The internal market was introduced but hedged with controls. The emphasis was much more on performance targets and accountability to the centre. Market testing was extended and PFI introduced. The need to improve public health was recognised, but with an emphasis mainly upon clinical prevention and individual responsibility for lifestyles. There was tight control of the NHS budget with tough efficiency targets.

4 *Early Blair Government*: tight control of the NHS budget continued, along with efficiency targets. Emphasis was given to equity of access, clinical quality and national standards. New national bodies were created, such as NICE and CHI. The purchaser–provider split was retained but with an emphasis on collaboration and equity. This was reflected in the abolition of GP fundholding, the introduction of longer-term service agreements, and duties of collaboration placed on NHS bodies and local government. Joined-up working became a key priority across healthcare, social care and public health. There was a broader acknowledgement of the socio-economic factors in ill health. Although the Government endorsed the use of the Private Finance Initiative in the NHS, uncertainty about the role of the independent sector remained. The tax relief on private health care for elderly people was ended and a new body established to regulate independent sector health and social care.

5 *Late Blair*: more generous public expenditure plans were announced, but pressure on providers to reduce costs continued. The commitment to a tax-funded NHS was reiterated but with greater plurality of provision, including greater reliance on the private sector. A strong emphasis on

patient-centred services emerged, initially focused on strengthened user-involvement, then on patient choice. Attempts were made to shift responsibility to local commissioners and service providers, culminating in the introduction of foundation hospitals. A tougher audit and inspection regime was introduced, with some rationalisation of responsibilities among the NHS regulatory bodies. Professional regulation was reformed with a new overarching body – the Council for the Regulation of Health Care Professionals. PFI was extended to primary care. There was also a revival of interest in the internal market, with resources following patients. Policies in social care highlighted the needs of groups such as the elderly and mentally ill people, but demonstrated impatience with agencies in health and social care, reflected in policies such as care trusts and cross-charging.

It can be seen from the above that there are elements of continuity between these phases. From one perspective this can be seen as a moving consensus (Rose and Davies, 1995), as Governments inherit policies from their predecessor, irrespective of party. Governments have to make decisions about priorities; which policies will they seek to reverse and which can they live with, at least for the short term. Indeed, new Governments can be quite opportunistic, and build on their predecessor's legislation – as happened with the 1997 Primary Care Act (see Chapter 10).

Eighteen years of Conservative Government could not be reversed immediately. Moreover, there was an element of path dependency (see Greener, 2004) in the system. Policies had already set in train various changes that could not be reversed without enormous legislative and political effort. The Blair Government did, however, have considerable legislative and political power. It had been elected with a huge majority, was very popular long after the initial honeymoon period usually enjoyed by new Governments. The Conservative opposition was in disarray, pulled apart by internal ideological forces that sought on the one hand to remain true to the Thatcherite legacy and, on the other, to develop a form of 'Caring Conservatism' more in tune with the times. The media was also initially supportive of 'New Labour', partly owing to the Party's well-honed media-management skills. But the newsworthiness of problems in the NHS in the end proved too tempting, and the Blair Government found itself in a corner amid allegations, yet again, that the service was in crisis.

The NHS crisis of 2000/1 proved a turning point for the Blair Government. It began to develop a tougher edge. Backbench MPs, particularly those of the 'old Labour' fraternity, became concerned about the direction of health policy. A rallying point was the Health Committee of the House of Commons, chaired by David Hinchliffe MP. This committee produced a series of critical reports of Government policies on topics including foundation hospitals, public and patient involvement and public health. Backbench discontent, coupled with opposition from the House of Lords, forced the Government into concessions, in order to secure the passage of key legislation. On two high-profile issues – the replacement of Community Health Councils with new bodies, and foundation hospitals – significant concessions were made, though it proved impossible to block the legislation.

Given that many policies do not require new legislation – they can be brought about by ministerial decisions based on existing powers – there is little that opponents of reform can do, apart from to try and persuade Government of the error of its ways, either through consultation processes or by enlisting media support. These arguments need not be confrontational. Indeed, they have greater chance of success when they are consistent with the Government's aims and objectives, and its general ideological stance.

Although there are important differences between the ideological orientation of the Thatcher, Major and Blair Governments, there has been a strong element of continuity in both the style and substance of policy-making in health care since 1979. All Governments in this period have endorsed the new public management approach, described in Chapter 3. They have pursued policies which adopt explicit standards and targets, use performance measurement and audit and emphasise strong accountability to central government. In this regard, the Blair Government has perhaps gone further than previous administrations.

But what about style? There were certainly important differences in style between the Thatcher and Major Governments. The style of the early Blair Government was very different to that which later developed. Taking the period as a whole, one would say that the dominant style of policy-making was one of authoritarianism combined with pragmatism. Governments took a strong position on most issues, but were prepared to modify their policies if they saw political advantage in doing so – for example to increase popularity, to diffuse strong opposition, to overcome implementation problems or to address problems caused by new policies.

The Impact of Reform since 1997

It is difficult to summarise the impact of the wide-ranging reforms that have been introduced since 1997, particularly as some policies have contradicted and undermined others. Many of the policies take the form of long-term strategies, which means that it is difficult to appraise them in the short term. In addition, the introduction of new policies before previous efforts have been fully implemented or evaluated, has made it difficult to assess their impact. This lack of evidence-based policy-making is ironic, given the Government's support for evidence-based clinical practice (Calman, Hunter and May, 2002). Similar criticisms could be made of the Conservative Government's reforms (Powell, 1997; see also Chapter 5). However, in spite of the difficulties, it is possible to come to a judgement on recent reforms.

Funding and Efficiency

More money is being spent on health care, largely as a result of the substantial increases generated by the Budgets since 2000. However, there is less information about how the additional funds are being spent. Although funds are earmarked for particular initiatives, for example the implementation of national service frameworks, it has been claimed that there has been some diversion to other uses.

Despite the increase in public funding for the NHS, its financial problems are far from settled. The Audit Commission (2003b) found that the majority of trusts were at high risk of not achieving financial balance. The continuation of deficits is the result of several factors, including poor financial management. Changes in resource-allocation formulas – disadvantaging some areas – have also played a part. Delays in securing service agreements were also identified as a key problem. The introduction of greater choice and competition in the NHS is likely to increase uncertainty within trusts about future income and deficits are expected. In addition, it must be acknowledged that some of the increase in spending has been absorbed by the cost of monitoring and regulation (see Leatherman and Sutherland, 2003).

The Blair Government has required NHS bodies to continue to make efficiency gains. The reference cost scheme provides a comparison, albeit flawed, of costs between different providers. But it has had little immediate impact on actual costs. In future, financial discipline is likely to come from market forces, as secondary providers compete with each other for resources under the new financial flows system. Meanwhile, the tax-funded model has survived, though with some modification. The additional National Insurance element introduced by the 2002 Budget raises funds from a different tax base. Meanwhile, other sources, such as charitable funding, the National Lottery, motor insurance and insurance against liabilities due to injury, are being increasingly exploited. Other co-payments for health care have been suggested, though no proposals have as yet emerged.

Public/Private Sector

Despite an inauspicious start, the Blair years have been fruitful for the independent health care sector. Although the British health care system remains for the time being a predominantly public service model, the independent sector has made important inroads. With regard to provision, the independent sector has established itself as a key player: a partner for the NHS in reducing waiting lists, a competitor for tax-payers' money, and an alternative to NHS management under franchising arrangements. At the moment the encouragement of plurality has been wholly on the supply side. It will be interesting to see whether independent sector organisations will be given a role in relation to the commissioning of NHS care – by franchising out PCTs to independent organisations for example.

In addition, the private sector has become more heavily involved in the NHS through the Private Finance Initiative (PFI). Critics believe the scheme subverts NHS priorities to commercial interests and allows tax-payers' money to subsidise company profits. They have also expressed doubts about the value for money of these projects, the appropriateness of facilities, and have criticised the secrecy surrounding the deals. The extension of private finance into primary care has been greeted with further alarm. However, although there is some evidence to fuel suspicion, the ideologically charged nature of this debate and the lack of data as a result of commercial secrecy make it difficult to arrive at an informed judgement about the threat posed to the public sector model of health care by greater reliance on private finance.

Quality of Service

There are many different aspects to quality. The Government has focused mainly on setting national standards and targets, and monitoring performance against these. In this narrow sense, there is evidence of service improvement – though considerable variation persists between different parts of the NHS (see Audit Commission, 2003b; CHI, 2003b; Leatherman and Sutherland, 2003). For example, there have been substantial difficulties in implementing the National Service Frameworks for mental health and older people (see Chapter 11 and Audit Commission, 2003b). Even within particular condition areas there are substantial variations in services. For example, it was found that the quality of services available to cancer patients varied according to the type of cancer (CHI/Audit Commission, 2001), and it has been suggested that patients with coronary heart disease receive a better service than patients with other heart problems (Siddall, 2002). Considerable differences in quality also persist both between service providers and within the same institutions (Audit Commission, 2003b; CHI, 2003b; *Heart*, 2002; National Confidential Enquiry into Perioperative Deaths, 2001; CHI/Audit Commission, 2001).

It is difficult to evaluate the impact of the new systems of quality assurance. There has certainly been substantial investment in these systems (NAO, 2003b; Leatherman and Sutherland, 2003). But as Chapters 7 and 9 suggested, quality assurance and performance management systems do not necessarily improve services. Indeed, crude targets may well have a perverse effect. Meanwhile, other initiatives have emphasised the prevention of errors, improved outcomes, shared learning and the importance of cultural change in NHS organisations.

These have great potential to improve standards of care in a wider sense. However, there are tensions between the organisational learning approach and regulatory models that need to be addressed. On balance, it is the latter approach that has predominated in recent years.

The Professions and the Workforce

The election of the Labour government in 1997 was warmly, if not enthusiastically, welcomed by most people working in the NHS. Staff have seen some positive changes, notably a substantial increase in NHS spending. Some staff have been offered new opportunities. For example, the introduction of modern matrons, nurse consultants, new primary care services, and changes to prescribing have extended the role of nurses. There has been more effort to involve staff, alongside commitments to improve the quality of working lives in the NHS. More specifically, improved conditions of work for some staff may arise from changes to junior doctors' hours and to primary care out-of-hours services. Efforts to improve professional education and training, continuing professional development and improved team-working were also long overdue.

On the other hand, low morale has continued (see Finlayson, 2002) and the pace of reform has been unrelenting. New regulatory systems and performance management systems have been criticised for creating huge burdens on staff and diverting resources from patient care. There has also been controversy over new contracts for professional staff, notably NHS consultants. These issues have continued the legacy of distrust that festered during the previous decades. Given the acknowledged relationship between organisational culture and performance, efforts to improve working relationships in the NHS must be redoubled.

Access, Fairness and Choice

Much activity has been geared to improving access to health services. Building on the previous Government's *Patient's Charter*, the Blair Government devised tougher targets for waiting times. Considerable success was achieved, though tainted by allegations of statistical massage and manipulation. New initiatives, such as NHS Direct, Walk-in Centres and Health Action Zones have been credited with improving access to services. With regard to the fairness of access, national standards were introduced in the form of the National Service Frameworks and NICE guidance. But the impact on equity of access is unknown, largely because there is no information on the extent to which these standards are being implemented across different populations. Anecdotally, however, it appears that there is variable implementation (see above) and that the so-called 'postcode' lottery persists (CHI, 2003b). Moreover, equity of access for different population groups remains a problem, given the experiences of people in deprived areas, elderly and disabled people, ethnic minorities and women (see Chapter 8).

The emphasis on fair access is somewhat at odds with the more recent emphasis of the Blair Government on patient choice. Giving patients greater choice is not a bad idea, providing they have the necessary information to make such choices. It is also important that the exercise of choice by one person does not disadvantage others, or undermine the efficiency and effectiveness of the health care system. This could happen if some people secure a better position than others to exercise choices or if they receive better information or have more alternatives to choose from. Another problem is that greater individual choice could absorb resources that could be spent on meeting the needs of all patients. The Blair Government has highlighted patient choice as its latest big idea for the NHS – reflected in the Command Paper status of its policy document on the subject (Cm 6079, 2003). It has sought to convince critics that choice and equity are not only compatible, but that the former can help achieve the latter. But apart from suggesting ways of levelling the playing field for consumers, by strengthening capacity in deprived communities for example, there is little in these proposals about how the very real tensions between choice and equity will be managed in practice.

Equity of access to high-quality care may also be threatened by other developments, such as the introduction of foundation hospitals and the new system of resource flows in the NHS. The idea of foundation trusts was criticised for its potential to create inequalities between providers. Although all hospitals are expected to become foundation trusts within the next few years, the earliest candidates may secure the greatest gains and a dominant position in the provision of health care. They will be best placed to respond to the new system of resource flows which will reward those providers that increase throughput through a standard tariff. As predicted by the inverse care law, this new fixed-price but nonetheless competitive market system is likely to increase inequalities between providers as those with deficits struggle to meet the necessary standards of care.

Accountability

As noted in Chapter 7, there are many different types of accountability in the NHS, and there are tensions between them. Since the mid-1980s Governments have opted for a stronger system of accountability to the centre. The emphasis was initially on managerial and financial accountability. This has changed to some extent since 1997. The Blair Government emphasised clinical accountability by imposing a duty of quality and introducing clinical governance. However, it has also strengthened managerial accountability through its Performance Assessment Frameworks and the emphasis on targets, indicators and star ratings.

The current mantra is shifting the balance of power back to the front line in the NHS. However, there are reasons for cynicism about this, given the enormous political and financial capital invested in the NHS in recent years. While there is no doubt that stronger accountability is needed to local communities, and that local NHS bodies must have greater freedom to meet local needs, this is at odds with the tax-funded nature of the NHS and its high political profile nationally. National politicians should not be able to avoid responsibility for the NHS. Arguments to depoliticise it by creating a separate agency will not resolve this, nor will the limited efforts so far to improve scrutiny and public involvement.

Public Involvement

Important changes have occurred in relation to patient and public involvement: a new statutory duty for the NHS to consult and involve the public, new statutory institutions at national and local level, local authority scrutiny of health, and the promise of a reformed complaints process directly linked to quality improvements. However, there has been much criticism of Government policy in this area. The decision to abolish CHCs in England was seen as vindictive. There are suspicions that the new system is too fragmented to be effective, and there are worries about a lack of resources. The system is also relatively inaccessible to patients and the public. The plethora of new bodies is confusing even to the expert. Others go further and see the system as a way of manipulating patient and public involvement, in order to endorse decisions made by service planners and providers.

Even though many of these criticisms are valid, it is far too early to assess the impact of this new regime. The system of patient and public involvement certainly has the potential to strengthen accountability and improve scrutiny of the NHS. But much will depend on how the national body (CPPIH) and the local patient and public involvement forums develop their role. A great deal will also depend on how effectively this system of representation works alongside other mechanisms for incorporating the views of patients, users and carers, such as PALS, complaints procedures, market research tools and the activities of the voluntary sector. It will also be interesting to see how it dovetails with the rather different model of public accountability and involvement embodied by the foundation trusts.

Primary Care

The Blair Government, like its predecessor, stressed the importance of a primary-care-led NHS. Although GP fundholding was abolished, primary care commissioning was retained in the form of primary care groups and subsequently PCTs. In addition, many new initiatives were introduced to encourage new ways of providing primary care services – such as NHS Direct for example – and these have been generally well-received, though doubts about cost-effectiveness remain. The introduction of new contractual arrangements for primary care professionals, notably for GPs, has been heralded as promoting further innovation and improvement in primary care services, but, as noted in Chapter 8, predictions here are particularly hazardous.

The move towards PCTs, with responsibility for the majority of the NHS budget, in theory created primary care authorities that could plan across the primary and secondary divide, and commission services accordingly. Subsequently, the location of the public health function in PCTs appeared to put primary care organisations in the driving seat with regard to health improvement. However, in reality acute and specialist services continued to dominate the agenda, and PCTs have had little room for manoeuvre. This may be reinforced by foundation trust status, which seems likely to strengthen the ability of hospitals to claim wider public support for their activities. PCTs have also had to struggle with an enormous agenda, with relatively limited management resources. They also lack expertise in key areas, with particular concern being expressed about their specialist resources in public health.

Health and Social Care

One of the worst aspects of the British health care system has been the poor levels of co-ordination between the NHS and social care agencies. This has been compounded by the low priority given to those groups that are the biggest users of health and social care: people with mental illness, learning disabilities, physical disabilities, and the elderly. Efforts have been made to improve the lot of these groups in recent years, with major policy initiatives and national standards, including the National Service Frameworks for mental health and older people. As in health care, there has been an effort to strengthen regulation in social care and to develop more effective systems of performance management, though similar caveats apply given the reliance on crude star ratings.

These 'Cinderella services' may now be at the ball. But their outfits are still not as plush as the more prestigious areas of health care. The two major priorities, cancer and heart disease, continue to dominate, as major reviews of performance and service quality confirm (Audit Commission, 2003b; CHI, 2003b). Services for older people and mental health continue to face severe resource constraints, in some cases because funds earmarked for service development have apparently been diverted elsewhere.

There are signs that working arrangements between the NHS and local government have improved. Important changes such as the creation of primary care organisations with local authority representation, the duty of co-operation, joint funding arrangements, improved planning arrangements and intermediate care all played a part in encouraging improved relationships between agencies. It remains to be seen whether integrated care trusts yield further advantages. However, time and again, the fundamental explanation for improved joint working comes through loud and clear. It is not structural reorganisation nor the imposition of statutory duties that is ultimately crucial. Rather, it is the development of trust and co-operation at the local level, often the result of specific historical and local circumstances, that seems to be the most important single factor.

Public Health and Inequalities

Building on the Major Government's *Health of the Nation* policy, the Blair Government sought to extend public health beyond efforts cajole individuals to improve their own lifestyles. It did appear willing to confront socio-economic factors in ill health and some of the commercial interests that profited from illness, injury and death. With regard to socio-economic factors, new initiatives were introduced to address deprivation at both an individual and community level. Policies included Health Action Zones, *Sure Start*, regeneration initiatives, a teenage pregnancy strategy, and changes to taxes and benefits. However, the underlying structure of British society remained unequal, which for some was the major obstacle to greater overall standards in health. After initial reluctance the Blair Government did adopt national health inequality targets, but these will be difficult to achieve given the persistence of underlying socio-economic inequalities in Britain.

Regarding the commercial interests in ill health, the Blair Government initially took on vested interests in the form of the tobacco industry. However, some credibility was lost as a result of the controversy over Formula One sponsorship. The ban on tobacco advertising took over five years to achieve. The Blair Government fought shy of the alcohol and food industries, though it did create a new Food Standards Agency. Moreover, at the time of writing, rising levels of alcohol abuse and an epidemic of obesity are placing pressures on Government to confront commercial interests about the health implications of their products and marketing activities.

Public health strategy continues to be disease-focused, emphasising reductions in mortality from the major killers. This has been reflected in National Service Frameworks and in health improvement plans at the local level. There has been some success: death rates for England and Wales fell by 14 per cent in men and 10 per cent in women between 1990 and 1999 (Office of Health Economics, 2003). Over the same period, death rates from the four biggest killers also fell: coronary heart disease (by 38 per cent in men and 32 per cent in women); stroke (by 30 and 26 per cent, respectively); lung cancer (32 and 9 per cent), breast cancer (24 per cent in women). Scotland and Northern Ireland have also seen reductions in the mortality rates from these diseases. It is difficult to attribute these to the Blair Government's health strategy given the multiple factors impinging on mortality rates, and the time lag between changing behaviour and death rates. Indeed, if anything, the previous Government's strategy should perhaps have been given some credit.

Public health has not been given as high a priority under the Blair Government that many hoped. Despite the initial emphasis on prevention and public health, the Governments' agenda has been dominated by acute sector issues and the reorganisation of the NHS. Similarly at local level, though important efforts have been made to secure health improvement, the delivery of the NHS Plan, with its emphasis on service delivery, has been central. Nonetheless, ministers have from time to time reiterated the importance of public health. At the time of writing the Government has promised a new White Paper on public health, expected in the autumn of 2004.

Devolution and Divergence

Devolution has created opportunities for different parts of the UK to reform the NHS in different ways. There have always been differences between the NHS in England, Scotland, Wales and Northern Ireland. These were mainly structural, or arose from time lags in the reform process. With devolution, the differences have become more pronounced, and not only in structural terms. For example, Scotland and Wales, and to some extent Northern Ireland too, have placed greater emphasis on public health and improving health and well-being than England. There are big differences in the approach to resource allocation within the NHS. In Scotland, the internal market was abolished and there has been a strong move towards integrated health care systems at local level. In Wales, commissioning was retained, but within a more overtly collaborative planning system. Early moves in this direction in England gave way to a market-style system with the promise of increased competition, extended patient choice and greater autonomy for hospitals. Substantial differences have emerged between England and Scotland and Wales on methods of performance management – the latter do not have the star rating system. In England, the independent sector has been seen as a key partner in NHS provision, while in other parts of the UK this is not the case. In addition, there are significant differences emerging in entitlement to free care. These include divergent policies on free personal care for the elderly between Scotland and other parts of the UK, while entitlements to free eye tests and dental checks have been extended in Wales.

There are, of course, many similarities. The stated priorities of the NHS in each country are similar. The challenges faced in each part of the UK are broadly similar: the need to improve efficiency, service quality, access, and to reduce health inequalities. Certain policies, such as changes to complaints systems and public and patient involvement, while different in detail, have been pursued across the UK. It will be interesting to see if the differences that have emerged are maintained. Indeed, it may well be that they create pressures for convergence, as different parts of the UK learn lessons from each other, and as people demand the same entitlements as NHS users in other parts of the UK.

The Future?

Speculating about future developments in health policy is a hazardous occupation. As recent events have shown, policy developments are often unpredictable. Important changes such as foundation trusts, extended patient choice and the revival of the internal market were not on the agenda in 1997. As this book will be published within a year of the next General Election, with the possibility of a closer contest than in 1997 and 2001, one needs to be a cautious tipster indeed.

Some things, however, are a safer bet than others. First, the crisis-driven nature of health care reform is certain to continue and the media will retain its role in driving the political agenda. Secondly, there is likely to be greater disquiet about the implications of the revival of the internal market in England, resulting in a more centralised and regulated approach than currently envisaged. There may also be concerns about the role of the independent sector, should issues of quality or unfair competition arise, and this may lead to greater regulation. Related to this, it will be very difficult for Government to relax its grip on the NHS, given the pressures for accountability already discussed. Meanwhile, pressures for the NHS in England to adopt policies in Wales and Scotland will grow, particularly where related to greater entitlements such as free personal care. There will also be increasing pressures to focus on health rather than health care. These will arise within Government – in an effort to reduce health service costs in the future – and be bolstered by campaigners from outside Government concerned about public health issues. Finally, the governance of health care – as in other areas of British Government policy-making – is likely to be dominated by a similar disregard for constructive criticism. For authoritarian pragmatism is not just a feature of health policy, nor is it the preserve of the Blair Government. It has become an established feature of the British political process.

Bibliography

Aanchawan, T. (1996) 'Room at the Top', *Health Service Journal*, 7 March, 26–8.

Abbott, A. (1988) *The System of Professions: An Essay in the Division of Expert Labour* (Chicago, Chicago University Press).

Abbott, S. and Gillam, S. (2000) 'Trusting to Luck', *Health Service Journal*, 18 May, 24–5.

Abbott, S., Florin, D., Fulop, N. and Gillam, S. (2001) *Primary Care Groups and Trusts: Improving Health* (London, King's Fund).

Abel-Smith, B. (1960) *History of the Nursing Profession* (London, Heinemann).

Abel-Smith, B. (1964) *The Hospitals 1800–1948* (London, Heinemann).

Abel-Smith, B. (1996) 'The Escalation of Health Care Costs: How Did We Get There', in *Health Care Reform: The Will To Change* (Paris, OECD), 17–30.

Acheson, D. (1981) *Primary Health Care in Inner London* (London, London Health Planning Consortium).

Ackroyd, S. (1995) 'Nurses, Management and Morale – A Diagnosis of Decline in the Hospital Service', in Soothill, K., Mackay, L. and Webb, C. (eds) *Interprofessional Relations in Healthcare* (London, Edward Arnold), 222–38.

Adams, C. (1995) 'OxDONS Syndrome: The Inevitable Disease of the NHS Reforms', *British Medical Journal*, 311, 1559–61.

Adams, J. (1995) 'With Complements', *Health Service Journal*, 1 June, 23.

Aggleton, P. (1990) *Health* (London, Routledge).

Agriculture Committee (1998) (HC 331) *4th Report 1997/98: Food Safety* (London, HMSO).

Ahmad, W. (ed.) (1993) *Race and Health in Contemporary Britain* (Buckingham, Open University Press).

Alaszewski, A. (1995) 'Restructuring Health and Welfare Professions in the United Kingdom: The Impact of Internal Markets on the Medical, Nursing and Social Work Professions', in Johnson, T., Larkin, G. and Saks, M. (eds) *Health Professions and the State in Europe* (London, Routledge), 55–74.

Alborz, A., Wilkin, D. and Smith, K. (2002) 'Are Primary Care Groups and Trusts Consulting Local Communities?', *Health and Social Care in the Community*, 10, 20–7.

Aldridge, J. and Becker, S. (1993) *Children Who Care: Insider World of Young Carers* (Loughborough, Loughborough University).

Aldridge, J. and Becker, S. (2003) *Children Caring for Parents with Mental Illness – The Perspectives of Young Carers, Parents and Professionals* (Bristol, Policy Press).

Alford, R. (1975) *Health Care Politics* (Chicago, IL, University of Chicago Press).

Alimo-Metcalfe, B. and Alban-Metcalfe, J. (2002) 'Half the Battle', *Health Service Journal*, 7 March, 26–7.

Allen, D. (1997) 'The Nursing-Medical Boundary – A Negotiated Order?', *Sociology of Health and Illness*, 19 (4), 498–520.

Allen, I. (1994) *Doctors and their Careers: A New Generation* (London, Policy Studies Institute).

Allen, I. (2001) *Stress Among Ward Sisters and Charge Nurses* (London, Policy Studies Institute).

Allen, P. (2002) 'Plus ça change, plus c'est la même chose: To the Internal Market and Back in the British NHS', *Applied Health Economics and Health Policy*, 1, 171–8.

Allsop, J. (1984) *Health Policy and the National Health Service* (Harlow, Longman).

Allsop, J. (1992) 'The Voice of the User in Health Care', in Beck, E., Lonsdale, S., Newman, S. and Paterson, D. (eds) *In the Best of Health?: The Status and Future of Health Care in the UK* (London, Chapman and Hall), 149–66.

Allsop, J. (1995) *Health Policy and the NHS – Towards 2000*, 2nd edn (Harlow, Longman).

Allsop, J. and May, A. (1986) *The Emperor's New Clothes. Family Practitioner Committees in the 1980s* (London, King's Fund).

Allsop, J., Baggott, R. and Jones, K. (2002) 'Health Consumer Groups and the National Policy Process', in Henderson, S. and Peterson, A. (eds) *Consuming Health: The*

Commodification of Health Care (London, Routledge), 48–65.

Allsop, J. and Mulcahy, L. (1996) *Regulating Medical Work: Formal and Informal Controls* (Buckingham, Open University Press).

Allsop, J. and Saks, M. (2002) *Regulating the Health Professions* (London, Sage).

Amu, O., Rajendran, S. and Bolaji, I. (1998) 'Maternal Choice Alone Should Not Determine Method of Delivery', *British Medical Journal*, 317, 463–5.

Anderson, P. (1988) 'Excess Mortality Associated with Alcohol Consumption', *British Medical Journal*, 297, 824–6.

Anderson, W., Florin, D., Gillam, S. and Mountford, L. (2002) *Every Voice Counts: Primary Care Organisations and Public Involvement* (London, King's Fund).

Andrews, K., Murphy, L., Munday, R. and Littlewood, C. (1996) 'Misdiagnosis of the Vegetative State: Retrospective Study in a Rehabilitation Unit', *British Medical Journal*, 313, 13–16.

Andrews, L., Stocking, C., Krizeck, T., Gottlieb, L., Krizek, C., Vargish, T. and Seigler, M. (1997) 'An Alternative Strategy for Studying Adverse Events in Medical Care', *Lancet*, 349, 309–12.

Annandale, E. (1998) *The Sociology of Health and Medicine. A Critical Introduction* (Cambridge, Polity Press, in association with Blackwell Publishers).

Annandale, E. and Hunt, K. (2000) *Gender Inequalities in Health* (Buckingham, Open University Press).

Appleby, J. (1999) 'The Modernisation Fund', in Appleby, J. and Harrison, A. (eds) *Health Care UK* (London, King's Fund), 152–8.

Appleby, J. (1999a) 'Government Funding of the UK NHS: What Does the Historical Record Reveal', *Journal of Health Services Research and Policy*, 4, 79–89.

Appleby, J. (2001) 'Cut and Run', *Health Service Journal*, 5 July, 33–4.

Appleby, J. (2002) 'US v UK', *Health Service Journal*, 21 February, 33.

Appleby, J. and Boyle, S. (2000) 'Blair's Billions: Where Will He Find the Money for the NHS', *British Medical Journal*, 320, 856–67.

Appleby, J. and Boyle, S. (2001) 'NHS Spending: The Wrong Target (Again)?', in Appleby, J. and Harrison, S. (eds) *Health Care UK*, Spring 2001 (London, King's Fund), 94–9.

Appleby, J. and Coote, A. (2002) *Five Year Health Check: A Review of Government Health Policy 1997–2002* (London, King's Fund).

Appleby, J. and Deeming, C. (2001) 'Inverse Care Law', *Health Service Journal*, 21 June, 37.

Appleby, J., Gillam, S., Harrison, A., Rosen, R., Dixon, M., Llewellyn, L., McNab, A. and Murray, T. (2001) *Public-Private Partnerships* (London, King's Fund).

Appleby, J., Harrison, A. and Devlin, N. (2003) *What is the Real Cost of More Patient Choice?* (London, King's Fund).

Appleby, J. and Mulligan, J. (2000) *How Well is the NHS Performing?* (London, King's Fund).

Appleby, J. and Rosete, A. (2003) 'The NHS: Keeping up with Public Expectations,' in Park, A., Curtice, J., Thomson, K., Jarvis, L., and Bromley, C. (eds) *British Social Attitudes. The 20th Report* (London, Sage).

Appleyard, B. (2000) *Brave New World – Genetics and the Human Experience* (London, Harper Collins).

Arason, V., Kristinnson, K., Sigurdsson, J. A., Stefansdottir, G., Molstad, S. and Gudmundsson, S. (1996) 'Do Antimicrobials Increase the Carriage Rate of Penicillin Resistant Pneumococci in Children? Cross Sectional Prevalence Study', *British Medical Journal*, 313, 387–91.

Armstrong, D. (1990) 'Medicine as a Profession: Times of Change', *British Medical Journal*, 301, 691–3.

Armstrong, D. (2002) 'Clinical Autonomy, Individual Collective: The Problem of Changing Doctors' Behaviour', *Social Science and Medicine*, 55, 1771–7.

Armstrong, P. W. (2000) 'Unrepresentative, Invalid and Misleading: Are Waiting Times for Elective Admission Wrongly Calculated?', *Journal of Epidemiology and Biostatistics*, 5, 117–23.

Arnesen, T. and Nord, E. (1999) 'The Value of DALY Life: Problems with Ethics and Validity of Disability Adjusted Life Years', *British Medical Journal*, 319, 1423–5.

Arrow, K. (1963) 'Uncertainty and the Welfare Economics of Medical Care', *American Economic Review*, 53, 941–73.

Ashburner, L. (1993) 'The Composition of NHS Trust Boards: A National Perspective', in Peck, E. and Spurgeon, P. (eds) *NHS Trusts in Practice* (London, Longman).

Ashmore, M., Mulkay, M. and Pinch, T. (1989) *Health and Efficiency: A Sociology of Health Economics* (Buckingham, Open University Press).

Ashton, J. (1992) 'The Origin of Healthy Cities', in Ashton, J. (ed.) *Healthy Citites* (Milton Keynes, Open University Press), 1–12.

Association of Community Health Councils for England and Wales (1998) *Medical Records: Restricted Access, Limited* Use (London, ACHCEW).

Association of Community Health Councils for England and Wales (2002) *Staffing for Patients' Forums: A Discussion Paper* (London, ACHCEW).

Atkinson, D. (1994) *A Common Sense of Community* (London, Demos).

Atkinson, S. (2002) 'Political Cultures, Health Systems and Health Policy', *Social Science and Medicine*, 55, 113–24.

Atrens, D. (1994) 'The Questionable Wisdom of a Low Fat Diet and Cholesterol Reduction', *Social Science and Medicine*, 39, 433–7.

Audit Commission (1986) *Making a Reality of Community Care* (London, HMSO).

Audit Commission (1989) *Developing Community Care for Adults with a Mental Handicap* (London, HMSO).

Audit Commission (1991) *Report and Accounts* (London, HMSO).

Audit Commission (1992) *Homeward Bound: A New Course for Community Health* (London, HMSO).

Audit Commission (1993a) *Their Health, Your Business: The Role of the District Health Authority* (London, HMSO).

Audit Commission (1993b) *Practices Make Perfect: The Role of the FHSA* (London, HMSO).

Audit Commission (1994a) *Annual Report and Accounts* (London, HMSO).

Audit Commission (1994b) *Taking Stock: Progress with Care in the Community* (London, HMSO).

Audit Commission (1995a) *Improving Your Image: How to Manage Radiology Services More Effectively* (London, HMSO).

Audit Commission (1995b) *A Price on their Heads. Measuring Management Costs in NHS Trusts* (London, HMSO).

Audit Commission (1995c) *The Doctor's Tale: The Work of Hospital Doctors in England and Wales* (London, HMSO).

Audit Commission (1995d) *Taken on Board: Corporate Governance in the NHS. Developing the Role of Non-Executives* (London, HMSO).

Audit Commission (1996a) *What the Doctor Ordered: A Study of GP Fundholders in England and Wales* (London, HMSO).

Audit Commission (1996b) *Balancing the Care Equation* (London, HMSO).

Audit Commission (1997a) *Take Your Choice: A Commissioning Framework for Community Care* (London, Audit Commission).

Audit Commission (1997b) *The Coming of Age* (London, Audit Commission).

Audit Commission (1999a) *A Healthy Balance: Financial Management in the NHS* (London, Audit Commission).

Audit Commission (1999b) *Children in Mind: Child and Adolescent Mental Health Services* (London, Audit Commission).

Audit Commission (1999c) *PCGs: An Early Review of Primary Care Groups in England* (London, Audit Commission).

Audit Commission (2000a) *Local Health Groups in Wales: The First Year* (London, HMSO).

Audit Commission (2000b) *Charging with Care. How Councils Charge for Home Care* (London, Audit Commission).

Audit Commission (2001a) *NHS Summarised Accounts 2000–2001* (London, The Stationery Office).

Audit Commission (2001b) *A Spoonful of Sugar – Medicines Management in NHS Hospitals* (London, The Stationery Office).

Audit Commission (2002a) *Acute Hospital Portfolio: Radiology* (London, HMSO).

Audit Commission (2002b) *Access to Care* (London, The Stationery Office).

Audit Commission (2002c) *Data Remember: Improving the Quality of Patient-based Information in the NHS* (London, The Stationery Office).

Audit Commission (2002d) *Pathways to Improved Social Services in Wales* (London, Audit Commission).

Audit Commission (2002e) *Integrated Services for Older People* (London, Audit Commission).

Audit Commission (2002f) *Primary Dental Care Services in England and Wales* (London, Audit Commission).

Audit Commission (2002g) *Tracking the Changes in Social Services in England* (London, The Stationery Office).

Audit Commission (2002h) *General Practice in England* (London, Audit Commission).

Audit Commission (2003a) *Targets in the Public Sector* (London, Audit Commission).

Audit Commission (2003b) *Achieving the NHS Plan* (London, Audit Commission).

Audit Commission (2003c) *Waiting List Accuracy* (London, DoH).

Audit Commission (2003d) *Primary Care Prescribing* (London, Audit Commission).

Audit Commission (2003e) *Personal Medical Services* (London, Audit Commission).

Audit Commission (2004a) *Quicker Treatment Closer to Home* (London, Audit Commission).

Audit Commission (2004b) *Transforming Primary Care* (London, Audit Commission).

Austin, D. (2002) 'The Buck Stops Here', *Health Service Journal*, 20 June, 32–3.

Austin, N. and Dopson, S. (1997) *The Clinical Directorate* (Oxford, Radcliffe Medical Press).

Austoker, J. (1994) 'Diet and Cancer', *British Medical Journal*, 308, 1611–14.

Avis, M. (1997) 'Incorporating Patients' Voices in the Audit Process', *Quality in Health Care*, 6, 69–91.

Babyak, M., Blumenthal, J., Herman, S., Khatri, P., Doraiswamy, M. et al. (2000) 'Exercise Treatment for Major Depression: Maintenance of Therapeutic Benefit at Ten Months', *Psychosomatic Medicine*, 62, 633–8.

Backett, K. C. and Davison, C. (1995) 'Lifecourse and Lifestyle – The Social and Cultural Location of Health Behaviours', *Social Science and Medicine*, 40 (5), 629–30.

Baeza, J. and Calnan, M. (1997) 'Implementing Quality: A Study of the Adoption and Implementation of Quality Standards in the Contracting Process in a General Practitioner Multifund', *Journal of Health Services Research and Policy*, 2, 205–11.

Baeza, J. I. (1999) 'Self-Regulation of Health Professionals: The Need for a Cohort Framework', in Appleby, J. and Harrison, A. (eds) *Health Care UK 1999/2000* (London, King's Fund), 115–18.

Baggott, R. and McGregor-Riley, V. (1999) 'Renewed Consultation or Continued Exclusion? Organised Interests and the Major Governments,' in Dorey, P. (ed.) *The Major Premiership: Politics and Policies Under John Major, 1990–97* (Basingstoke, Macmillan), 68–86.

Baggott, R. (1994) 'Reforming the British Healthcare System: A Permanent Revolution?', *Policy Studies*, 15, 35–47.

Baggott, R. (1997) 'Evaluating Health Care Reform: The Case of the NHS Internal Market', *Public Administration*, 75, 283–306.

Baggott, R. (2000) *Public Health, Policy and Politics* (Basingstoke, Palgrave).

Baggott, R., Allsop, J. and Jones, K. (2004) *Speaking for Patients and Carers: Health Consumer Groups and the Policy Process* (London, Palgrave).

Baggott, R. and Buchanan, R. (2002) *George Eliot Hospital NHS Trust: Patient Advice and Liaison Service* (Leicester, Health Policy Research Unit, De Montfort University).

Baggs, J., Schmitt, M., Mushlen, A., Mitchell, P., Eldridge, D., Oakes, D. and Hutson, A. (1999) 'Associations between Nurse Physician Collaboration and Patient Outcomes in Three Intensive Care Units', *Critical Care Medicine*, 27, 1991–7.

Bailey, S. and Bruce, A. (1994) 'Funding the NHS: The Continuing Search for Alternatives', *Journal of Social Policy*, 23 (4), 489–516.

Baker, C. and Lorimer, A. (2000) 'Cardiology: The Development of a Managed Clinical Network', *British Medical Journal*, 321, 1152–3.

Bakwin, H. (1945) 'Pseudoxia Pediatrica', *New England Journal of Medicine*, 232, 691–7.

Balarajan, R. and Soni Raleigh, V. (1995) *Ethnicity and Health in England* (London, HMSO).

Baldwin, S. and Lunt, N. (1996) *Charging Ahead: Local Authority Charging Policies for Community Care* (Bristol, Policy Press).

Ball, R., Heafey, M. and King, D. (2000) 'Private Finance Initiative: A Good Deal to the Public Purse or a Drain on Further Generations', *Policy and Politics*, 29, 95–108.

Balloch, S. and Taylor, M. (2001) *Partnership Working: Policy and Practice* (Bristol, Policy Press).

Balogh, R. (1996) 'Exploring the Role of Localities in Health Commissioning: A Review of the Literature', *Social Policy and Administration*, 30 (2), 99–113.

Bamford, T. (2001) *Commissioning and Purchasing* (London, Routledge).

Banks, P. (2001) 'Patient and Public Involvement Beyond Chapter 10', in Appleby, J. and Harrison, A. (eds) *Health Care UK 2001* (London, King's Fund), 4–18.

Banks, P. (2002) *Partnerships Under Pressure* (London, King's Fund).

Banks, P. and Roberts, E. (2001) *More Breaks for Carers* (London, King's Fund).

Barham, P. (1992) *Closing the Asylum: Mental Patients in Modern Society* (Harmondsworth, Penguin).

Barker, J., Bullen, M. and De Ville, J. (1997) *Reference Manual for Public Involvement* (Bromley Health Authority; West Kent Health Authority; Lambeth, Lewisham and Southwark Health Authority).

Barnes, M. (1997) *Care, Communities and Citizens* (Harlow, Addison Wesley Longman).

Barnes, M., Harrison, S., Mort, M. and Shardlow, P. (1999) *Unequal Partners: User Groups and Community Care* (Bristol, Policy Press).

Barnes, M., Sullivan, H. and Matka, E. (2001) *Building Capacity for Collaboration: The National Evaluation of Health Action Zones. Context, Strategy and Capacity* (Birmingham, University of Birmingham).

Barnet Health Authority (1997) *Report of the Review Panel into the Deaths of Eight Patients Following their Transfer from Napsbury Hospital to Elmstead House Nursing Home* (London, Barnet Health Authority).

Bartley, M., Montgomery, S., Cook, D. and Wadsworth, M. (1996) 'Health and Work Insecurity in Young Men', in Blane, D., Brunner, E. and Wilkinson, R. (eds) *Health and Social Organisation* (London, Routledge), 255–71.

Bartley, M. and Owen, C. (1996) 'Relation between Socioeconomic Status, Employment and Health during Economic Change 1979–83', *British Medical Journal*, 313, 445–9.

Bartley, M., Popay, J. and Plewis, I. (1992) 'Domestic Conditions, Paid Employment and Women's Experience of Ill Health', *Sociology of Health and Illness*, 14 (3), 313–45.

Bartrip, P. (1996) *Themselves Writ Large: The BMA 1832–1966* (London, BMJ).

Bate, P. (2000) 'Changing the Culture of a Hospital from Hierarchy to Networked Community', *Public Administration*, 78, 485–512.

Bate, P., Robert, G. and McLeod, H. (2002) *Report on the Breakthrough Collaborative Approach to Quality and Service Improvement within Four Regions of the NHS* (Birmingham, HSMC).

Batt, S. (1994) *Patient No More: The Politics of Breast Cancer* (London, Scarlett Press).

Batty, D. (2002) 'Fresh Doubts Cast on NHS League', *The Guardian*, 24 October. http://society.guardian.co.uk/nhsperformance/story/0,8150,818626,00.html

Batty, D. and Thune, I. (2000) 'Does Physical Activity Prevent Cancer?', *British Medical Journal*, 321, 1424.

Bauld, L., Chesterman, J., Davies, B., Judge, K. and Mangabe, R. (2000) *Caring for Older People: An Assessment of Community Care in the 1990s* (Aldershot, Ashgate).

Bauld, L. and Judge, K. (2002) *Learning from Health Action Zones* (Chichester, AKD Press).

Baxter, K., Shepherd, J., Weiss, M. and Le Grand, J. (2002) 'Ready Steady Stop', *Health Service Journal*, 14 March, 28–9.

BBC (2002) 'NHS Managers Keep Quiet Rather than Tell it as it is', http://news.bbc.co.uk/1/ow/health/2299291.stm

BBC News (2003) *GPs Losing Faith with NHS Reforms*, www.news.bbc.co.uk, 4 August.

Beaglehole, R. and Bonita, R. (1997) *Public Health at the Crossroads: Achievements and Prospects* (Cambridge, Cambridge University Press).

Becker, S., Dearden, C. and Aldridge, J. (2001) 'Children's Labour of Love – Young Carers and Care Work', in Mizen, P., Pole, E. and Bolton, A. (eds) *Hidden Hands: International Perspectives on Children's Work and Labour* (Brighton, Routledge Falmer), 70–87.

Bennett, C. and Ferlie, E. (1996) 'Contracting in Theory and Practice: Some Evidence from the NHS', *Public Administration*, 74, 49–66.

Bennett, F. (2000) 'Should the NHS Be Funded by a Hypothecated Tax? No' *Fabian Review*, Winter, 9.

Ben-Shlomo, Y., White, I. and Marmot, M. (1996) 'Does Variation in the Socio-Economic Characteristics of an Area Affect Mortality?', *British Medical Journal*, 312, 1013–14.

Benson, L., Boyd, A. and Walshe, K. (2004) *Learning from CHI: The Impact of Healthcare Regulation* (University of Manchester).

Benzeval, M., Judge, K. and Shouls, S. (2001) 'Understanding the Relationship between Income and Health: How Much Can Be Gleaned from Cross-Sectional Data', *Social Policy and Administration*, 35, 376–96.

Beresford, P. (1988) 'Consumer Views: Data Collection or Democracy?', in Allen, I. (ed.) *Hearing the Voice of the Consumer* (London, Public Studies Institute), 37–51.

Berridge, V. and Blume, S. (eds) (2003) *Social Inequality Before and After the Black Report* (London, Frank Cass).

Berwick, D. M., Enthoven, A. and Bunker, J. P. (1992) 'Quality Management in the NHS: The Doctors' Role', *British Medical Journal*, 304, 235–9.

Besley, T., Hall, J. and Preston, I. (1996) *Private Health Insurance and the State of the NHS* (London, Institute for Fiscal Studies).

Best, G. (1997) 'The Rationing Debate: Confusion or Conspiracy?', *Health Director*, 35, 12.

Bethune, A. (1996) 'Economic Activity and Mortality of the 1981 Census Cohort in the OPCS Longitudinal Study', *Population Trends*, 83, 37–41.

Better Regulation Task Force (1998) *Long Term Care* (London, Central Office of Information).

Bevan, G., Holland, W., Maynard, A. and Mays, N. (1988) *Reforming UK Health Care to Improve Health: The Case for Research and Experiment* (University of York, Centre for Health Economics).

Bines, W. (1994) *The Health of Single Homeless People*, Discussion Paper 9 (York, Centre for Housing Policy, University of York).

Bjorkman, J. W. (1989) 'Politicising Medicine and Medicalising Politics: Physician Power in the

United States', in Freddi, G. and Bjorkman, J. W. (eds) *Controlling Medical Professionals: The Comparative Politics of Health Governance* (London, Sage), 28–73.

Black, D. (1984) *An Anthology of False Antitheses* (London, Nuffield Provincial Hospitals Trust).

Black, D. (1987) *Recollections and Reflections* (London, BMJ).

Black, D., Birchall, A. and Trimble, I. (1994) 'Non-Fundholding in Nottingham: A Vision of the Future', *British Medical Journal*, 308, 930–2.

Black, N. (1996) 'Why We Need Observational Studies to Evaluate the Effectiveness of Healthcare', *British Medical Journal*, 312, 1215–18.

Black, N., Langam, S. and Petticrew, M. (1995) 'Coronary Revascularisation – Why Do Rates Vary Geographically in the UK', *Journal of Epidemiology and Community Health*, 49, 408–12.

Black, N. and Thompson, E. (1993) 'Obstacles to Medical Audit: British Doctors Speak', *Social Science and Medicine*, 36 (7), 849–56.

Blackhurst, C. (1995) 'Finance Watchdog Prescribes Cure for Unhealthy NHS', *Independent*, 24 August, 10.

Blane, D., Smith, G. D. and Bartley, M. (1990) 'Social Class Differences in Years of Potential Life Lost: Size, Trends and Principal Causes', *British Medical Journal*, 301, 29–32.

Blaxter, M. (1990) *Health and Lifestyles* (London, Tavistock/Routledge).

Blendon, R., Schoen, C., Des Roches, C. and Zapert, K. (2003) 'Common Concerns Amid Diverse Systems: Health Care Experiences in Five Countries', *Health Affairs*, 22 (3), 106–21.

Bloor, K. and Maynard, A. (1998) *Clinical Governance: Clinician Heal Thyself* (London, Institute for Health Service Management Paper).

BMA (British Medical Association) (1929) *A General Medical Service for the Nation* (London, BMA).

BMA (British Medical Association) (1942) *Draft Interim Report of the Medical Planning Commission* (London, BMA).

BMA (British Medical Association) (1962) *Report of the Medical Services Review Committee* (The Porritt Report) (London, BMA).

BMA (British Medical Association) (1986) *Alternative Therapy* (London, BMA).

BMA (British Medical Association) (1993) *Complementary Medicine: New Approaches to Good Practice* (Oxford, Oxford University Press).

BMA (British Medical Association) (1995) *Inequalities in Health*. Board of Science and Education Occasional Paper (London, BMA).

BMA (British Medical Association) (1997) *Options for Funding Health Care* (London, BMA, Health Policy and Economic Research Unit).

BMA (British Medical Association) (1999) *Growing Up in Britain* (London, BMA).

BMA (British Medical Association) (2001) *Healthcare Funding Review* (London, BMA).

BMA (British Medical Association) (2002) *Press Release – Mori Poll for BMA Finds Many Patients Willing to Travel Abroad for Treatment* (London, BMA).

BMA (British Medical Association) (2003) *Housing and Health – Building for the Future* (London, BMA).

Boaden, N. (1997) *Primary Care: Making the Connections* (Buckingham, Open University Press).

Bogle, I. (2002) *Speech from the Chairman of Council–Dr Ian Bogle* (London, BMA), 1st July.

Bojke, C., Gravelle, H. and Wilkin, D. (2001) 'Is Bigger Better for Primary Care Groups and Trusts', *British Medical Journal*, 322, 599–602.

Bolton, M. (2000) 'Cancel That Taxi, It's NHS Net', *Health Service Journal*, 28 October, 20–1.

Bond, M. (2002) 'Nurture not Nature', *Health Service Journal*, 21 February, 30–1.

Bone, M., Bebbington, A., Jagger, C., Morgan, K. and Nicholaas, G. (1995) *Health Expectancy and its Uses* (London, HMSO).

Boreham, K. and Shaw, A. (eds) (2001) *Smoking, Drinking and Drug Use Among Young People in England in 2000: Summary of Findings* (London, The Stationery Office).

Borooah, V. K. (1999) 'Occupational Class and the Probability of Long-Term Limiting Illness', *Social Science and Medicine*, 49, 253–66.

Bosanquet, N. (1986) 'GPs as Firms: Creating an Internal Market for Primary Care', *Public Money and Management*, 6 (1), 53–62.

Bosanquet, N. (2003) 'NICE to See You', *Health Service Journal*, 16 June, 30–1.

Botting, B. (1997) 'Mortality in Childhood', in Drever, F. and Whitehead, M. (eds) *Health Inequalities: Decennial Supplement* (London, The Stationery Office), 83–95.

Bowie, C., Richardson, A. and Sykes, W. (1995) 'Consulting the Public about Health Service Priorities', *British Medical Journal*, 311, 1155–8.

Bowling, A. (1997) *Measuring Health – A Review of Quality of Life Measurement Scales*, 2nd edn (Buckingham, Open University Press).

Boyle, D. (2000) *The Tyranny of Numbers: Why Counting Can't Make Us Happy* (London, Harper Collins).

Boyne, G. (2001) 'Planning, Performance and Public Services', *Public Administration*, 79, 73–88.

Brand, J. L. (1965) *Doctors and the State: The British Medical Profession and Government Action on Public Health: 1870–1912* (Baltimore MD, Johns Hopkins University Press).

Brazier, M., Lovecy, J., Moran, M. and Potton, M. (1993) 'Falling from a Tightrope? Doctors and Lawyers between the Market and State', *Political Studies*, 41 (2), 197–213.

Brechin, E., Brown, H. and Eby, M. (1999) *Critical Practice in Health and Social Care* (Buckingham, Open University Press).

Brewin, T. (1985) 'Orthodox and Alternative Medicine', *Scottish Medical Journal*, 30, 203–5.

Bridgwood, A., Lilly, R., Thomas, M., Bacon, J., Sykes, W. and Morris, S. (2000) *Living in Britain: Results from the 1998 General Household Survey* (London, Office for National Statistics, The Stationery Office).

British Association of Medical Managers (1996) *Putting Principles into Practice: The Involvement of Clinical Staff on the Management of NHS Trusts* (Manchester, BAMM).

British Association of Medical Managers, BMA, IHSM and RCN (1993) *Managing Clinical Services: A Consensus Statement of Principles for Effective Clinical Management* (London, IHSM).

British Dental Association (1999) *Access to Dental Services and Recruitment of Salaried GDPs – A Survey of Health Authority* (London, BDA).

British Medical Journal (1999) 'The Impact of New Technologies in Medicine', Volume 319(S).

British Medical Journal (2000) 'The Public Still Trusts Doctors', Volume 320, 653.

Bristol Royal Infirmary Inquiry (2001a) *The Inquiry into the Management of Care of Children Receiving Complex Heart Surgery at the Bristol Royal Infirmary – Removal and Retention of Human Material* (London, The Stationery Office).

Bristol Royal Infirmary Inquiry (2001b) *The Inquiry into the Management of Care of Children Receiving Complex Heart Surgery at the Bristol Royal Infirmary – Final Report* (London, The Stationery Office).

British Thoracic Society (2003) *Press Release, NHS Priorities Threaten Care of Patients with Respiratory Disease*, 16 April.

Britton, A., McKee, M., Black, N., Sanderson, C. and Bain, C. (1999) 'Threats to Applicability of Randomised Trials: Exclusions and Selective Participation', *Journal of Health Services Research and Policy*, 4, 112–21.

Broadbent, J. (1998) 'Practice Nurses and the Effects of the New GP Contract in the British NHS: The Advent of a Professional Project', *Social Science and Medicine*, 47, 4, 497–506.

Brooks, R., Regan, S. and Robinson, P. (2002) *A New Contract for Retirement* (London, IPPR).

Brown, C., Belfield, C. and Field, S. (2002) 'Cost Effectiveness of Continuing Professional Development in Health Care: A Critical Review of the Evidence', *British Medical Journal*, 324, 652–5.

Brown, G. (2002) Chancellor of the Exchequer's Budget Statement. House of Commons *Hansard*, 17 April vol. 383, Col. 577–92.

Brown, I. (1999) 'Patient Participation Groups in General Practice in the NHS', *Health Expectations*, 2, 169–78.

Brown, L., Tucker, C. and Domokos, T. (2003) 'Evaluating the Impact of Integrated Health and Social Care Teams in Older People Living in the Community', *Health and Social Care in the Community*, 11, 85–94.

Brown, M., Fallon, M., Favell, T., Forth, E., Hamilton, N., Heathcoat-Amory, D., Howarth, G., Jones, G., Leigh, E., Redwood, J., Stewart, A. and Twinn, I. (1988) *The NHS: A Suitable Case for Treatment* (London, Conservative Political Centre).

Bruster, S., Jarman, B., Bosanquet, N., Weston, D., Erens, R. and Delbanco, T. (1994) 'National Survey of Hospital Patients', *British Medical Journal*, 309, 1542–9.

BSE Inquiry, The (2000) *The Report* (London, The Stationery Office).

Buchan, J. (2002) 'Rallying the Troops', *Health Service Journal*, 30 May, 24–5.

Buchanan, D. (1996) *Representing Process: The Re-engineering Frame*, Occasional Paper 37 (Leicester, Leicester Business School).

Buchanan, D., Jordan, S., Preston, D. and Smith, A. (1997) *Doctor in the Process – Engaging Doctors in Hospital Management* (Leicester Business School, Occasional Paper No. 40).

Buchanan, D. and Wilson, B. (1996) *Re-engineering Operating Theatres: The Perspective Assessed* (Leicester Business School, Occasional Paper No. 34).

Buck, N., Devlin, B. and Lunn, J. N. (1987) *Report of a Confidential Inquiry into Perioperative Deaths* (London, Nuffield Hospitals Provincial Trust).

Bunker, J., Frazier, H. and Mostelle, F. (1994) 'Improving Health: Measuring Effects of Medical Care', *Milbank Quarterly*, 72 (2), 225–58.

Butler, E. and Pirie, M. (1988) *The Health Alternatives* (London, Adam Smith Institute).

Butler, J. (1992) *Patients, Policies and Politics: Before and After 'Working for Patients'* (Buckingham, Open University Press).

Butler, P. (1995) 'Trusts Aim to Streamline ECR System', *Health Service Journal*, 21 September, 6.

Bynum, W. (1994) *Science and the Practice of Medicine in the Nineteenth Century* (Cambridge, Cambridge University Press).

Byrne, P. S. and Long, B. E. (1976) *Doctors Talking to Patients* (London, HMSO).

Cabinet Office (2000) *Out of Hours* (London, Cabinet Office).

Cabinet Office, Prime Minister's Strategy Unit (2004) *Alcohol Harm Reduction Strategy for England* (London, Cabinet Office).

Cadbury, A. (1992) *Report of the Committee on the Financial Aspects of Corporate Governance* (The Cadbury Report) (London, Gee and Co.).

Cairns, J. (1996) 'Measuring Health Outcomes', *British Medical Journal*, 313, 6.

Calman, C., Hunter, D. and May, A. (2002) *Make or Break Time: A Commentary on Labour's Health Policy Two Years into the NHS Plan* (Durham, University of Durham).

Calnan, M. (1987) *Health and Illness. The Lay Perspective* (London, Tavistock).

Calnan, M., Cant, S. and Gabe, J. (1993) *Going Private: Why People Pay for their Health Care* (Buckingham, Open University Press).

Cameron, C. and Bernardes, J. (1998) 'Gender and Disadvantage in Health: Men's Health for a Change', *Sociology of Health and Illness*, 20, 673–93.

Cameron, H. M. and McCoogan, E. (1981) 'A Prospective Study of 1152 Hospital Autopsies', *Journal of Pathology*, 133, 273–85.

Campbell, B. (1995) 'Old Fogies and Angry Young Men: A Critique of Communitarianism', *Soundings*, 1, 47–64.

Campbell, E. J. M., Scadding, J. G. and Roberts, R. S. (1979) 'The Concept of Disease', *British Medical Journal*, 2, 757–62.

Campbell, S., Roland, M. and Wilkin, D. (2001) 'PCGs – Improving the Quality of Care through Clinical Governance', *British Medical Journal*, 322, 1580–2.

Campling, E. A., Devlin, H. B., Hoile, R. and Lunn, J. A. (1995) *The National Confidential Enquiry into Perioperative Deaths 1992/3* (London, NCEPOD).

Campling, E. A., Lunn, J. N., Hoile, R. and Devlin, H. B. (1992) *The National Confidential Enquiry into Perioperative Deaths 1990* (London, NCEPOD).

Cancer BACUP (2002) *Funding for Cancer Services. An Independent Audit of Cancer Networks in England* (London, Cancer BACUP).

Cant, S. and Sharma, U. (1999) *A New Medical Pluralism?* (London, UCL Press).

Capewell, S. (1996) 'The Continuing Rise in Emergency Admissions', *British Medical Journal*, 312, 991–2.

Carers National Association (1997) *In on the Act? Social Services Experience of the First Year of the Carer's Act* (London, CNA).

Carers UK (2002) *Without Us* (London, Carers UK).

Carers UK (2003) *Missed Opportunities: The Impact of New Rights for Carers* (London, Carers UK).

Carlisle, D. (2002) 'For Better or Worse?', *Health Service Journal*, 20 June, 40.

Carlisle, D. (2003a) 'Independent DTCs May Use NHS Consultants', *Health Service Journal*, 21 August, 9.

Carlisle, D. (2003b) 'Patient Choice "Gaming" Leaves Beds Empty', *Health Service Journal*, 24 July, 5.

Carlisle, D. (2003c) 'Dereliction of Duty', *Health Service Journal*, 2 October, 12–15.

Carpenter, L. (1987) 'Some Observations on the Healthy Worker Effect', *British Journal of Industrial Medicine*, 44, 289–91.

Carr-Hill, R. (1987) 'The Inequalities in Health Debate: A Critical Review of the Literature', *Journal of Social Policy*, 16 (4), 509–42.

Carr-Hill, R. (1991) 'Allocating Resources to Health Care: Is the Qaly a Technical Solution to a Political Problem?', *International Journal of Health Services*, 21 (2), 351–63.

Carr-Hill, R. and Morris, J. (1991) 'Current Practice in Obtaining the Q in Qalys: A Cautionary Note', *British Medical Journal*, 303, 699–701.

Carrier, J. and Kendall, I. (1990) *Socialism and the NHS* (Aldershot, Avebury).

Carruthers, J., Fillingham, D., Ham, C. and James, J. (1995) *Purchasing in the NHS: The Story So Far* (Birmingham, Health Services Management Centre).

Carstairs, V. and Morris, R. (1989) 'Deprivation: Explaining Differences in Mortality between Scotland and England and Wales', *British Medical Journal*, 299, 886–9.

Cattell, V. (2001) 'Poor People, Poor Places, and Poor Health: The Mediating Role of Social

Networks and Social Capital', *Social Science and Medicine*, 52, 1501–46.

Cd 4499 (1909) *Royal Commission on the Poor Laws and Relief of Distress*, Minority Report (London, HMSO).

Chadwick, E. (1842) *Report on the Sanitary Condition of the Labouring Population of Great Britain* (London, Poor Law Commission).

Chan, A. (2000) *A Guide to Public Involvement for Health Services in Leicester, Leicestershire and Rutland* (Leicester, Leicestershire Health).

Chandola, T., Bartely, M., Sacker, A., Jenkinson, C. and Marmot, M. (2003) 'Health Selection in the Whitehall II Study, UK', *Social Science and Medicine*, 56, 2059–72.

Chapman, J. (2002) *System Failure – Why Government Must Learn to Think Differently* (London, Demos).

Chappel, D., Miller, P., Parkin, D. and Thompson, R. (1999) 'Models of Commissioning Health Services in the British NHS', *Journal of Public Health Medicine*, 21, 221–7.

Chapple, A., Halliwell, S., Sibbald, B., Roland, M. and Rogers, A. (2000) 'A Walk-in? Now You're Talkin', *Health Service Journal*, 4 May, 28–9.

Charities Aid Foundation (2001) *Philanthropic Funds in London's Health Care* (Tonbridge, Charities Aid Foundation).

Charlesworth, J., Clarke, J. and Cochrane, A. (1996) 'Tangled Webs? Managing Local Mixed Economies of Care', *Public Administration*, 74 (1), 67–88.

Charlton, J. (1996) 'Which Areas are the Healthiest?', *Population Trends*, 83, 17–24.

Charlton, J., Wallace, M. and White, M. (1994) 'Long-term Illness: Results from the 1991 Census', *Population Trends*, 75, 18–25.

Chaturvedi, N. and Ben-Shlomo, Y. (1995) 'From the Surgery to Surgeon: Does Deprivation Influence Consultation and Operation Rates?', *British Journal of General Practice*, 45, 127–31.

Chaturvedi, N., Rai, H. and Ben-Shlomo, Y. (1997) 'Lay Diagnosis and Health Care Seeking Behaviour for Chest Pain among South Asians and Europeans', *Lancet*, 350, 1578–83.

CHI (Commission for Health Improvement) (2002) *Emerging Themes from 175 Clinical Governance Reviews* (London, CHI).

CHI (Commission for Health Improvement) (2003a) *What CHI Has Found in Ambulance Trusts* (London, CHI).

CHI (Commission for Health Improvement) (2003b) *Getting Better? A Report on the NHS* (London, CHI).

CHI (Commission for Health Improvement) (2003c) *What CHI Has Found In: NHS Direct Services. Sector Report* (London, CHI).

CHI (Commission for Health Improvement) (2003d) *What CHI Has Found in Mental Health Trusts* (London, CHI).

CHI (Commission for Health Improvement) (2004) *What CHI Has Found in Primary Care Trusts* (London, CHI).

CHI (Commission for Health Improvement)/ Audit Commission (2001) *NHS Cancer Care in England and Wales* (London, CHI and Audit Commission).

Child Accident Prevention Trust (1991) *Safe As Houses: Guidelines for the Safety of Children in Temporary Accommodation* (London, CAPT).

Child Poverty Action Group and Carers UK (2001) *Paying the Price: Carers, Poverty and Social Exclusion* (London, CPAG).

Chrisafis, A. (2002) 'Widespread Cheating Devalues School Tests', *The Guardian*, 28 October, 1.

Christie, S. and Fone, D. (2003) 'Equity of Access to Tertiary Hospitals in Wales: A Travel Time Analysis', *Journal of Public Health Medicine,* 25(4), 344–50.

Clark, J. and Newman, J. (1997) *The Managerial State: Power, Politics and Ideology: The Remaking of Social Welfare* (London, Routledge).

Clarke, A., McKee, M. and Appleby, J. (1993) 'Efficient Purchasing', *British Medical Journal*, 307, 1436–7.

Clarke, J. and Newman, J. (1997) *The Managerial State: Power, Politics and Ideology in the Remaking of Social Welfare* (London, Sage).

Clarke, K., Gray, D., Keating, N. and Hampton, J. (1994) 'Do Women with Acute Myocardial Infarction Receive the Same Treatment as Men?', *British Medical Journal*, 309, 563–6.

Clatworthy, M. and Mellet, H. (1997) 'Managing Health and Finances. Conflict or Convergence?', *Public Policy and Management*, 17, 41–6.

Clinical Standards Advisory Group (1998a) *Clinical Effectiveness Report of the Clinical Standards Advisory Group* (London, The Stationery Office).

Clinical Standards Advisory Group (1998b) *Community Health Care for Elderly People* (London, CSAG).

Cm 249 (1987) *Promoting Better Health* (London, HMSO).

Cm 289 (1988) *Public Health in England*, Report of the Acheson Committee of Inquiry into the

Future Development of the Public Health Function (London, HMSO).

Cm 555 (1989) *Working for Patients* (London, HMSO).

Cm 849 (1989) *Caring for People* (London, HMSO).

Cm 1599 (1992) *The Citizen's Charter* (London, HMSO).

Cm 1986 (1992) *The Health of the Nation: A Strategy for Health in England* (London, HMSO).

Cm 2625 (1994) *Improving NHS Dentistry* (London, HMSO).

Cm 2850 (1995) *Report of the Committee on Standards in Public Life* (London, HMSO).

Cm 3242 (1996) *A New Partnership for Old Age* (London, HMSO).

Cm 3390 (1996) *Choice and Opportunity. Primary Care: The Future* (London, HMSO).

Cm 3512 (1996) *Primary Care: Delivering the Future* (London, HMSO).

Cm 3807 (1997) *The New NHS: Modern, Dependable* (London, HMSO).

Cm 3841 (1998) *NHS Wales: Putting Patients First* (London, The Stationery Office).

Cm 3852 (1998) *Our Healthier Nation* (London, The Stationery Office).

Cm 3854 (1998) *Working for a Healthier Scotland. A Consultation Document* (London, The Stationery Office).

Cm 3922 (1998) *Better Health: Better Wales. A Consultation Document* (London, The Stationery Office).

Cm 3945 (1998) *Tackling Drugs to Build a Better Britain* (London, The Stationery Office).

Cm 4014 (1998) *Modernising Local Government – In Touch with the People* (London, The Stationery Office).

Cm 4169 (1998) *Modernising Social Services: Promoting Independence, Improving Protection, Raising Standards* (London, The Stationery Office).

Cm 4177 (1998) *Smoking Kills* (London, The Stationery Office).

Cm 4192 (1999) *With Respect to Old Age: Long Term Care – Rights and Responsibilities. A Report by the Royal Commission on Long Term Care* (London, The Stationery Office).

Cm 4269 (1999) *Towards a Healthier Scotland* (London, The Stationery Office).

Cm 4386 (1999) *Saving Lives* (London, The Stationery Office).

Cm 4818 (2000) *NHS Plan: A Plan for Investment, A Plan for Reform* (London, The Stationery Office).

Cm 5086 (2001) *Valuing People: A New Strategy for Learning Disability for the 21st century* (London, DoH).

Cm 5403 (2002) *Expenditure Plans 2002–03 to 2003–04* (Department of Health – Departmental Report) (London, HMSO).

Cm 5503 (2002) *Delivering the NHS Plan: Next Steps on Investment, Next Steps on Reform* (London, The Stationery Office).

Cm 5730 (2003) *The Victoria Climbié Inquiry* (London, The Stationery Office).

Cm 5860 (2003) *Every Child Matters* (London, The Stationery Office).

Cm 6079 (2003) *Building on the Best: Choice, Responsiveness and Equity in the NHS* (London, The Stationery Office).

Cmd 693 (1920) *Interim Report on the Future Provision of Medical and Allied Services* (The Dawson Report) (London, HMSO).

Cmd 2596 (1926) *Report of the Royal Commission on National Health Insurance* (London, HMSO).

Cmd 6404 (1942) *Social Insurance and Allied Services* (The Beveridge Report) (London, HMSO).

Cmd 6502 (1944) *A National Health Service* (London, HMSO).

Cmd 9663 (1956) *Report of the Committee of Inquiry into the Cost of the National Health Service* (The Guillebaud Report) (London, HMSO).

Cmnd 1604 (1962) *A Hospital Plan for England and Wales* (London, HMSO).

Cmnd 1973 (1963) *Health and Welfare: The Development of Community Care. Plans for the Health and Welfare Services of the Local Authorities in England and Wales* (London, HMSO).

Cmnd 4683 (1971) *Better Services for the Mentally Handicapped* (London, HMSO).

Cmnd 5055 (1972) *National Health Service Reorganisation: England* (London, HMSO).

Cmnd 6018 (1975) *Report of the Committee of Inquiry into the Regulation of the Medical Profession* (London, HMSO).

Cmnd 6233 (1975) *Better Services for the Mentally Ill* (London, HMSO).

Cmnd 7047 (1977) *Prevention and Health* (London, HMSO).

Cmnd 7615 (1979) *Report of the Royal Commission on the NHS* (The Merrison Commission) (London, HMSO).

Cmnd 8173 (1981) *Growing Older* (London, HMSO).

Cmnd 9771 (1986) *Primary Health Care: An Agenda for Discussion* (London, HMSO).

Coast, J. (1997) 'Rationing in the NHS: The Case Against', *British Medical Journal*, 314, 1118–22.

Coburn, D. (1992) 'Freidson Then and Now. An Internalists' Critique of Freidson's Past and Present Views of the Medical Profession', *International Journal of Health Services*, 25 (3), 497–512.

Cochrane, A. L. (1971) *Effectiveness and Efficiency: Random Reflections on Health Services* (London, Nuffield Provincial Hospital Trust).

Cochrane, R. and Bal, S. (1989) 'Mental Hospital Admission Rates of Immigrants to England: A Comparison of 1971 and 1981', *Social Psychiatry and Psychiatric Epidemiology*, 24, 2–11.

Cohen, G., Forbes, J. and Garroway, M. (1996) 'Can Different Patient Satisfaction Survey Methods Yield Consistent Results. Comparison of Three Surveys', *British Medical Journal*, 313, 841–4.

Cole, A. (2002a) 'Mix and Match', *Health Service Journal*, 24 October, 26–9.

Cole, A. (2002b) 'Take Me to Your Leader', *Health Service Journal*, 28 November, 24–9.

Cole, A. (2003) 'Devil's Advocacy', *Health Service Journal*, 12 June, 26–8.

Coleman, M. P. (1999) *Cancer Survival Trends in England and Wales 1971–95: Deprivation and NHS Region* (London, The Stationery Office).

Colhoun, H., Ben-Shlomo, Y., Dong, W., Bost, L. and Marmot, M. (1997) 'Ecological Analysis of Collectivity of Alcohol Consumption in England. Importance of the Average Drinker', *British Medical Journal*, 314, 1164–8.

Colhoun, H. and Prescott-Clarke, P. (1996) *Health Survey for England 1994* (London, HMSO).

Collier, J. (1989) *The Health Conspiracy* (London, Century Hutchinson).

Colyer, H. and Kamath, P. (1997) 'Evidence Based Practice. A Philosophical and Political Analysis: Some Matters for Consideration by Professional Practitioners', *Journal of Advanced Nursing*, 29, 188–93.

COMA (Committee on Medical Aspects of Food Policy) (1994) *Nutritional Aspects of Cardiovascular Disease* (London, HMSO).

Consumers' Association (2001) *National Institute for Clinical Excellence: A Patient Centred Inquiry* (London, Which?).

Conway, J. (ed.) (1988) *Prescription for Poor Health: The Crisis for Homeless Families* (London, London Food Commission, The Maternity Alliance, SHAC, Shelter).

Conway, J. (1995) 'Housing as an Instrument of Health Care', *Health and Social Care in the Community*, 3, 141–50.

Cooper, L., Coote, A., Davis, A. and Jackson, C. (1995) *Voices Off: Tackling the Democratic Deficit in Health* (London, IPPR).

Cope, R. (1989) 'The Compulsory Detention of Afro-Caribbeans Under the Mental Health Act', *New Community*, 15 (3), 343–56.

Corby, S. and Mathieson, H. (1997) 'The NHS and the Limits to Flexibility', *Public Policy and Administration*, 12, 60–72.

Cosgrave, P. (1990) *The Lives of Enoch Powell* (London, Pan Books).

Coulter, A. (1995) 'General Practice Fundholding: Time for a Cool Appraisal', *British Journal of General Practitioners*, 45, 119–20.

Coulter, A. (1997) 'Partnerships with Patients: The Pros and Cons of Shared Decision Making', *Journal of Health Services Research and Policy*, 2, 112–21.

Coulter, A. (2002) 'After Bristol: Putting Patients at the Centre', *British Medical Journal*, 324, 648–51.

Coulter, A. and Ham, C. (eds) (2000) *The Global Challenge of Health Care Rationing* (Buckingham, Open University Press).

Council of Europe, Committee of Ministers (2000) *Recommendation No. 5 of the Committee of Ministers on the Development of Structures for Citizen and Patient Participation* (Council of Europe).

Craft, N. (1994) 'Secrecy in the NHS', *British Medical Journal*, 309, 1640–5.

Crail, M. (1995) 'Most Trust Managers Claim NHS Secrecy has Increased, *Health Service Journal*, 2 February, 5.

Crawshaw, P., Bunton, R. and Killen, K. (2003) 'Health Action Zones and the Problem of Community', *Health and Social Care in the Community*, 11, 36–44.

Crinson, I. (1998) 'Putting Patients First: The Continuity of the Consumerists Discourse in Health Policy, from the Radical Right to New Labour', *Critical Social Policy*, 18, 227–34.

Cross, M. (2000) 'As Not Seen on TV', *Health Service Journal*, 9 March, 26–7.

Croxson, B. (1999) *Organisational Costs in the New NHS: An Introduction to the Transaction Costs and Internal Costs of Delivering Healthcare* (Association of the British Pharmaceutical Industry, Office of Health Economics).

Culyer, A. (1991) 'The Promise of a Reformed NHS: An Economist's Angle', *British Medical Journal*, 302, 1253–6.

Culyer, A. J., Brazier, J. E. and O'Donnell, O. (1988) *Organising Health Service Provision. Drawing on Experience* (London, Institute for Health Service Management).

Curtis, S., Southall, H., Congdon, P. and Dodgeon, B. (2003) 'Area Effects on Health Variations over the Life Course: Analyses of the Longitudinal Study Sample in England Using New Data on Area of Residence in Childhood', *Social Service and Medicine*, 58, 57–74.

Cutler, T. and Waine, B. (2003) 'Advancing Public Accountability? The Social Services "Star" Ratings', *Public Money and Management*, 23, 125.

Dally, A. (1991) *Women Under the Knife* (London, Hutchinson).

Daly, M. (1979) *Gynaecology: The Metaethics of Radical Feminism* (London, The Women's Press).

Davey Smith, G., Blane, D. and Bartley, M. (1994) 'Explanations for Socio-Economic Differentials in Mortality', *European Journal of Public Health*, 4, 131–44.

Davey Smith, G. and Egger, M. (1994) 'Who Benefits from Medical Interventions?', *British Medical Journal*, 308, 71–5.

Davey Smith, G., Shipley, M., Batty, G., Morris, J. and Marmot, M. (2000) 'Physical Activity and Cause-Specific Mortality in the Whitehall Study', *Public Health*, 114, 308–15.

Davies, A. (2000) 'Don't Trust Me, I'm a Doctor – Medical Regulation and the 1999 NHS Reforms', *Oxford Journal of Legal Studies*, 20, 437–56.

Davies, C. (1995) *Gender and the Professional Predicament in Nursing* (Buckingham, Open University Press).

Davies, H., Hodges, C. and Rundall, T. (2003) 'Views of Doctors and Managers on the Doctor – Manager Relationship in the NHS', *British Medical Journal*, 326, 626–8.

Davies, H. and Nutley, S. (1999) 'The Rise and Rise of Evidence in Health Care', *Public Money and Management*, 19, 9–16.

Davies, M. and Nutley, S. (2000) 'Developing Learning Organisations in the NHS', *British Medical Journal*, 320, 998–1001.

Davies, H. T. O., Nutley, S. M. and Mannion, R. (2000) 'Organisational Culture and Quality of Health Care', *Quality of Health Care*, 9, 111–19.

Davis, H. and Daly, G. (1999) 'Extended Viewpoint: Achieving Democratic Potential in the NHS', *Public Money and Management*, 59–62.

Davison, C., MacIntyre, S. and Davey Smith, G. (1994) 'The Potential Impact of Predictive Genetic Testing for Susceptibility to Common Chronic Diseases: A Review and Proposed Research Agenda', *Sociology of Health and Illness*, 16 (3), 340–71.

Dawson, D. (2001) 'The Private Finance Initiative: A Public Finance Illusion', *Health Economics*, 10, 479–86.

Dawson, D. and Jacobs, R. (2003) 'Do We Have a Redundant Set of Cost Efficiency Targets in the NHS?', *Public Money and Management*, 23(1), 67–71.

Dawson, D. and Street, A. (2000) 'Comparing NHS Hospitals Unit Costs', *Public Money and Management*, 20, 58–62.

Day, P. and Klein, R. (1987) *Accountabilities: Five Public Services* (London, Tavistock).

Day, P. and Klein, R. (1997) *Steering but not Rowing – The Transformation of the NHS* (Bristol, Policy Press).

Day, P. and Klein, R. (2001) 'Commission for Health Improvement Invents Itself', *British Medical Journal*, 322, 1502–3.

Day, P. and Klein, R. (2004) *The NHS Improvers: A Study of the Commission for Health Improvement* (London, King's Fund).

De Luc, K. (2001) *Developing Care Pathways: The Tool Kit* (Oxford, Radcliffe Medical Press).

Deakin, N. (1991) 'Government and the Voluntary Sector in the 1990s', *Policy Studies*, 12 (3), 11–21.

Deakin, N. (1994) 'Accentuating the Apostrophe: The Citizen's Charter', *Policy Studies*, 15, 48–58.

Deeming, C. and Keen, J. (2001) 'The Politics of Long-Term Care', in Appleby, J. and Harrison, A. (eds) *Health Care UK* , Spring, 78–87.

Deffenbaugh, J. (2002) 'And Ne'er the Twain Shall Meet', *Health Service Journal*, 16 May, 28–9.

Degner, L., Kristjanson, L., Bowman, D., Sloan, J., Carriere, K. and O'Neil, J. (1997) 'Information Needs and Decisional Preferences in Women with Breast Cancer', *Journal of the American Medical Association*, 277, 1485–92.

Department of the Environment, Transport and the Regions (DETR) (2001) *Supporting People: Policy and Practice* (London, DETR).

Dewar, S. (1999) *Clinical Governance under Construction: Problems of Design and Difficulties in Practice* (London, King's Fund).

Dewar, S. (2003) *Government and the NHS: Time for a New Relationship* (London, King's Fund).

Dewar, S. and Finlayson, B. (2002) 'The "I" in the New CHAI', *British Medical Journal*, 325, 848–9.

DHSS (Department of Health and Social Security) (1970) *National Health Service. The Future Structure of the National Health Service in England* (London, HMSO).

DHSS (Department of Health and Social Security) (1971) *National Health Service Reorganisation: A Consultative Document* (London, DHSS).

DHSS (Department of Health and Social Security) (1976a) *Priorities for Health and Personal Social Services in England: A Consultative Document* (London, HMSO).

DHSS (Department of Health and Social Security) (1976b) *Report of the Regional Chairmen's Enquiry into the Working of the DHSS, in Relation to Regional Health Authorities* (London, DHSS).

DHSS (Department of Health and Social Security) (1976c) *Prevention and Health: Everybody's Business* (London, HMSO).

DHSS (Department of Health and Social Security) (1977) *The Way Forward* (London, HMSO).

DHSS (Department of Health and Social Security) (1980) *Report of the Working Group on Inequalities in Health* (The Black Report) (London, DHSS).

DHSS (Department of Health and Social Security) (1981a) *The Primary Care Team: Report of a Joint Working Group* (The Harding Report) (London, HMSO).

DHSS (Department of Health and Social Security) (1981b) *Care in Action* (London, HMSO).

DHSS (Department of Health and Social Security) (1983) *NHS Management Inquiry* (The Griffiths Management Report) (London, DHSS).

DHSS (Department of Health and Social Security) (1986) *Neighbourhood Nursing: A Focus for Care. Report of the Community Nursing Review* (The Cumberlege Report) (London, HMSO).

DHSS (Department of Health and Social Security) (1988) *Community Care: Agenda for Action* (The Griffiths Community Care Report) (London, HMSO).

Dixon, A. and Mossialos, E. (2001) 'Funding Healthcare in Europe: Recent Experiences', *Health Care UK*, Spring (London, King's Fund).

Dixon, J. (2001) 'Health Care: Modernising the Leviathan', *Political Quarterly*, 72, 30–8.

Dixon, J. and Glennerster, H. (1995) 'What Do We Know about Fundholding in General Practice?', *British Medical Journal*, 311, 727–30.

Dixon, J., Harrison, A. and New, B. (1997) 'Is the NHS Underfunded?', *British Medical Journal*, 314, 58–61.

Dobson, B., Beardsworth, A., Keil, T. and Walker, R. (1994) *Diet, Choice and Poverty* (London, Family Policy Studies Centre).

DoH (Department of Health) (1991) *The Patient's Charter* (London, HMSO).

DoH (Department of Health) (1993) *Hospital Doctors. Training for the Future* (The Calman Report) (London, DoH).

DoH (Department of Health) (1994a) *The Operation of the Internal Market: Local Freedoms, National Responsibilities* (London, DoH).

DoH (Department of Health) (1994b) *Supporting Research and Development in the NHS* (The Culyer Report) (London, HMSO).

DoH (Department of Health) (1994c) *Being Heard: Report of a Review Committee on NHS Complaints Procedures* (The Wilson Committee) (London, DoH).

DoH (Department of Health) (1995a) *A Policy Framework for the Commissioning of Cancer Services* (London, DoH).

DoH (Department of Health) (1995b) *Variations in Health: What Can the Department of Health and NHS Do?* (London, DoH).

DoH (Department of Health) (1995c) *NHS Responsibilities for Meeting Continuing Health Care Needs*, HSG (95) 8 (London, DoH).

DoH (Department of Health) (1995d) *Acting on Complaints* (London, DoH).

DoH (Department of Health) (1995e) *An Accountability Framework for GP Fundholding* (London, DoH).

DoH (Department of Health) (1996a) *The Patient's Charter and You* (London, DoH).

DoH (Department of Health) (1996b) *Patient Partnership: Building a Collaborative Strategy* (London, DoH).

DoH (Department of Health) (1997a) *Better Services for Vulnerable People* EL 97 (62) (London, DoH).

DoH (Department of Health) (1997b) *Report of the Review of Patient Identifiable Information*, Caldicott Committee (London, DoH).

DoH (Department of Health) (1998a) *The New NHS: Modern and Dependable: A National Framework for Assessing Performance. Consultation Document. NHS Executive* (London, The Stationery Office).

DoH (Department of Health) (1998b) *A First Class Service: Quality in the New NHS* (London, DoH).

DoH (Department of Health) (1998c) *Paediatric Intensive Care – A Framework for the Future: Report from National Paediatric Intensive Care Coordinating Group* (London, DoH).

DoH (Department of Health) (1998d) *Modernising Health and Social Services: National Priorities Guidance 1999–2000/ 2001–2002* (London, DoH).

DoH (Department of Health) (1998e) *Information for Health* (London, DoH).

DoH (Department of Health) (1998f) *Partnership in Action: New Opportunities for Joint Working between Health and Social Services. A Discussion Document* (London, DoH).

DoH (Department of Health) (1998g) *Modernising Mental Health Services, Safe, Sound and Supportive* (London, The Stationery Office).

DoH (Department of Health) (1998h) *The Health of the Nation: A Policy Assessed* (London, The Stationery Office).

DoH (Department of Health) (1999a) *Making a Difference* (London, DoH).

DoH (Department of Health) (1999b) *Modern Standards and Service Models: Mental Health National Service Frameworks* (London, DoH).

DoH (Department of Health) (1999c) *The NHS Performance Assessment Framework* (London, DoH).

DoH (Department of Health) (1999d) *Clinical Governance: Quality in the New NHS* (London, DoH).

DoH (Department of Health) (1999e) *Supporting Doctors, Protecting Patients. A Consultation Paper on Preventing, Recognising and Dealing with Poor Performance of Doctors in the NHS in England* (London, DoH).

DoH (Department of Health) (1999f) *Patient and Public Involvement in the New NHS* (London, DoH).

DoH (Department of Health) (1999g) *Better Care – Higher Standards. A Charter for Long Term Care* (London, DoH).

DoH (Department of Health) (2000a) *A Health Service of All the Talents: Developing the NHS Workforce* (London, DoH).

DoH (Department of Health) (2000b) *Continuing Professional Development: Quality in the New NHS* (London, DoH).

DoH (Department of Health) (2000c) *Shaping the Future NHS: Long Term Planning for Hospitals and Related Services. Consultation Document on the Findings of the National Beds Inquiry* (London, DoH).

DoH (Department of Health) (2000d) *National Service Framework: Coronary Heart Disease* (London, DoH).

DoH (Department of Health) (2000e) *The NHS Cancer Plan* (London, DoH).

DoH (Department of Health) (2000f) *Research and Development for a First Class Service: R & D Funding in the New NHS* (London, DoH).

DoH (Department of Health) (2000g) *An Organisation with a Memory: Report of an Expert Group on Learning from Adverse Events in the NHS Chaired by the Chief Medical Officer* (London, The Stationery Office).

DoH (Department of Health) (2000h) *The Management and Control of Hospital Acquired Infection HSC 2000/2002* (London, DoH).

DoH (Department of Health) (2000i) *UK Antimicrobial Resistance Strategy and Action Plan* (London, DoH).

DoH (Department of Health) (2000j) *Pharmacy in the Future: Implementing the NHS Plan* (London, DoH).

DoH (Department of Health) (2000k) *Modernising NHS Dentistry: Implementing the NHS Plan* (London, DoH).

DoH (Department of Health) (2000l) *Quality Strategy for Social Care* (London, DoH).

DoH (Department of Health) (2001a) *Report of the CFS/ME Working Group: Report to the Chief Medical Officer of an Independent Working Group* (London, DoH).

DoH (Department of Health) (2001b) *Working Together, Learning Together: A Framework for Lifelong Learning in the NHS* (London, DoH).

DoH (Department of Health) (2001c) *The Essence of Care: Patient Focused Benchmarking for Health Care Practitioners* (London, DoH).

DoH (Department of Health) (2001d) *Shifting the Balance of Power within the NHS: Securing Delivering* (London, DoH).

DoH (Department of Health) (2001e) *National Service Framework for Older People* (London, DoH).

DoH (Department of Health) (2001f) *Research Governance Framework for Health and Social Care* (London, DoH).

DoH (Department of Health) (2001g) *Report of a Census of Organs and Tissues Retained by Pathology Services in England: Conducted in 2000 by the Chief Medical Officer* (London, The Stationery Office).

DoH (Department of Health) (2001h) *Building a Safer NHS for Patients* (London, DoH).

DoH (Department of Health) (2001i) *Assuring the Quality of Medical Practice* (London, DoH).

DoH (Department of Health) (2001j) *Continuing Care: NHS and Local Councils Responsibilities* HSC 2001/015 (London, DoH).

DoH (Department of Health) (2001k) *Care Trusts: An Emerging Framework* (London, DoH).

DoH (Department of Health) (2001l) *Your Guide to the NHS* (London, DoH).

DoH (Department of Health) (2001m) *Reference Guide to Consent for Examinations or Treatment* (London, DoH).

DoH (Department of Health) (2001n) *Good Practice in Consent Implementation Guide* (London, DoH).

DoH (Department of Health) (2001o) *Involving Patients and the Public in Health Care: A Discussion Document* (London, DoH).

DoH (Department of Health) (2001p) *Involving Patients and the Public in Health Care: Responses to the Listening Exercise* (London, DoH).

DoH (Department of Health) (2001q) *The Expert Patient: A New Approach to Chronic Disease Management for the 21st Century* (London, DoH).

DoH (Department of Health) (2001r) *National Service Framework for Diabetes: Standards* (London, DoH).

DoH (Department of Health) (2001s) *Better Prevention, Better Services, Better Sexual Health* (London, The Stationery Office).

DoH (Department of Health) (2001t) *Fair Access to Care Services: Guidance on Eligibility Criteria for Adult Social Care* (London, DoH).

DoH (Department of Health) (2001u) *Extending Choice for Patients* (London, DoH).

DoH (Department of Health) (2002a) *Hospital Public Health Medicine and Community Health Services Medical and Dental Staff in England: 1991–2001* (London, DoH).

DoH (Department of Health) (2002b) *The New NHS 2001 Reference Costs* (London, DoH).

DoH (Department of Health) (2002c) *New Figures Show There is Less Inequality in the NHS* Press Release, Ref: 2002/0449 (London, DoH).

DoH (Department of Health) (2002d) *Growing Capacity: A New Role for External Healthcare Providers* (London, DoH).

DoH (Department of Health) (2002e) *A Guide to NHS Foundation Trusts* (London, DoH).

DoH (Department of Health) (2002f) *Improvement, Expansion and Reform: The Next Three Years Priorities and Planning Framework 2003–06* (London, DoH).

DoH (Department of Health) (2002g) *Planning and Priorities Framework 2003–06* (London, DoH).

DoH (Department of Health) (2002h) *Managing Excellence in the NHS* (London, DoH).

DoH (Department of Health) (2002i) *Reforming NHS Financial Flows: Introducing Payments by Results* (London, DoH).

DoH (Department of Health) (2002j) *Modern Matrons in the NHS: A Progress Report* (London, DoH).

DoH (Department of Health) (2002k) *A Framework for Personal Medical Pilot Agreements* (London, DoH).

DoH (Department of Health) (2002l) *NHS Dentistry: Options for Change* (London, DoH).

DoH (Department of Health) (2002m) *NSF for Older People – Intermediate Care: Moving Forward* (London, DoH).

DoH (Department of Health) (2002n) *Pharmacy Workforce in the New NHS* (London, DoH).

DoH (Department of Health) (2002o) *Care Homes for Older People. National Minimum Standards* (London, The Stationery Office).

DoH (Department of Health) (2002p) *Supporting the Implementation of Patient Advice and Liaison Services* (London, DoH).

DoH (Department of Health) (2002q) *Securing Service Delivery – Commissioning Freedoms of Primary Care Trusts* (London, DoH).

DoH (Department of Health) (2003a) *Payment by Results. Consultation: Preparing for 2005* (London, DoH).

DoH (Department of Health) (2003b) *Tackling Health Inequalities: A Programme for Action* (London, DoH).

DoH (Department of Health) (2003c) *Winning Ways: Working Together to Reduce Health-care Associated Infection in England. Report from the Chief Medical Officer* (London, DoH).

DoH (Department of Health) (2003d) *A Vision for Pharmacy in the New NHS* (London, DoH).

DoH (Department of Health) (2003e) *Care Standards Act 2000: Domiciliary Care National Minimum Standards Regulations* (London, DoH).

DoH (Department of Health) (2003f) *National Service Framework for Older People: A Report of Progress and Future Challenges* (London, DoH).

DoH (Department of Health) (2003g) *Getting the Right Start: National Service Framework for Children. Standards for Hospital Services* (London, DoH).

DoH (Department of Health) (2003h) *NHS Complaints Reform: Making Things Right* (London, DoH).

DoH (Department of Health) (2003i) *PALS Core National Standards and Evaluation Framework* (London, DoH).

DoH (Department of Health) (2003j) *Families and Post Mortems: A Code of Practice* (London, DoH).

DoH (Department of Health) (2003k) *Strengthening Accountability: Involving Patients and the Public* (London, DoH).

DoH (Department of Health) (2003l) *Making Partnership Work for Patients, Carers and Service Users* (London, DoH).

DoH (Department of Health) and Department for Work and Pensions (2002) *Fairer Charging Policies for Home Care and Other Non-Residential Social Services. Practical Guidance* (London, DoH).

DoH (Department of Health) and Welsh Assembly Government (2002) *Human Bodies: Human Choices The Law on Human Organs and Tissue in England and Wales. A Consultation Report* (London, DoH).

DoH (Department of Health) and Welsh Assembly Government (2003) *The Use of Human Organs and Tissue. An Interim Statement* (London, DoH).

DoH (Department of Health) Department for Education and Employment, Home Office (2001a) *Report of a Census of Organs and Tissues Retained by Pathology Services in England: Conducted in 2000 by the Chief Medical Officer* (London, The Stationery Office).

DoH (Department of Health) Department for Education and Employment, Home Office (2001b) *The Removal, Retention and Use of Human Organs and Tissue from Post Mortem Examinations* (London, The Stationery Office).

DoH (Department of Health), Welsh Office, Scottish Office and Department of Health and Social Services, Northern Ireland (1998) *Why Mothers Die: Report on Confidential Enquiries into Maternal Deaths in the UK 1994–96* (London, DoH).

DoH (Department of Health) and FSA (2000) *Vol 1: Report of the Diet and Nutrition Survey. National Diet and Nutrition Survey: Young People Aged 4–18 years* (London, The Stationery Office).

Doll, R. and Peto, R. (1981) 'The Causes of Cancer', *Journal of the National Cancer Institute*, 66, 1191–308.

Doll, R., Peto, R., Wheatley, R., Gray, R. and Sutherland, I. (1994) 'Mortality in Relation to Smoking: 40 Years Observation on Male British Doctors', *British Medical Journal*, 309, 901–11.

Donaldson, L. (1994) 'Doctors with Problems in the NHS Workforce', *British Medical Journal*, 308, 1277–82.

Donelan, K., Blendon, R., Schoen, C., Davis, K. and Binns, K. (1999) 'The Cost of Health System Change: Public Discontent in Five Nations', *Health Affairs*, 18, 206–16.

Donkin, A., Goldblatt, P. and Lynch, K. (2002) 'Inequalities in Life Expectancy by Social Class', *Health Statistics Quarterly*, 15, 5–15.

Donnison, J. (1988) *Midwives and Medical Men: A History of Interprofessional Rivalries and Women's Rights* (London, Heinemann).

Dopson, S. and Locock, L. (2002) 'The Commissioning Process in the NHS: The Theory and the Application', *Public Management Review*, 4, 209–30.

Dopson, S., Locock, L. and Stewart, R. (1999) 'Regional Offices in the New NHS: An Analysis of the Effects and Significance of Recent Change', *Public Administration*, 77, 91–110.

Dowling, B. (1997) 'Effect of Fundholding on Waiting Times: A Database Study', *British Medical Journal*, 315, 290–2.

Dowling, B. and Glendinning, C. (2003) *New Primary Care* (Buckingham, Open University Press).

Dowling, S., Martine, R., Skidmore, Doyal, L., Cameron, A. and Lloyd, S. (1996) 'Nurses Taking on Junior Doctors' Work – A Confusion of Accountability', *British Medical Journal*, 312, 1211–14.

Doyal, L. (1979) *The Political Economy of Health* (London, Pluto).

Doyal, L. (1994) 'Waged Work and Well-being', in Wilkinson, S. and Kitzinger, C. (eds) *Women and Health* (London, Taylor and Francis), 65–84.

Doyal, L. (1995) *What Makes Women Sick?* (London, Macmillan).

Doyal, L. (ed.) (1998) *Women and Health Services: An Agenda for Change* (Buckingham, Open University Press).

Doyal, L. (2000) 'Gender Equity in Health Debates and Dilemmas', *Social Science and Medicine*, 51, 931–9.

Doyal, L. (2001) 'Sex, Gender and Health: The Need for a New Approach', *British Medical Journal*, 323, 1061–3.

Doyal, L., Dowling, S. and Cameron, A. (1998) *Challenging Practice: An Evaluation of Four Innovatory Nursing Posts in the South West* (Bristol, Policy Press).

Doyle, Y. (2001) 'Equity in the New NHS: Hard Lessons from Implementing a Local Healthcare Policy on Donepezil', *British Medical Journal*, 323, 222–4.

Doyle, Y. and Bull, A. (2000) 'Roll of the Private Sector in the United Kingdom Healthcare System', *British Medical Journal*, 321, 563–5.

Draper, M., Cohen, P. and Buchan, H. (2001) 'Seeking Consumer Views: What Use Are Results of Hospitals Satisfaction Surveys', *International Journal of Quality in Health Care*, 13, 463–8.

Drennan, V., Iliffe, S., Haworth, D., Tai, S., Lenitian, P. and Deave, T. (2003) 'A Picture of Health', *Health Service Journal*, 24 April, 22–4.

Drever, F. and Whitehead, M. (1995) 'Mortality in Regions and Local Authority Districts in the 1990s: Exploring the Relationship with Deprivation', *Population Trends*, 82, 19–27.

Drever, F., Whitehead, M. and Roder, M., 'Current Patterns and Trends in Male Mortality by Social Class', *Population Trends*, 86, 15–20.

Driver, S. and Martell, L. (1997) 'New Labour's Communitarians', *Critical Social Policy*, 17, 27–46.

Driver, S. and Martell, L. (2002) *Blair's Britain* (Cambridge, Polity Press).

Drummond, M., O'Brien, B., Stoddart, G. and Torrance, G. (1997) *Methods for the Economic Evaluation of Health Care Programmes*, 2nd edn (Buckingham, Open University Press).

Duhl, L. J. (1986) 'The Health City: Its Function and its Future', *Health Promotion*, 1, 55–60.

Duncan, G. and Brooks Gunn, J. (1997) *The Consequence of Growing Up Poor* (New York, Russell Sage Foundation).

Dunman, P. (2001) 'Winning Ways', *Health Service Journal*, 10 May, 20–3.

Dunnell, K. (1995) 'Population Review (2): Are We Healthier?', *Population Trends*, 82, 12–18.

Durward, L. and Evans, R. (1990) 'Pressure Groups and Maternity Care', in Garcia, J., Kilpatrick, R. and Richards, M. (eds) *The Politics of Maternity Care Services for Childbearing Women in 20th Century Britain* (Oxford, Oxford University Press).

Dyer, C. and Boseley, S. (1999) 'A Matter of Life and Death', *Guardian*, 16 July, 3.

Dyke, G. (1998) *The New NHS Charter A Different Approach: Report on the New NHS Charter* (London, DoH).

Edwards, A. and Elwyn, G. (eds) (2001) *Evidence-Based Patient Choice* (Oxford, Oxford University Press).

Edwards, B. (1993) *The National Health Service: A Manager's Tale 1946–92* (London, Nuffield Provincial Hospitals Trust).

Edwards, G. (ed.) (1994) *Alcohol Policy and the Public Good* (Oxford, Oxford University Press).

Edwards, L. (2001) 'Walk in Centres Checked Out', *Which?*, January, 7–9.

Edwards, N., Kornacki, M. and Silversin, J. (2002) 'Unhappy Doctors: What Are the Causes and What Can Be Done?', *British Medical Journal*, 324, 835–8.

Edwards, N. E. (2000) 'Barrier Grief', *Health Service Journal*, 30 March, 28.

Egger, G. and Swinburn, B. (1997) 'An Ecological Approach to the Obesity Pandemic', *British Medical Journal*, 315, 477–80.

Elcock, H. and Haywood, S. (1980) 'The Centre Cannot Hold', *Public Administration Bulletin*, 36, 53–62.

Elizabeth, S., Davies, S. and Hanley, B. (1998) *Ordinary Wisdom – Reflection on an Experiment in Citizenship and Health* (London, King's Fund).

Elliott, P., Stamler, J., Nichols, R., Dyer, A. et al. (1996) 'Intersalt Revisited: Further Analyses of 24 Hour Sodium Excretion and Blood Pressure Within and Across Populations', *British Medical Journal*, 312, 1249–53.

Elofsson, S., Unden, A. and Krakau, I. (1998) 'Patient Charges – A Hindrance to Financially and Psychosocially Disadvantaged Groups Getting Care', *Social Science and Medicine*, 46, 1375–80.

Elston, M. (1991) 'The Politics of Professional Power: Medicine in a Changing Health Service', in Gabe, J., Calnan, M. and Bury, M. (eds) *The Sociology of the Health Service* (London, Routledge), 58–88.

Emmerson, C., Frayne, C. and Goodman, A. (2002) *How Much Would It Cost to Increase UK Health Spending to the European Union Average?* (London, IFS).

Engel, G. (1977) 'The Need for a New Medical Model: A Challenge for Biomedicine', *Science*, 196, 129–36.

Ennew, C., Whynes, D., Jolleys, J. and Robinson, P. (1998) 'Entrepreneurship and Innovation among GP fundholders', *Public Policy and Management*, 18, 59–65.

Enthoven, A. (1985) *Reflections on the Management of the National Health Service* (London, Nuffield Provincial Hospital Trust).

Ermisch, J. (1990) *Fewer Babies, Longer Lives* (York, Joseph Rowntree Foundation).

Ettore, E. (1997) *Women and Alcohol* (London, Women's Press).

Etzioni, A. (1993) *The Spirit of Community* (New York, Random House).

European Observatory on Health Care Systems (2002) *Health Care Systems in Eight Countries – Trends and Challenges* (London, London School of Economics).

European Union (1997) *The Treaty of Amsterdam* (Luxembourg, European Commission).

Eurostat (2000) *Health in the EU under the Microscope. A First Statistical Guide* (Luxembourg, Office for Official Publications of the European Communities).

Ewles, L. (1993) 'Hope Against Hype', *Health Service Journal*, 26 August, 30–1.

Exworthy, M. and Powell, M. (1999) 'Markets, Bureaucracy and Public Management. The NHS Quasi Market, Quasi Hierarchy or Quasi Network?', *Public Money and Management*, 19, 15–22.

Exworthy, M. and Powell, M. (2000) 'Variations on a Theme: New Labour, Health Inequalities and Policy Failure', in Hann, A. (ed.) *Analysing Health Policy* (Aldershot, Ashgate), 45–62.

Exworthy, M., Powell, M. and Mohan, J. (1999) 'The NHS Quasi-Market, Quasi-Hierarchy and Quasi-Network', *Public Money and Management*, 19, 15–22.

Fabian Society (2000) *Paying for Progress: A New Politics of Tax for Public Spending* (London, Fabian Society).

Fahey, T., Montgomery, A., Barnes, J. and Protheroe, J. (2003) 'Quality of Care for Elderly Residents in Nursing Homes and Elderly People Living at Home: Controlled Observational Study', *British Medical Journal*, 326, 580–3.

Fairfield, G., Hunter, D. J., Mechanic, D. and Rosleff, F. (1997) 'Implications of Managed Care for Health Systems, Clinicians and Patients', *British Medical Journal*, 314, 1895–8.

Falkingham, J. (1989) 'Dependence and Ageing in Britain: A Re-examination of the Evidence', *Journal of Social Policy*, 18, 211–33.

Farrell, C., Levenson, R. and Snape, D. (1998) *The Patient's Charter: Past and Future* (London, King's Fund).

Farrell, C., Robinson, J. and Fletcher, P. (1999) *A New Era for Community Care? What People Want from Health, Housing and Social Services* (London, King's Fund).

Fatchett, A. (1998) *Nursing in the New NHS: Modern, Dependable* (London, Baillière Tindall).

Fentem, P. H. (1994) 'Benefits of Exercise in Health and Disease, *British Medical Journal*, 308, 1291–5.

Ferguson, P. (2002) 'Doctors Contract–Letter', *The Independent*, 6 November, 15.

Ferlie, E. (1994) 'The Creation and Evolution of Quasi-Markets in the Public Sector: Early Evidence From the National Health Service', *Policy and Politics*, 22 (2), 105–22.

Ferlie, E., Ashburner, L. and Fitzgerald, L. (1993) 'Movers and Shakers', *Health Service Journal*, 18 November, 24–6.

Ferlie, E., Pettigrew, A., Ashburner, L. and Fitzgerald, L. (1996) *The New Public Management in Action* (Oxford, Oxford University Press).

Ferrie, J. E., Martikainen, P., Shipley, M., Marmot, M., Stansfeld, S. and Davey Smith, G. (2001) 'Employment Status and Health after Privatisation: White Collar Civil Servants Prospective Cohort Study', *British Medical Journal*, 322, 647.

Ferrie, J. E., Shipley, M. J., Marmot, M. G., Stansfeld, S. and Davey Smith, G. (1995) 'Health Effects of Anticipation of Job Change and Non-Employment: Longitudinal Data from the Whitehall II Study', *British Medical Journal*, 311, 1264–9.

Fielder, H., Poon-King, C., Palmer, S., Moss, N. and Coleman, G. (2000) 'Assessment of Impact on Health of Residents Living near Nant-y-Gwyddon Landfill Site: Retrospective Analysis', *British Medical Journal*, 320, 19–22.

Finlayson, A. (1999) 'Third Way Theory', *Political Quarterly*, 70, 42–51.

Finlayson, B. (2002) 'Singing the Blues', *Health Service Journal*, 4 April, 30–1.

Fisher, C. and Best, A. (1995) 'Management and Medics: How Professionals Adapt to Management', *Public Money and Management*, 15 (2), 48–54.

Fisher, K. and Collins, J. (eds) (1993) *Homelessness, Health Care and Welfare Provision* (London, Routledge).

Fitzgerald, L. and Dufour, Y. (1997) 'Clinical Management as Boundary Management Comparative Analysis of Canadian and UK Health Institutions', *International Journal of Public Sector Management*, 10, 5–20.

Fitzgerald, L. and Reeves, S. (1999) *An Exploratory Examination of the Management of Four Clinical Directorates* (London, Internal Report, City University, St Bartholomew School of Nursing and Midwifery).

Fitzherbert, L. (1992) *Charity and NHS Reform* (London, Directory of Social Change).

Fitzherbert, L. and Giles, S. (1990) *Charity and The National Health: A Report on the Extent and Potential of Charitable Funds within the NHS* (London, The Directory of Social Change).

Fitzhugh Directory, The (2002) *Independent Healthcare and Long Term Care* (London, Health Care Information Service).

Fitzhugh, W. (1995) *The Fitzhugh Directory: Independent Health Care in Long Term Care 1995/6* (London, Health Care Information Services).

Fitzpatrick, M. (2001) *The Tyranny of Health: Doctors and the Regulation of Lifestyle* (London, Routledge).

Fitzpatrick, R. (1984) 'Lay Concepts of Illness', in Fitzpatrick, R., Hinton, J., Newman, S., Scambler, G. and Thompson, J. (eds) *The Experience of Illness* (London, Tavistock).

Flynn, R. (1992) *Structures of Control in Health Management* (London, Routledge).

Flynn, R., Williams, G. and Pickard, S. (1996) *Markets and Networks: Contracting in Community Health Services* (Buckingham, Open University Press).

Food Standards Agency/Welsh Assembly Government (2003) *Food and Wellbeing* (London and Cardiff, Food Standards Agency and Welsh Assembly Government).

Forder, J., Knapp, M. and Wistow, G. (1994) 'Competition in the Mixed Economy of Care', *Journal of Social Policy*, 25, 201–22.

Foreman, A. (1996) 'Health Needs Assessment', in Percy-Smith, J. (ed.) *Needs Appraisal and Public Policy* (Buckingham, Open University Press).

Foresight Health Care Panel (2000) *HealthCare 2020* (London, Department of Trade and Industry).

Foster, P. (1995) *Women and the Health Care Industry: An Unhealthy Relationship* (Buckingham, Open University Press).

Fotaki, M. (1998) 'The Impact of Market-Oriented Reforms on Patient Choice and Information: A Case Study of Outer London and Stockholm', *Social Science and Medicine*, 48, 1415–32.

Foucault, M. (1973) *The Birth of the Clinic* (London, Tavistock).

Foucault, M. (1979) 'On Governmentality', *Ideology and Consciousness*, 6, 5–22.

Fox, J., Goldblatt, P. and Jones, D. (1990) 'Social Class Mortality Differentials: Artefact, Selection, or Life Circumstances?', in Goldblatt, P. (ed.) *Longitudinal Study: Mortality and Social Organisation 1971–81*, OPCS LS 6 (London, HMSO), 100–8.

Frankel, S., Ebrahim, S. and Davey Smith, G. (2000) 'The Limits to Demand for Health Care', *British Medical Journal*, 321, 40–5.

Freddi, G. and Bjorkman, J. (1989) *Controlling Medical Professionals: The Comparative Politics of Health Governance* (London, Sage).

Freeman, A. C. and Sweeney, K. (2001) 'Why General Practitioners Do Not Implement Evidence: Qualitative Study', *British Medical Journal*, 323, 1100–2.

Freeman, R. (2000) *The Politics of Health in Europe* (Manchester, Manchester University Press).

Freemantle, N. (1992) 'Spot the Flaw', *Health Service Journal*, 9 July, 122–3.

Freidson, E. (1988) *Profession of Medicine* (London, University of Chicago Press).

Friedman, M. (1962) *Capitalism and Freedom* (Chicago, University of Chicago Press).

Fuchs, C., Giovannucci, E., Colditz, G., Hunter, J., Stampfer, M., Rosner, B., Speizer, F. and Willet, W. (1999) 'Dietary Fiber and the Risk of Colorectal Cancer and Adenoma in Women', *New England Journal of Medicine*, 340, 169–76.

Fuchs, V. (1974) *Who Shall Live?* (New York, Basic Books).

Fuchs, V. (1996) 'Economics, Values and Health Care Reform', *American Economic Review*, 86, 1–24.

Gabe, J. and Williams, P. (1993) 'Women, Crowding and Mental Health', in Burridge, R. and Ormandy, S. (eds) *Unhealthy Housing: Research, Remedies and Reform* (London, E. and F. N. Spon), 191–208.

Gaines, A. (1979) 'Definitions and Diagnoses: Cultural Implications of Psychiatric Help Seeking and Psychiatrists' Definitions of the Situation in Psychiatric Emergencies', *Culture, Medicine and Psychiatry*, 3 (4), 381–428.

Gamarnikow, E. (1978) 'Sexual Division of Labour: The Case of Nursing' in Kahn, A. and Wolpe, A. M. (eds) *Feminism and Materialism* (London, Routledge and Kegan Paul), 96–123.

Gamble, A. (1994) *The Free Economy and the Strong State. The Politics of Thatcherism*, 2nd edn (London, Macmillan).

Garrett, L. (1995) *The Coming Plague: Newly Emerging Diseases in a World Out of Balance* (Harmondsworth, Penguin).

Gattellari, M., Butow, P. and Tattersall, M. (2001) 'Sharing Decisions in Cancer Care', *Social Science and Medicine*, 52, 1865–78.

Gazdar, C. and Pettit, R. (2000) *Out in the Open Breaking Down the Barriers for Older People* (London, DoH).

Geddes, M. and Martin, S. (2000) 'The Policy and Politics of Best Value: Currents, Cross Currents and Undercurrents in the New Regime', *Policy and Politics*, 28, 379–95.

Geller, R. (2001) 'The First Year of Health Improvement Programmes: Views from Directors of Public Health', *Journal of Public Health Medicine*, 23, 57–64.

Giddens, A. (1998) *The Third Way: The Renewal of Social Democracy* (Cambridge, Polity Press).

Giddings, P. (1993) 'Complaints, Remedies and the Health Service Commissioner', *Public Administration*, 71 (3) 377–94.

Gilchrist, C. (1999) *Turning Your Back on Us: Older People and the NHS* (London, Age Concern).

Gillam, S., Abbott, S. and Banks-Smith, J. (2001) 'Can Primary Care Groups and Trusts Improve Health?', *British Medical Journal*, 323, 89–92.

Gillam, S. and Brooks, F. (2001) *New Beginnings: Towards Patient and Public Involvement in Primary Health Care* (London, King's Fund).

Ginzberg, E. (1990) *The Medical Triangle: Physicians and the Public* (Cambridge, MA, Harvard University Press).

Gladstone, D. (1992) *Opening up the Medical Monopoly: Consumer Choice Versus Professional Power* (London, Adam Smith Institute).

Gladstone, D. (ed.) (1997) *How to Pay for Health Care: Public and Private Alternatives* (London, IEA Health and Welfare Unit).

Glasby, J. (2003) *Hospital Discharge: Integrating Health and Social Care* (Oxford, Radcliffe Medical Press).

Glasby, J. and Littlechild, R. (2004) *The Health and Social Care Divide – The Experiences of Older People*, 2nd edn (Bristol, Policy Press).

Glasby, J. and Peck, E. (2003) *Care Trusts: Partnership Working in Action* (Abingdon, Radcliffe Medical Press).

Glendinning, C. (1999) 'GPs and Contracts: Bringing General Practice into Primary Care', *Social Policy and Administration*, 33, 115–31.

Glendinning, C., Abbott, S. and Coleman, A. (2001) 'Bridging the Gap: New Relationships between Primary Care Groups and Local Authorities', *Social Policy and Administration*, 25, 411–25.

Glendinning, C. and Bailey, J. (2000) 'The Private Sector and the NHS: The Case of Capital Developments in Primary Health Care', *Policy and Politics*, 26, 387–99.

Glendinning, C., Powell, M. and Rummery, K. (2003) *Partnerships, New Labour and the Governance of Welfare* (Bristol, Policy Press).

Glendinning, C. and Rummery, K. (1997) *Working Together Primary Care Involvement in Commissioning Social Care Services* (Manchester, University of Manchester).

Glendinning, C., Rummery, K. and Clarke, R. (1998) 'From Collaboration to Commissioning: Developing Relationship Between Primary Health and Social Services', *British Medical Journal*, 317, 122–5.

Glennerster, H., Matsaganis, M. and Owens, P. (1994) *Implementing GP Fundholding: Wild Card or Winning Hand?* (Buckingham, Open University Press).

GMC (1998) *Seeking Patients Consent: The Ethical Considerations* (London, GMC).

GMC (2001) *Good Medical Practice* (London, GMC).

GMC (2002) *Withholding and Withdrawing Life-Prolonging Treatments: Good Practice in Decision Making* (London, GMC).

Goddard, M., Mannion, R. and Smith, P. (2000) 'The Performance Framework: Taking Account of Economic Behaviour', in Smith, P. C. (ed.) *Reforming Markets in Health Care* (Buckingham, Open University Press), 139–61.

Goddard, M. and Smith, P. (2001) 'Equity of Access to Health Care Services: Theory and Evidence from the UK', *Social Science and Medicine*, 53, 1149–62.

Godden, S. and Pollock, A. (2000) 'Information on Community Health Services', *British Medical Journal*, 320, 265.

Godden, S., Pollock, A. and Player, S. (2001) 'Capital Investment in Primary Care: The Funding and Ownership of Primary Care Premises', *Public Money and Management*, 21 (4), 43–50.

Godt, P. (1987) 'Confederation, Consent and Corporation: State Strategies and the Medical Profession in France, Great Britain and West Germany', *Journal of Health Politics, Policy and Law*, 12 (3), 459–80.

Goffman, E. (1961) *Asylums: Essays on the Social Situation of Mental Patients and Other Inmates* (New York, Anchor/Doubleday).

Goffman, E. (1968) *Stigma: Notes on the Management of Spoiled Identity* (Harmondsworth, Penguin).

Goldacre, M. and Harris R. (1980) 'Mortality, Morbidity, Resource Allocation and Planning: A Consideration of Disease Classification', *British Medical Journal*, 281, 1515–19.

Goldblatt, P. (1989) 'Mortality by Social Class 1971–85', *Population Trends* (London, HMSO).

Goldblatt, P., Fox, J. and Leon, D. (1990) 'Mortality of Employed Men and Women', in Goldblatt, P. (ed.) *Longitudinal Study: Mortality and Social Organisation*, 1971–81, OPCS LS 6 (London, HMSO), 67–80.

Goldsmith, M. and Willetts, D. (1988) *Managed Health Care Organisations: A New System for a Better Health Service* (London, Centre for Policy Studies).

Goldstein, H. and Spiegelhalter, D. (1996) 'League Tables and their Limitations: Statistical Issues in Comparisons of Institutional Performance', *Journal of the Royal Statistical Society*, 159 (3), 385–443.

Goodchild, B. (1998) 'Poor Housing: Poor Health', *International Journal of Health Promotion and Education*, 36 (3) 84–6.

Goodfellow, P. and Claydon, P. (2001) 'Students Sitting Medical Finals: Ready to be House Officers?', *Journal of the Royal Society of Medicine*, 94, 516–20.

Goodman, N. W. (1998) 'Clinical Governance', *British Medical Journal*, 317, 1725–27.

Goodwin, N., Mays, N., McLeod, H., Malbon, G. and Raftey, J. (1998) 'Evaluation of Total Purchasing Pilots in England and Scotland and Implications for Primary Care Groups in England: Personal Interviews and Analysis of Routine Data', *British Medical Journal*, 317, 256–9.

Graffy, J. and Williams, J. (1994) 'Purchasing for All: An Alternative to Fundholding', *British Medical Journal*, 308, 391–4.

Graham, B., Normand, C. and Goodall, Y. (2002) *Proximity to Death and Acute Health Care Utilisation* (Information and Statistics Division, ISD, NHS Scotland website, www.show.scot.nhs.uk).

Graham, H. (1993) *Hardship and Health in Women's Lives* (Brighton, Harvester Wheatsheaf).

Graham, H. (ed.) (2000) *Understanding Health Inequalities* (Buckingham, Open University Press).

Grant, C., Nicholas, R., Moore, L. and Salisbury, C. (2002) 'An Observational Study Comparing Quality of Care in Walk-in Centres with General Practice Using Standardised Patients', *British Medical Journal*, 324, 1556–62.

Gravelle, H. (1998) 'How Much of the Relation Between Population Mortality and Unequal Distribution of Income is a Statistical Artefact', *British Medical Journal*, 316, 382–5.

Gray, D., Hampson, J., Bernstein, S., Kosekoff, J. and Brook, R. (1990) 'Clinical Practice: The Appropriateness of Performing Coronary Artery Bypass Grafts', *Lancet*, 335, 1317–20.

Gray, J. (1993) *Beyond the New Right: Markets Government and the Common Environment* (London, Routledge).

Grayson, L. (1997) *Evidence Based Medicine* (London, The British Library).

Green, D. (1990) 'A Missed Opportunity', in Green, D., Neuberger, J., Lord Young of Darlington, and Burstall, M. (eds) *The NHS Reforms: What Ever Happened to Consumer Choice* (London, Institute for Economic Affairs, Health Unit).

Green, D. G. (1986) 'Joint Finance: An Analysis of the Reasons for its Limited Success', *Policy and Politics*, 14 (2), 209–20.

Green, D. G. and Irvine, B. (2001) *Health Care in France and Germany* (London, Civitas; Institute for the Study of Civil Society).

Greener, I. (2003) 'Performance in the NHS: The Insistence of Measurement and Confusion of Content', *Public Performance and Management Review*, 26, 237–50.

Greener, I. (2004) 'Path Dependency and the Creation and Reform of the NHS', in Smythe, N. (ed.) *Healthcare in Transition*, vol. 3 (Hauppage, NY, Norascience).

Greener, I. and Powell, J. (2003) 'Health Authorities, Priority Setting and Resource Allocation: A Study in Decision Making in New Labour's NHS', *Social Policy and Administration*, 37, 35–48.

Gregory, P., Malka, E., Kostis, J., Wilson, A., Arora, J. and Rhodes, G. (2000) 'Impact of Geographic Proximity to Cardial Revascularisation Services on Service Utilisation', *Medical Care*, 38, 45–57.

Grembowski, D. E., Cook, K. S., Patrick, D. and Roussel, A. (2002) 'Managed care and the US Health Care System: A Social Exchange Perspective', *Social Science and Medicine*, 54, 1167–80.

Grey-Turner, E. and Sutherland, F. M. (1982) *History of the BMA Part 2, 1932–81* (London, BMA).

Griffiths, D. (1971) 'Inequalities and Management in the NHS', *The Hospital*, July, 229–33.

Griffiths, L. and Hughes, D. (2000) 'Talking Contracts and Taking Care: Managers and Professionals in the British NHS Internal Market', *Social Science and Medicine*, 51, 209–22.

Griffiths, S. and Hunter, D. (eds) (1999) *Perspectives in Public Health* (Oxford, Radcliffe Medical).

Griggs, E. (1991) 'The Politics of Health Care Reform in Britain', *Political Quarterly*, 62 (4), 419–30.

Grindey, S. (1997) *Losing Sight of Blindness: Campaign Report 2* (London, Royal National Institute for the Blind).

Gronback, M., Deis, A., Sorenson, T. I. A., Becker, U., Schnohr, P. and Jenson, G. (1995) 'Mortality Associated with Moderate Intakes of Wine, Beer or Spirits', *British Medical Journal*, 310, 1165–9.

Grout, P., Jenkins, A. and Propper, C. (2000) *Benchmarking and Incentives in the NHS* (London, Office of Health Economics).

Groves, T. (1990) 'The Future of Community Care', *British Medical Journal*, 300, 923–4.

Guadagnoli, E. and Ward, P. (1998) 'Patient Participation in Decision Making', *Social Science and Medicine*, 47, 329–39.

Gulliford, M., Hughes, D., Figeroa-Minnoz, J., Hudson, N, and Connel, P. (2001) *Access to Health Care: Report of a Scoping Exercise* (London, NCCSDO).

Hacking, J. (2003) 'Beggars Belief', *Health Service Journal*, 10 April, 28–30.

Hadley, R. and Clough, R. (1996) *Care in Chaos: Frustration and Challenge in Community Care* (London, Cassell).

Hadley, R. and Forster, D. (1993) *Doctors as Managers: Experiences from the Front Line* (London, Longman).

Hadley, T. and Goldman, H. (1995) 'Effect of Recent Health and Social Service Policy Reforms on Britain's Mental Health System', *British Medical Journal*, 311, 1556–8.

Hall, C. (1999) 'Junior Doctor Hours Rising Out of Control', *Daily Telegraph*, 17 December, 7.

Halladay, M. and Bero, L. (2000) 'Implementing Evidence Based Practice in Health Care', *Public Money and Management*, 20, 43–50.

Hallam, L. and Henthorne, K. (1998) *Executive Summary 8: GP Cooperatives and Primary Care Emergency Centres Organisations and Impact* (Manchester, National Primary Care Research and Development Centre).

Ham, C. (1986) *Managing Health Services: Health Authority Members in Search of a Role* (University of Bristol, School for Advanced Urban Studies).

Ham, C. (1999a) *Health Policy in Britain*, 4th edn (Basingstoke, Palgrave).

Ham, C. (1999b) 'Improving NHS Performance: Human Behaviour and Health Policy', *British Medical Journal*, 319, 1490–92.

Ham, C. (2000) *The Politics of NHS Reform 1988–97 – Metaphor or Reality?* (London, King's Fund).

Ham, C. and Alberti, K. (2002) 'The Medical Profession, the Public and the Government', *British Medical Journal*, 324, 834–42.

Ham, C. and McIver, S. (2000) *Contested Decisions – Priority Setting in the NHS* (London, King's Fund).

Ham, C. and Pickard, S. (1998) *Tragic Choices in Health Care: The Case of Child B* (London, King's Fund).

Ham, C. and Robert, G. (2003) *Reasonable Rationing: International Experience of Priority Setting in Health Care* (Buckingham, Open University Press).

Hambleton, R. (1983) 'Health Planning – A Second Chance', *Policy and Politics*, 11 (2), 198–201.

Hamblin, R. (1998) 'Trusts' in Le Grand, J., Mays, N. and Mulligan, J. (eds) Learning from the NHS Internal Market: A Review of Evidence (London, King's Fund), 100–16.

Hamer, L. (2000) *A National Review and Analysis of Health Improvement Programmes 1999–2000* (London, Health Development Agency).

Hamer, L., and Easton, N. (2002) *Planning Across the LSP: Case Studies of integrating Commissioned Strategies and Health Improvement* (London, Health Development Agency).

Hammer, M. and Champy, J. (1993) *Re-engineering the Corporation: A Manifesto for Business Revolution* (London, Harper Collins).

Hancock, G. and Carim, E. (1987) *AIDS: The Deadly Epidemic* (London, Gollancz).

Hancock, T. (1985) 'The Mandala of Health: A Model of the Human Ecosystem', *Family and Community Health*, 8, 1–10.

Hann, A. (1996) *The Politics of Breast Cancer Screening* (Aldershot, Avebury).

Hansard (2002) *House of Commons Written Answers*, part 25, Column 1217, 11 June.

Harding, S. and Maxwell, R. (1997) 'Differences in the Mortality of Migrants', in Drever F. and Whitehead, M. (eds) *Health Inequalities: Decennial Supplement* (London, The Stationery Office), 108–21.

Harker, L. (1998) 'A National Childcare Strategy: Does it Meet the Childcare Challenge?', *Political Quarterly*, 69, 458–63.

Harrison, A., Dixon, J., New, B. and Judge, K. (1997) 'Can the NHS Cope in Future', *British Medical Journal*, 314, 139–42.

Harrison, A. and New, B. (2000) 'Rationing Access to Elective Care: The Way Forward', in Appleby, J. and Harrison, A. (eds) *Health Care UK* (London, King's Fund), 129–38.

Harrison, S. (1998) 'The Politics of Evidence Based Healthcare in the UK', *Policy and Politics*, 26, 15–31.

Harrison, S. (1999) 'Clinical Autonomy and Health Policy: Past and Future', in Exworthy, M. and Halford, S. (eds) *Professionals and the New Managerialism in the Public Sector* (Buckingham, Open University Press), 50–64.

Harrison, S. (2001) 'Right a Bit More', *Health Matters*, 44, 5–8.

Harrison, S. and Ahmad, W. (2000) 'Medical Autonomy and the UK State 1975 to 2005', *Sociology*, 34, 129–46.

Harrison, S. and Hunter, D. (1994) *Rationing Health Care* (London, Institute for Public Policy Research).

Harrison, S., Hunter, D. J., Marnoch, G. and Pollitt, C. (1992) *Just Managing: Power and Culture in the National Health Service* (London, Macmillan).

Harrison, S. and Mort, M. (1998) 'Which Champions, Which People? Public and User Involvement in Health Care as a Technology of Legitimacy', *Social Policy and Administration*, 32, 60–70.

Harrison, S and Pollitt, C. (1994) *Controlling Health Professionals* (Buckingham, Open University Press).

Harrison, S. and Wood, B. (1999) 'Designing Health Service Organisation in the UK 1968 to 1998: From Blueprint to Bright Idea and Manipulated Emergence', *Public Administration*, 77, 751–68.

Harrow, J. (1991) 'Local Authority Health Strategies', in McNaught, A. (ed.) *Managing Community Health Services* (London, Chapman and Hall), 3–16.

Hart, C. (2004) *Nurses and Politics: The Impact of Power and Practice* (London, Palgrave).

Hart, C. L., Davey Smith, G. and Blane, D. (1998) 'Social Mobility and 21 Year Mortality in a Cohort of Scottish Men', *Social Science and Medicine*, 47 (8), 1121–30.

Hart, C., Smith, G., Hole, D. and Hawthorne, V. (1999) 'Alcohol Consumption and Mortality from All Causes, Coronary Heart Disease and Stroke: Results from a Prospective Cohort study of Scottish Men with 21 years of Follow-up', *British Medical Journal*, 318, 1725–9.

Hartley, H. (2002) 'The System of Alignment Challenging Physicians Professional Dominance: An Elaborated Theory of Countervailing Powers', *Sociology of Health and Illness*, 24, 178–207.

Harvard Medical Practice Study (1990) *Patients, Doctors and Lawyers: Medical Injury Malpractice and Patient Compensation in New York* (Boston, Harvard Medical Practice Study).

Hastings, G., Stedd, M., McDermott, L., Forsyth, A. et al. (2003) *Review of Research on the Effects of Food Promotion to Children* (Glasgow, Centre for Social Marketing, University of Strathclyde).

Hattersley, L. (1997) 'Expectation of Life by Social Class', in Drever, F. and Whitehead, M. (eds) *Health Inequalities: Decennial Supplement* (London, TSO), 73–82.

Hawley, K. and Hudson, B. (1996) *Community Care and the Prospects for Service Development* (London, King's Fund).

Haycox, A., Bagust, A. and Walley, T. (1999) 'Clinical Guidelines the Hidden Costs', *British Medical Journal*, 318, 391–3.

Hayek, F. (1944) *Road to Serfdom* (London, Routledge and Kegan Paul).

Hayes, B. and Prior, P. M. (2003) *Gender and Healthcare in the UK* (Basingstoke, Palgrave).

Haynes, R. (1991) 'Inequalities in Health and Health Service Use. Evidence from the General Household Survey', *Social Science and Medicine*, 33, 361–8.

Haynes, R., Bentham, G., Lovett, A. and Gale, S. (1999) 'Effects of Distances to Hospital and GP Surgery on Hospital Inpatient Episodes, Controlling for Needs and Provision', *Social Science and Medicine*, 49, 425–33.

Haynes, R. B., Sackett, D., Guyatt, G. and Cook, D. (1997) 'Transferring Evidence for Research to Practice: Overcoming Barriers to Application', *Evidence Based Medicine*, 2, 68–9.

Hayward, J. (1999) 'NHS Dentistry', in Appleby, J. and Harrison, A. (eds) *Health Care UK 1999/2000* (London, King's Fund), 98–107.

Hayward, S. and Fee, E. (1992) 'More in Sorrow than in Anger: The British Nurses' Strike of 1988', *International Journal of Health Services*, 22 (3), 397–416.

Haywood, S. (1990) 'Efficiency and the NHS', *Public Money and Management*, 10 (2), 51–4.

Haywood, S. and Alaszewski, A. (1980) *Crisis in the Health Service* (London, Croom Helm).

He, J., Vupputuri, S., Allen, K., Prerost, M., Hughes, J. and Whelton, P. (1999) 'Passive Smoking and the Risk of Coronary Heart Disease – A Meta-Analysis of Epidemiologic Studies', *New England Journal of Medicine*, 340, 920–6.

HEA (Health Education Authority) (1991) *The Smoking Epidemic: Counting the Costs in England* (London, HEA).

HEA (Health Education Authority) (1997) *Guidelines: Promoting Physical Activity with Black and Minority Ethnic Groups* (London, HEA).

Headrick, L., Wilcock, P. and Batazdan, P. (1998) 'Interprofessional Working and Continuing Medical Education', *British Medical Journal*, 316, 771–4.

Health Advisory Service (1998) *Not Because They Are Old – Independent Inquiry into the Care of Older People on Acute Wards in General Hospitals* (London, Health Advisory Service).

Health Care Financial Management Association (2001) *NHS Finance in the UK*, 5th edn (London, NHSE and HFMA).

Health Committee (1988) (HC 613) *5th Report 1987/88. The Future of the NHS* (London, HMSO).

Health Committee (1993) (HC 264-1) *4th Report 1992/3. Dental Services* (London, HMSO).

Health Committee (1995a) (HC 134) *1st Report 1994/95. Priority Setting in the NHS* (London, HMSO).

Health Committee (1995b) (HC 19) *1st Report 1995/96. Long-term Care: NHS Responsibilities for Meeting Continuing Healthcare Needs* (London, HMSO).

Health Committee (1999a) (HC 318) *4th Report 1998/99. The Long Term Care of the Elderly* (London, The Stationery Office).

Health Committee (1999b) (HC 281–I) *5th Report 1998/99. The Regulation of Private and Other Independent Healthcare* (London, The Stationery Office).

Health Committee (1999c) (HC 549) *6th Report 1999/2000. Procedures Related to Adverse Clinical Incidents and Outcome in Medical Care* (London, The Stationery Office).

Health Committee (1999d) (HC 74–I) *1st Report 1998/99. The Relationship between Health and Social Services* (London, HMSO).

Health Committee (2000a) (HC 586) *3rd Report 1999/2000. Consultants' Contracts* (London, The Stationery Office).

Health Committee (2000b) (HC 373) *4th Report 1999/2000. Provision of NHS Mental Health Services* (London, The Stationery Office).

Health Committee (2001a) (HC 30) *2nd Report 2000/01. Public Health* (London, The Stationery Office).

Health Committee (2001b) (HC 247) *1st Report 2000/01. Access to NHS Dentistry* (London, The Stationery Office).

Health Committee (2002a) (HC 308–I) *1st Report 2001/02. The Role of the Private Sector in the NHS* (London, HMSO).

Health Committee (2002b) (HC 833i) *Minutes of Evidence for Wednesday 15 May 2002 Role and Functioning of the NHS Appointments Commission* (London, HMSO).

Health Committee (2002c) (HC 515-I) *2nd Report 2001/02. National Institute for Clinical Excellence* (London, The Stationery Office).

Health Committee (2002d) (HC 617) *3rd Report 2001/02. Delayed Discharges* (London, The Stationery Office).

Health Committee (2003a) (HC 395-I) *2nd Report 2002/03. Foundation Trusts* (London, The Stationery Office).

Health Committee (2003b) (HC 697) *7th Report 2002/03. Patient and Public Involvement* (London, The Stationery Office).

Health Committee (2003c) (HC 69) *3rd Report 2002/3. Sexual Health* (London, TSO (The Stationery Office)).

Health Service Commissioner (1994) (HC 197) *2nd Report 1993/4. Failure to Provide Long Term Care for a Brain Damaged Patient* (London, HMSO).

Health Service Commissioner (1996a) (HC 87) *2nd Report 1996/7. Selected Investigations Completed April to September* (London, HMSO).

Health Service Commissioner (1996b) (HC 62) *1st Report 1996/7. Selected Investigations. Access to Official Information in the NHS* (London, HMSO).

Health Service Commissioner for England (2002) (HC 887) *Annual Report 2001–02* (London, The Stationery Office).

Health Service Commissioner for England (2003a) (HC 399) Session 2002/03 *NHS Funding for Long Term Care of Older and Disabled People* (London, The Stationery Office).

Health Service Commissioner for England (2003b) *Annual Report 2002/03* (London, The Stationery Office).

Health Service Journal (1995) 'Manager Doctor Relations are Fine', *Health Service Journal*, 2 March, 8.

Health Service Journal (2001) 'Public Still Has Faith in Doctors Despite Scandals', *Health Service Journal*, 29 March.

Health Service Journal (2003) 'Reducing Health Inequalities Local Government and the NHS Working Together', *Health Service Journal* (Supplement), 13 March, 14.

Health Services Management Unit (1996a) *The Future Healthcare Workforce* (Manchester, HSMU).

Health Services Management Unit (1996b) *The Evaluation of the NHS Resource Management Programme in England* (Manchester, HSMU).

Healthcare 2000 (1995) *UK Health and Healthcare Services: Challenges and Policy Options* (London, Healthcare 2000).

Heart (2002) 'Fifth Report on the Provision of Services for Patients with Heart Disease', *Heart*, 8 (3), 1–59.

Heath, I. (2002) 'Long Term Care for Older People', *British Medical Journal*, 324, 1534–55.

Heaton, J. and Sloper, T. (2003) *National Survey of Patient Advice and Liaison Services in England: Children, Young People and Parents' Access to and Use of PALS* (York, Social Policy Research Unit, University of York).

Hedges, A. and Bromley, C. (2000) *Public Attitudes towards Taxation* (London, Fabian Society).

Helman, C. (1990) *Culture, Health and Illness*, 2nd edn (London, Wright).

Hemingway, H., Crook, A., Feder, G., Banerjee, S., Dawson, R. et al. (2001) 'Under Use of Coronary Revascularisation Procedures in Patients Considered Appropriate Candidates for Revascularisation', *New England Journal of Medicine*, 344 (9), 645–94.

Henderson, S. and Petersen, A. (2002) *Consuming Health: The Commodification of Healthcare* (London, Routledge).

Henke, N., Murray, R. and Nelson, C. (2002) 'Expectations of the 2020 UK Healthcare System', *Health Europe*, (Düsseldorf, McKinsey and Co), 10–23.

Hensher, M. and Fulop, N. (1999) 'The Influence of Health Needs Assessment on Healthcare Decision Making in London Health Authorities', *Journal of Health Services Research and Policy*, 4, 90–5.

Henwood, M. (1995) *Making a Difference?: Imlementation of the Community Care Reforms Two Years On* (London, King's Fund).

Henwood, M. (2001) *Future Imperfect* (London, King's Fund).

Her Majesty's Government (1999) *Caring About Carers: A National Strategy for Carers* (London, The Stationery Office).

Her, M. and Rehm, J. (1998) 'Alcohol and All Cause Mortality in Europe 1982–90: A Pooled Cross-Section Time Series Analysis', *Addiction*, 93 (9), 1335–40.

Herzlich, C. and Pierret, J. (1985) 'The Social Construction of the Patient: Patients and Illnesses in Other Ages', *Social Science and Medicine*, 25, 1019–32.

Hewson, B. (2000) 'Why the Human Rights Act Matters to Doctors', *British Medical Journal*, 321, 780–1.

Higgins, J. (1989) 'Defining Community Care: Realities and Myths', *Social Policy and Administration*, 23 (1), 3–16.

Higgins, J. (2001a) 'Let's Drink to That', *Health Service Journal*, 11 January, 22–3.

Higgins, J. (2001b) 'Back to the Future', *Health Service Journal*, 21 June, 26–7.

Hill, J. O. and Peters, J. C. (1998) 'Environmental Contributions to the Obesity Epidemic', *Science*, 280, 1371–4.

Hill, R. and Marks, W. (2003) *A Friend in Deed? A Survey of Patient Advice and Liaison Services (PALS)* (London, Association of Community Health Councils for England and Wales).

Himmelstein, D. H., Woolhandler, I. and Wolfe, S. (1999) 'Quality of Care in Investor-Owned versus Not For Profit HMOs', *Journal of the American Medical Association*, 282, 159–63.

Himsworth, R. L. and Goldacre, M. J. (1999) 'Does Time Spent in Hospital in the Final 15 Years of Life Increase with Age at Death. A Population-Based Study'. *British Medical Journal*, 319, 338–9.

Hippisley-Cox, J., Hardy, C., Pringle, M., Fielding, K., Carlisle, R. and Chilver, C. (1997) 'The Effect of Deprivation on Variations in General Practitioners Referral Rates: A Cross Sectional Study of Computerised Data on New Medical and Surgical Out Patient Referrals in Nottinghamshire', *British Medical Journal*, 314, 458–61.

Hiscock, J. and Pearson, M. (1999) 'Looking Inwards, Looking Outwards: Dismantling the "Berlin Wall" Between Health and Social Services', *Social Policy and Administration*, 33, 150–63.

Ho, S., Chan, L. and Kidwell, R. (1999) 'The Implementation of Busniess Process Re-engineering in American and Candian Hospitals', *Health Care Management Review*, 24, 19–31.

Hodgkinson, R. (1967) *The Origins of the NHS: The Medical Services of the New Poor Law* (London, Wellcome Foundation).

Hoffenberg, R. (1987) *Clinical Freedom* (London, Nuffield Provincial Hospital Trust).

Hogg, C. (1986) *Community Health Councils: A Review of Their Role and Structure* (London, ACHCEW).

Hogg, C. (1999) *Patients, Power and Politics* (London, Sage).

Hogg, C. (2002) *National Service Frameworks: Involving Patients and the Public* (London, The Patients Forum).

Hogg, C. and Williamson, C. (2001) 'Whose Interests Do Lay People Represent? Towards an Understanding of the Role of Lay People as Members of Committees', *Health Expectations*, 4, 2–9.

Holtzman, N. (2001) 'Putting the Search for Genes in Perspective', *International Journal of Health Services*, 31 (2), 445–61.

Honigsbaum, F. (1979) *The Division in British Medicine* (London, Kogan Page).

Honigsbaum, F. (1989) *Health, Happiness and Security: The Creation of the NHS* (London, Routledge and Chapman and Hall).

Honigsbaum, F. (1990) 'The Evolution of the NHS', *British Medical Journal*, 301, 694–9.

Honigsbaum, F. (1992) *Who Shall Live? Who Shall Die?, Oregon's Health Financing Proposals* (London, King's Fund).

Honigsbaum, F. (1995) *Priority Setting Processes for Health Care in Oregon, USA, New Zealand, The Netherlands, Sweden and the UK* (Oxford, Radcliffe Medical Press).

Hope, T., Hicks, N., Reynolds, D., Crisp, R. and Griffiths, S. (1998) 'Rationing and the Health Authority', *British Medical Journal*, 317, 1067–9.

Hopkins, J. (1999) 'Apo E4 Gene Linked to Breast Cancer', *British Medical Journal*, 319, 662.

Hopton, J. and Heaney, D. (1999) 'The Development of Local Healthcare Cooperatives in Scotland', *British Medical Journal*, 313, 1185–7.

Hornby, S. (ed.) (2000) *Collaborative Care: Interprofessional, Interagency and Interpersonal* (Oxford, Blackwell Science).

Horrobin, D. (1977) *Medical Hubris: A Reply to Illich* (London, Churchill Livingstone).

Horrocks, S., Anderson, E. and Salisbury, C. (2002) 'Systematic Review of Whether Nurse Practitioners Working in Primary Care Can Provide Equivalent Care to Doctors', *British Medical Journal*, 324, 819–23.

Horton, S. and Farnham, D. (1999) *Public Management Britain* (Basingstoke, Palgrave).

Hospital HealthcareCom (2002) *European Surgery Costs Revealed in New Research from Hospital Healthcare* (London, Campden Publishing).

House of Lords (2000) (HL 123) *6th Report of the Science and Technology Committee 1999/2000: Complementary and Alternative Medicine* (London, The Stationery Office).

House of Lords (2001) (HL 56) *3rd Report of the Science and Technology Committee 2000/2001: Resistance to Antibiotics* (London, The Stationery Office).

Howie, J., Heaney, D. and Maxwell, M. (1995) *General Practice Fundholding Shadow Project and Evaluation* (Edinburgh, University of Edinburgh).

Hudson, B. (1995) 'Joint Commissioning: Organisational Revolution or Misplaced Enthusiasm?', *Policy and Politics*, 23 (3), 233–49.

Hudson, B. (1998) 'Circumstances Change Cases: Local Government and the NHS', *Social Policy and Administration*, 32, 71–86.

Hudson, B. (ed.) (2000) *The Changing Role of Social Care* (London, Jessica Kingsley).

Hudson, B. (2002) 'Integrated Care and Structural Change: The Case of Care Trusts', *Policy Studies*, 23, 77–95.

Hudson, B. (2003) 'New Kid on the Block', *Health Service Journal*, 17 April, 24–5.

Hudson, B., Exworthy, M., Peckham, S. and Callaghan, G. (1999) *Locality Partnerships: The Early PCG Experience* (Leeds, Nuffield Institute for Health).

Hudson, B., Hardy, B., Glendinning, C. and Young, R. (2002) *National Evaluation of Use of the Section 31. Partnership Flexibilities of the Health Act 1999 Final Project Report* (Leeds and Manchester, National Primary Care Research and Development Centre, Nuffield Institute).

Hudson, B., Hardy, B., Henwood, M. and Wistow, G. (1997) 'Working Across Professional Boundaries: Primary Health Care and Social Care', *Public Money and Management*, 26–30.

Hudson, B. and Henwood, M. (2002) 'The NHS and Social Care: The Final Countdown', *Policy and Politics*, 30, 153–66.

Hughes, D. (1998) 'When Nurse Knows Best: Some Aspects of Nurse-Doctor Interaction in a Casualty Department', *Sociology of Health and Illness*, 10, 1–22.

Hughes, D. (2001) *Nursing and the Division of Labour* (Basingstoke, Palgrave).

Hughes, D. and Griffiths, L. (1999) 'On Penalties and the *Patient's Charter*: Centralism and Decentralised Governance in the NHS', *Sociology of Health and Illness*, 21, 71–94.

Huisman, M., Kunst, A. and Mackenbach, J. (2003) 'Socioeconomic Inequalities in Morbidity among the Elderly: A European Overview', *Social Science and Medicine*, 57, 861–73.

Humphrey, J. (2003) 'New Labour and the Regulatory Reform of Social Care', *Critical Social Policy*, 23, 5–24.

Hunt, G. (1995) *Whistleblowing in the Health Service – Accountability, Law and Professional Practice* (London, Edward Arnold).

Hunt, K., Ford, G., Harkins, L. and Wyke, S. (1999) 'Are Women More Ready to Consult then Men? Gender Differences in Family Practitioner Consultation for Common Chronic Conditions', *Journal of Health Services Research*, 4 (2), 96–100.

Hunt, S. (1997) 'Housing-Related Disorders' in Charlton, J. and Murphy, M. (eds) *The Health of Adult Britain 1841–1994 Volume 1* (London, The Stationery Office), 156–70.

Hunter, D. (1997) *Desperately Seeking Solutions: Rationing Health Care* (London, Longman).

Hunter, D. (2003) *Public Health Policy* (Oxford, Polity Press).

Hunter, D. J. (2000) 'Managing the NHS', in Appleby, J. and Harrison, A. (eds) *Health Care UK, Winter* (London, King's Fund), 69–76.

Hunter, H. (1995) 'CHCs Challenge Attempt to Undermine Autonomy', *Health Service Journal*, 14 July, 8.

Huntington, J., Walsh, N., Barnes, M., Rogers, H. and Baines, D. (2000) 'This is Your Pilot Speaking', *Health Service Journal*, 3 August, 30–1.

Hurwitz, B. (1999) 'Legal and Political Considerations of Clinical Practice Guidelines', *British Medical Journal*, 318, 661–4.

Hutton, W. (1996) *The State We're In* (London, Vintage).

Hutton, W. (2000) *New Life for Health: The Commission on the NHS* (London, Vintage).

Illich, I. (1975) *Limits to Medicine* (Harmondsworth, Penguin).

Illsley, R. (1986) 'Occupational Class Selection and the Production of Inequalities in Health', *Quarterly Journal of Social Affairs*, 2 (2), 151–65.

Independent (1997) 'Cigarettes Set to Kill 10 million by 2005', *The Independent*, 11 March, 6.

Independent Healthcare Association and DoH (2000) *For the Benefit of Patients: A Concordat with the Private and Voluntary Health Care Provider* (London, DoH).

Independent Inquiry into Inequalities in Health (1998) *Report (Acheson Report)* (London, The Stationery Office).

Independent Inquiry into the Misuse of Drugs Act 1971 (2000) *Drugs and the Law* (London, Police Foundation).

Independent Scientific Committee on Smoking and Health (1988) *4th Report* (London, HMSO).

Inglis, B. (1965) *A History of Medicine* (London, Weidenfeld and Nicolson).

Inglis, B. (1981) *The Diseases of Civilisation* (London, Hodder and Stoughton).

Insight Management Consulting (1996) *Resourcing and Performance Management in Community Health Councils* (London, DoH).

IPPR (1995a) *Primary Health Care: A Prognosis* (London, IPPR).

IPPR (1995b) *Voices Off: Tackling the Democratic Deficit in Health* (London, IPPR).

IPPR (1996) *Paying for Long Term Care* (London, IPPR).

IPPR (2001) *Building Better Partnerships: The Final Report from the Commission on Public Private Partnerships* (London, IPPR)

Jack, R. (ed.) (1998) *Residential versus Community Care: The Role of Institutions in Welfare Provision* (London, Macmillan).

Jacobs, A. (1999) 'Seeing Difference: Market Health Reform in Europe', *Journal of Health Politics, Policy and Law*, 23, 1–33.

Jacobs, L., Marmor, T. and Oberlander, T. (1999) 'The Oregon Health Plan and the Political Paradox of Rationing: What Advocates and Critics Have Claimed and What Oregon Did', *Journal of Health Politics, Policy and Law*, 24, 161–80.

Jacobson, B., Smith, A. and Whitehead, M. (1991) *The Nation's Health: A Strategy for the 1990s*, 2nd edn (London, King's Fund).

James, C., Dixon, M. and Sonanja, M. (2002) *Refocusing Commissioning for Primary Care Trusts* (Retford, NHS Alliance).

James, W., Nelson, M., Ralph, A. and Leather, S. (1997) 'The Contribution of Nutrition to Inequalities in Health', *British Medical Journal*, 314, 1545–9.

Jankowski, R. (2001) 'Implementing National Guidelines at Local Level', *British Medical Journal*, 26 May, 1258–9.

Jansen, M. C., Bueno-de-Mesquista, H. B., Buzina, R., Fidanza, F., Menotti, A., Blackburn, H., Nissiner, A. M., Kok, F. J. and Kromhout, D. (1999) 'Dietary Fibre and Plant Foods in Relation to Colorectal Cancer Mortality: The 7 Countries Study', *International Journal of Cancer*, 81 (2) 174–9.

Janzon, K., Law, S., Watts, A. and Pollock, A. (2000) 'Lost and Confused: Inappropriate Admission to Nursing and Residential Care', *Health Service Journal*, 9 November, 26–9.

Jarvis, C., Hancock, R., Askham, J. and Tinker, A. (1996) *Getting Around After 60: A Profile of Britain's Older Population* (London, HMSO).

Jeffreys, M. (1998) 'General Practitioners and the Other Caring Professions', in Loudon, I., Horder, J. and Webster, G. (eds) *General Practice Under the National Health Service 1948–97. The First Fifty Years* (Oxford, Clarendon).

Jenkins, C. (1999) 'Personal Medical Services Pilots – New Opportunities', in Lewis, R. and Gillam, S. (eds) *Transforming Primary Care Personal Medical Services in the New NHS: National Primary Care Research and Development Centre* (London, King's Fund), 20–8.

Jenkins, J. (1985) *Caring for Women's Health* (London, Search Press).

Jenkins, P. (1987) *Mrs Thatcher's Revolution: The Ending of the Socialist Era* (London, Jonathan Cape).

Jenkins, R. (1993) 'Defining the Problem. Stress, Depression and Anxiety: Causes, Prevalence and Consequences', in Jenkins, R. and Warman, D. (eds) *Promoting Mental Health Policies in the Workplace* (London, HMSO).

Jervis, P. and Hazell, R. (1998) 'Separate Ways', *Health Service Journal*, 26 November, 26–7.

Johnson, P., Conrad, C. and Thomson, D. (1989) *Workers versus Pensioners* (London, Centre for Economic Policy Research).

Johnson, T. (1972) *Professions and Power* (London, Macmillan).

Johnson, T. (1995) 'Governmentality and the Institutionalisation of Expertise', in Johnson, T., Larkin, G. and Saks, M. (eds) *Health Professions and the State in Europe* (London, Routledge), 7–24.

Jones, A. and Duncan, A. (1995) *Hypothecated Health Taxes: An Evaluation of Recent Proposals* (London, Office of Health Economics).

Jones, B. (1994) 'Nursing, Obstetrics and Gynaecology', in Burrows, M., Dyson, R., Jackson, P. and Saxton, H. (eds) *Management for Hospital Doctors* (Oxford, Butterworth-Heinemann).

Jones, D. (1999) 'Nurse led PMS Pilots', in Lewis, R. and Gillam, S. (eds) *Transforming Primary Care Personal Medical Services in the New NHS: National Primary Care Research and Development Centre* (London, King's Fund).

Jones, I. and Higgs, P. (1990) 'Putting People before Logic', *Health Service Journal*, 31 May, 814–5.

Jones, J., Wilson, A., Parker, H., Wynn, A., Jagger, C., Spiers, N. and Parker, G. (1999) 'Economic Evaluation of Hospital at Home versus Hospital Care: Cost Minimisation Analysis from Randomised Controlled Trial' *British Medical Journal*, 319, 1547–50.

Jones, K. (1998) 'We Need the Bed – Continuing Care and Community Care' in Jack, R. (ed.) *Residential versus Community Care: The Role of Institutions in Welfare Provision* (London, Macmillan).

Jones, L., Sidell, M. and Douglas, J. (2002) *The Challenge of Promoting Health*, 2nd edn (Basingstoke, Palgrave).

Jones, M. (2000) 'Walk in Primary Care Centres: Lessons from Canada', *British Medical Journal*, 321, 928–31.

Jones, R., Rubin, G. and Hungin, P. (2001) 'Is the Two Week Rule for Cancer Referrals Working', *British Medical Journal*, 322, 1555–6.

Jones, T. (2001) *Health and Healthcare in the EU: A Financial Perspective* (London, The Association of Chartered and Certified Accountants).

Joseph Rowntree Foundation (1996) *Inquiry into Meeting the Cost of Continuing Care* (York, York Publishing Services).

Joseph Rowntree Foundation (2003) *Monitoring Poverty and Social Exclusion* (York, JRF).

Joss, R. and Kogan, M. (1995) *Advancing Total Quality: Total Quality Management in the National Health Service* (Buckingham, Open University Press).

Judge, K. (1995) 'Income Distribution and Life Expectancy: A Critical Appraisal', *British Medical Journal*, 311, 1282–5.

Kahan, J., Bernstein, S. and Leape, L. (1994) 'Measuring the Necessity of Medical Procedures', *Medical Care*, 32, 357–63.

Kahn, R., Wise, P., Kennedy, B. and Kawacki, I. (2000) 'State Income Inequality, Household Income and Maternal Mental and Physical Health: Cross Sectional National Survey', *British Medical Journal*, 321, 1311–15.

Kammerling, R. and Kinnear, A. (1996) 'The Extent of the Two Tier Service for Fundholders', *British Medical Journal*, 312, 1399–1401.

Kanavos, P. and McKee, M. (2000) 'Cross-Border Issues in the Provision of Health Services: Are We Moving towards a European Health Care Policy?', *Journal of Health Services Research and Policy*, 5, 231–6.

Kaplan, G., Pamuk, E., Lynch, J., Cohen, R. and Balfour, J. (1996) 'Inequality in Income and Mortality in the United States', *British Medical Journal*, 312, 999–1003.

Kavanagh, S. and Knapp, M. (1998) 'The Impact on General Practitioners of the Changing Balance of Care for Elderly People Living in Institutions', *British Medical Journal*, 317, 322–7.

Kawachi, I. and Kennedy, B. (1997) 'Health and Social Cohesion. Why Care About Income Inequality?', *British Medical Journal*, 314, 1037–40.

Kawachi, I., Kennedy, B., Lochner, K. and Prothrow-Stith, D. (1997) 'Social Capital, Income Inequality and Mortality', *American Journal of Public Health*, 87 (9), 1491–8.

Keen, J. (1999) 'NHS Networks: Rational Technology or Triffid?' in Appleby, J. and Harrison, A. (eds) *Health Care UK 1999/2000* (London, King's Fund), 111–14.

Keen, J., Light, D. and Mays, N. (2001) *Public-Private Relations in Healthcare* (London, King's Fund).

Keen, J. and Malby, R. (1992) 'Nursing Power and Practice in the UK NHS', *Journal of Advanced Nursing*, 17, 863–70.

Kelleher, D. and Hillier, S. (1996) *Researching Cultural Differences in Health* (London: Routledge).

Kelly, S. and Baker, A. (2000) 'Healthy Life Expectancy in Great Britain 1980–1996', *Health Statistics Quarterly*, 7, 32–7.

Kelner, M., Wellman, B., Pecosolido, B. and Saks, M. W. (eds) (2000) *Complementary and Alternative Medicine: Challenge and Change* (Amsterdam, Harwood Academic Press).

Kendall, L. (1998) *Local Inequalities Targets* (London, King's Fund).

Kendall, L. (2001) *The Future Patient* (London, Institute for Public Policy Research).

Kendrick, K., Weir, P. and Rosser, E. (1995) *Innovations in Nursing Practice* (London, Edward Arnold).

Kennedy, B., Kawachi, I. and Proterow-Stith, D. (1996) 'Income Distribution and Mortality: Cross Sectional Ecological Study of the Robin Hood Index in the United States', *British Medical Journal*, 312, 1004–7.

Kennedy, I. (1981) *The Unmasking of Medicine* (London, Allen and Unwin).

Kerrison, S. and Pollock, A. (2001) 'Caring for Older People in the Private Sector in England', *British Medical Journal*, 323, 566–9.

Key, T., Thorogood, M., Appleby, P. and Burr, M. (1996) 'Dietary Habits and Mortality in 11000 Vegetarians and Health Conscious People: Results of a 17 Year Follow-up', *British Medical Journal*, 313, 775–9.

Keys, A. (1980) *Seven Countries: A Multi Analysis of Death and Coronary Heart Disease* (Cambridge, MA, Harvard University Press).

Kickbusch, I. (2000). 'The Development of International Health Policy – Accountability Intact', *Social Science and Medicine*, 51, 979–89.

King's Fund (1999) *Briefing: Learning Disabilities from Care to Citizenship* (London, King's Fund).

King's Fund (2002) *The Future of the National Health Service: A Framework for Debate* (London, King's Fund).

King's Fund/NHS Alliance (2001) *Public Private Partnerships and Primary Care* (London and Retford, King's Fund, NHSA).

Kirkcaldy, A., Robinson, J. and Perkins, L. (2003) *An Evaluation of PALS Pathfinder Projects in the North West* (Liverpool, University of Liverpool, Department of Health).

Kitzinger, S. (1994) *The Experience of Childbirth* (Harmondsworth, Penguin).

Klein, R. (1983) *The Politics of the National Health Service* (London, Longman).

Klein, R. (1990) 'The State and the Profession: The Politics of the Double Bed', *British Medical Journal*, 301, 700–2.

Klein, R. (1991) 'Making Sense of Inequalities: A Response to Peter Townsend', *International Journal of Health Services*, 21 (1), 75–81.

Klein, R. (1995) *The New Politics of the NHS*, 3rd edn (London, Longman).

Klein, R. (1998) 'Competence, Professional Self Regulation and the Public Interest', *British Medical Journal*, 316, 1740–42.

Klein, R. (1999) 'Has the NHS a Future?', in Appleby, J. and Harrison, A. (eds) *Health Care UK* (London, King's Fund), 1–5.

Klein, R. (2000) *The New Politics of the NHS*, 4th edn (London, Prentice-Hall).

Klein, R. (2003) 'Governance for NHS Foundation Trusts', *British Medical Journal*, 326, 174–5.

Klein, R. and Day, P. (1992) 'Constitutional and Distributional Conflict in British Medical Politics: The Case of General Practice 1911–1991', *Political Studies*, 40 (3), 462–78.

Klein, R., Day, P. and Redmayne, S. (1996) *Managing Scarcity. Priority-Setting and Rationing in the NHS* (Buckingham, Open University Press).

Klein, R. and Lewis, J. (1976) *The Politics of Consumer Representation* (London, Centre for Studies in Social Policy).

Kleinman, A. (1978) 'Concepts and a Model for the Comparison of Medical Systems as Cultural Systems', *Social Science and Medicine*, 12 (2B), 85–93.

Knapp, M., Hardy, B. and Forder, J. (2001) 'Commissioning for Quality: Ten Years of Social Care Markets in England', *Journal of Social Policy*, 30, 283–306.

Kohn, L. T., Corrigan, J. M. and Donaldson, M. S. (eds) (1999) *To Err is Human: Building a Safer Health System* (Washington DC, National Academy Press).

Kramer, A., Hahn, S., Cohen, N., Banich, M., McAuley, E., Harrison, C. R., Chason, J., Vakil, E., Bardell, L., Boileau, R. and Colcombe, A. (1999) 'Ageing, Fitness and Neurocognitive Function', *Nature*, 400, 418–9.

Kumpers, S., Van Raak, A., Hardy, B., and Mur, I. (2002) 'The Influence of Institutions and Culture on Health Politics: Different Approaches to Integrated Care in England and the Netherlands', *Public Administration*, 80 (2), 339–58.

Kunkler, I. (2000) 'Managed Clinical Networks: A New Paradigm for Clinical Medicine', *Journal of the Royal College of Physicians*, 34, http://www.rcplondon.ac.uk/pubs/journal/journ_34_may_ed4.htm

Kunst, A. E., Groenhof, F. and Mackenbach, J. (1990) 'Occupational Class and Cause Specific Mortality in Middle Aged Men in 11 European Countries: Comparison of Population Based Studies', *British Medical Journal*, 30 May, 1636–42.

Kunst, A., Groenhof, J., Mackenbach, J. and EU Working Group on Socioeconomic Inequalities in Health (1998) 'Occupational Class and Case-specific Mortality in Middle-aged Men in 11 European Countries: Comparision of

Population-based Studies', *British Medical Journal*, 316, 1636–42.

Kunzli, N., Kaiser, R., Medina, S., Studnicka, M., Chanel, O., Filliger, P., Herry, M., Horak Jr, F., Puybonnieux-Texier, V., Quenet, P., Schneider, J., Seethaler, R., Vergnaud, J-C. and Sommer, H. (2000) 'Public Health Impact of Outdoor and Traffic-Related Air Pollution: A European Assessment', *The Lancet*, 356, 795–801.

Labour Party (1992) *No Previous Experience Required: A Survey of 3rd Wave Trusts* (London, Labour Party).

Labour Research Department (1994) 'The NHS: Unelected Tory Quangos', *Labour Research*, December.

Laing, W. (1996) *Laing's Review of Private Health Care 1996* (London, Laing and Buisson).

Laing and Buisson (2001) *Laing's Healthcare Market Review 2001/2002* (London, Laing and Buisson Publications).

Lakin, C. (2001) 'The Effects of Taxes and Benefits on Household Income. 1999–2000', *Economic Trends*, 569, April, 35–74.

Langham, S. and Black, N. (1995) 'The Evolution of a Public Sector Market for Cardiac Services in the UK 1991–4', *Public Money and Management*, 15 (3), July–September, 31–8.

Larkin, G. (1983) *Occupational Monopoly and Modern Medicine* (London, Tavistock).

Larson, E. (1999) 'The Impact of Physician-Nurse Interaction on Patient Care', *Holistic Nursing Practice*, 13, 38–47.

Larson, M. (1977) *The Rise of Professionalism* (Berkeley, CA, University of California Press).

Lattimer, V., George, S., Thompson, F., Thomas, E., Mullee, M., Turnbull, J., Smith, H., Moore, M., Bond, H. and Glasper, A. (1998) 'Safety and Effectiveness of Nurse Telephone Consultation in Out of Hours Primary Care: Randomised Controlled Trial', *British Medical Journal*, 317, 1054–9.

Laurance, J. (2003) 'Thousands Set for Free Surgery abroad after NHS Ruling', *The Independent*, 2 October, 5.

Law, M. and Wald, N. (1999) 'Why Heart Disease Mortality is Low in France: The Time Lag Explanation', *British Medical Journal*, 318, 1471–6.

Lawrence, M. (ed.) (1987) *Fed Up and Hungry: Women, Oppression and Food* (London, Women's, Press).

Lawson, N. (1992) *The View from Number 11. Memoirs of a Tory Radical* (London, Bantam Press).

Le Fanu, J. (1999) *The Rise and Fall of Modern Medicine* (London, Abacus).

Le Grand, J. (2000) 'Should the NHS be Funded by a Hypothecated Tax? Yes', *Fabian Review*, Winter, 8.

Le Grand, J., Mays, N. and Dixon, J. (1998) 'The Reforms; Success or Failure or Neither?', in Le Grand, J., Mays, N. and Mulligan, J. (eds) *Learning From the NHS Internal Market: A Review of the Evidence* (London, King's Fund), 117–43.

Le Grand, J., Mays, N. and Mulligan, J. (eds) (1998) *Learning from the NHS Internal Market: A Review of Evidence* (London, King's Fund).

Leape, L., Park, R., Bashore, T., Harrison, J., Davidson, C. and Brook, R. (2000) 'Effect of Variability in the Interpretation of Coronary Angiograms on the Appropriateness of Coronary Revascularisation Procedures', *American Heart Journal*, 139 (1), 106–13.

Lear, J., Lawrence, I., Pohl, J. and Burden, A. (1994) 'Myocardial Infarction and Thrombolysis: A Comparison of the Indian and European Populations on a Coronary Care Unit', *Journal of the Royal College of Physicians*, 28, 143–7.

Leatherman, S. and Sutherland, K. (2003) *The Quest for Quality in the NHS* (London, Nuffield Trust).

Leavey, R., Wilkin, D. and Metcalfe, D. (1989) 'Consumerism and General Practice', *British Medical Journal*, 298, 737–9.

Lee, C. D., Blair, S. N. and Jackson, A. J. (1999) 'Cardiorespiratory Fitness, Body Composition, and All Cause and Cardiovascular Disease Mortality in Men', *American Journal of Clinical Nutrition*, 69 (3), 373–80.

Lee-Potter, J. (1997) *A Damn Bad Business: The NHS Deformed* (London, Indigo).

Leese, B. (1996) 'Dr Livingstone I Presume?', *Health Service Journal*, 5 December, 24–6.

Leese, B. and Bosanquet, N. (1995a) 'Change in General Practice and its Effects on Service Provision in Areas with Different Socioeconomic Characteristics', *British Medical Journal*, 311, 546–7.

Leese, B. and Bosanquet, N. (1995b) 'Family Doctors and Change in Practice Strategy Since 1986', *British Medical Journal*, 310, 705–8.

Leeson, J. and Gray, J. (1978) *Women and Medicine* (London, Tavistock).

Leichter, H. M. (1999) 'Oregon's Bold Experiment Whatever Happened to Rationing?', *Journal of Health Policy and Law*, 24, 147–60.

Lenaghan, J. (1996) *Rationing and Rights in Health Care* (London, Institute for Public Policy Research).

Lennane, K. (1993) 'Whistleblowing: A Health Issue', *British Medical Journal*, 307, 667–7.

Levenson, R., Joule, N. and Russell, J. (1997) *Developing Public Health in the NHS: The Multidisciplinary Contribution* (London, King's Fund).

Levitt, R., Wall, A. and Appleby, J. (1995) *The Reorganised National Health Service* (London, Chapman and Hall)

Lewis, C., Eaton, L. and Carlisle, D. (2002) 'Mental Health and the National Service Framework', *Health Service Journal*, 20 June, 35–40.

Lewis, J. (1986) *What Price Community Medicine?* (Brighton, Wheatsheaf).

Lewis, J. (1998) 'The Medical Profession and the State: GPs and the GP contract in the 1960s and the 1990s', *Social Policy and Administration*, 32, 132–50.

Lewis, J., Bernstock, P., Bovell, V. and Wookey, F. (1996) 'The Purchaser–Provider Split in Social Care: Is it Working?', *Social Policy and Administration*, 30 (1), 1–19.

Lewis, J. and Glennerster, H. (1996) *Implementing the New Community Care* (Buckingham, Open University Press).

Lewis, R. (2001a) *Nurse-Led Primary Care: Learning from PMS Pilots* (London, King's Fund).

Lewis, R. (2001b) 'High Street Lows', *Health Service Journal*, 23 August, 27.

Lewis, R., Dixon, J. and Gillam, S. (2003a) *Future Directions for Primary Care Trusts* (London, King's Fund).

Lewis, R., Dixon, J. and Gillam, S. (2003b) 'Outside Chance', *Health Service Journal*, 8 May, 24–6.

Lewis, R. and Gillam, S. (eds) (1999) *Transforming Primary Care Personal Medical Services in the New NHS: National Primary Care Research and Development Centre* (London, King's Fund).

Lewis, R. and Gillam, S. (2002) 'Personal Medical Services', *British Medical Services*, 325, 1126–7.

Lewis, R. and Gillam, S. (2003) 'Back to the Market: Yet More Reform of the National Health Service', *International Journal of Health Services*, 33, 77–84.

Lewis, R., Malbon, G. and Gillam, S. (2000) 'A Future for Primary Care Groups', in Appleby, J. and Harrison, A. (eds) *Health Care UK 1999/2000* (London, King's Fund), 9–14.

Ley, P. (1982) 'Satisfaction, Compliance and Communication', *British Journal of Clinical Psychology*, 21, 241–54.

Liberal Democrats (2003) *Government Hospital Ratings*, Press Release, 4 August.

Light, D. (1991) 'Professionalism as Countervailing Power', *Journal of Health Politics, Policy and Law*, 16, 499–506.

Llewellyn, S. and Northcott, D. (2002) *The Average Hospital: From Markets to Metrics in Health Care*, accessed from http://aux. zicklin.baruch.cuny.edu/critical/html2/8031 llewellyn.html

Lloyd, L. (2000) 'Caring About Carers: Only Half the Picture?', *Critical Social Policy*, 20 (1), 136–50.

Lobmayer, P. and Wilkinson, R. (2000) 'Income Inequality and Mortality in 14 Developed Countries', *Sociology of Health and Illness*, 22 (4), 401–14.

Local Government Association (2000) *Partnership with Health: A Survey of Local Authorities* (London, Local Government Association).

Lockhart-Wood, K. (2000) 'Collaboration between Nurses and Doctors in Clinical Practice', *British Journal of Nursing*, 9, 276–80.

Locock, L. (2000) 'The Changing Nature of Rationing in the UK NHS', *Public Administration*, 78, 91–110.

Loewy, E. H. (1980) 'Cost Should Not Be A Factor In Medical Care', *New England Journal of Medicine*, 302, 697.

Lord Sutherland of Houndwood et al. (2003) *Long Term Care: Statement By Royal Commissioners*.

Loudon, I., Horder, J. and Webster, C. (eds) (1998) *General Practice under the NHS 1948–1997* (London, Clarendon Press).

Loveland, I. (1999) 'Incorporating the European Convention on Human Rights into UK Law', *Parliamentary Affairs*, 52, 112–27.

Loveridge, R. and Starkey, K. (1992) *Continuity and Crisis in the NHS* (Buckingham, Open University Press).

Low, J. (2001) *Lay Perspectives on the Efficacy of Alternative and Complementary Therapies: The Experiences of People Living with Parkinson's Disease* (Leicester, De Montfort University).

Lowe, R. (1997) *The Welfare State in Britain Since 1945* (Basingstoke, Macmillan).

Lowry, S. (1991) *Housing and Health* (London, BMJ).

Luke, C. (1998) 'Accident and Emergency', *Alcohol Alert*, 3, 2–4.

Lugon, M. and Secker-Walker, J. (1998) *Clinical Governance: Making it Happen* (London, Royal Society of Medicine).

Lundberg, G. D. (1998) 'Low Tech Autopsies in an Era of High Tech Medicine–Continued Value for Quality Assurance and Patient Safety', *Journal of American Medicine Association*, 280, 1273–4.

Lupton, C., Peckham, S. and Taylor, P. (1998) *Managing Public Involvement in Commissioning for Health* (Buckingham, Open University Press).

Lupton, D., Donaldson, C. and Lloyd, P. (1991) 'Caveat Emptor or Blissful Ignorance? Patients and the Consumerists Ethos', *Social Science and Medicine*, 33, 559–68.

de Lusignan, S. (2003) 'Commentary: Improve the Quality of the Consultation', *British Medical Journal*, 326, 205.

Lynch, J. and Kaplan, G. (1997) 'Understanding How Inequality in the Distribution of Income Affects Health', *Journal of Health Psychology*, 2 (3), 297–314.

MacIntyre, A. (1981) *After Virtue* (London, Duckworth).

MacIntyre, S. and Hunt, K. (1997) 'Socioeconomic Position, Gender and Health', *Journal of Health Psychology*, 2, 315–34.

MacIntyre, S., Hunt, K. and Sweeting, H. (1996) 'Gender Differences in Health: Are Things Really as Simple as They Seem?', *Social Science and Medicine*, 42, 617–24.

MacIntyre, S., McIver, S., and Soomans, A. (1993) 'Area, Class and Health: Should We Be Focusing on Places or People?', *Journal of Social Policy*, 22, 213–34.

Mackay, L. (1993) *Conflicts in Care: Medicine and Nursing* (London: Chapman and Hall).

Mackenbach, J. P., Kunst, A., Cavelaars, A., Groenhof, F., Guerts, J. and EU Working Group on Socioeconomic Inequalities in Health (1997) 'Socioeconomic Inequalities in Morbidity and Mortality in Western Europe', *Lancet*, 349, 1655–9.

Macran, S., Clark, L. and Joshi, H. (1996) 'Women's Health: Dimensions and Differentials', *Social Science and Medicine*, 42, 1203–16.

MAFF (1998) *National Food Survey* (London, The Stationery Office).

Maher, J. and Green, H. (2002) *Carers 2000* (London, The Stationery Office).

Maile, S. and Hoggett, P. (2001) 'Best Value and the Politics of Pragmatism', *Policy and Politics*, 29 (4), 509–19.

Majeed, A. (2003) 'Ten Ways to Improve Information Technology in the NHS', *British Medical Journal*, 326, 202–6.

Major, J. (2000) *The Autobiography* (London, Harper Collins).

Malby, R. (1996) 'Nursing Development Units in the UK', *Advanced Practice Nursing Quarterly*, 1 (4), 20–7.

Maniadakis, N., Hollingsworth, B. and Thanassoulis, E. (1999) 'The Impact of the Internal Market on Hospitals Efficiency, Productivity and Service Quality', *Health Care Management Science*, 2, 75–85.

Manias, E. and Street, A. (2000) 'The Interplay of Knowledge and Decision-Making between Doctors and Nurses in Critical Care', *International Journal of Nursing Studies*, 38, 129–40.

Mannion, R. and Goddard, M. (2001) 'Impact of Published Clinical Outcomes Data: Case Study in NHS Hospital Trusts', *British Medical Journal*, 323, 260–3.

Manton, K. Stalland, E. and Corder, L. (1995) 'Changes in Morbidity and Chronic Disability in the US Elderly Population. Evidence from 1982, 1984 and 1989 National Long Term Care Survey', *Journal of Gerontology*, 50B, S104–204.

Marinker, M. (ed.) (1990) *Medical Audit and General Practice* (London, British Medical Journal).

Marinker, M. (ed.) (1994) *Controversies in Health Care Practice* (London, British Medical Journal).

Marks, D. (1995) 'Balancing Act', *Health Service Journal*, 13 April, 26–7.

Marks, L. (1988) *Promoting Better Health: An Analysis of the Government's Programme for Improving Primary Care*, Briefing Paper no. 7 (London, King's Fund).

Marmot, M. and Shipley, M. (1996) 'Do Socioeconomic Differences in Mortality Persist After Retirement? 25 Year Follow Up of Civil Servants from the First Whitehall Study', *British Medical Journal*, 313, 1177–80.

Marmot, M. G., Davey-Smith, G., Stansfeld, S., Patel, C., North, F., Head, J., White, I., Brunner, E. and Feeney, A. (1991) 'Health Inequalities among British Civil Servants: The Whitehall II Study', *Lancet*, 337, 1387–93.

Marnoch, G. (1996) *Doctors and Management in the NHS* (Buckingham, Open University Press).

Marsh, A., Gordon, D., Pantazis, C. and Heslop, P. (1999) *Home Sweet Home: The Impact of Poor Housing on Health* (Bristol, Policy Press).

Marsh, D., and Rhodes, R. (1992) *Implementing Thatcherite Policies* (Buckingham, Open University Press).

Martin, C. (1992) 'Attached, Detached or New Recruits?', *British Medical Journal*, 305, 348–50.

Martin, D., Pater, J. and Singer, P. (2001) 'Priority-Setting Decisions for New Cancer Drugs: A Qualitative Case Study', *The Lancet*, 358, 1676–81.

Martin, J. (1984) *Hospitals in Trouble* (Oxford, Blackwell).

Martin, R., Sterne, J., Ebrahim, S., Davey Smith, G., and Frankel, S. (2003) 'NHS Waiting Lists and Evidence of National and Local Failure: Analysis of Health Service Data', *British Medical Journal*, 326, 188–92.

Marx, K. and Engels, F. (1976) *The Communist Manifesto* (Harmondsworth, Penguin).

Mason, J., Freemantle, N. and Browning, G. (2001) 'Impact of Effective Healthcare Bulletin on Treatment of Persistent Glue Ear in Children: Time Series Analysis', *British Medical Journal*, 323, 1096–7.

Mathiason, N. (2000) 'New Hospitals Pose Health Risk', *Observer*, 20 August, 8.

Matka, E., Barnes, M. and Sullivan, H. (2002) 'Health Action Zones: Creating Alliances to Achieve Change', *Policy Studies*, 23, 97–106.

Mathew, C. (2001) 'Postgenomic Technologies: Hunting the Genes from Common Disorders', *British Medical Journal*, 322, 1031–4.

Maxwell, R. J. (1988) 'Financing Health Care. Lessons from Abroad', *British Medical Journal*, 296, 1423–6.

Mays, N. and Bevan, G. (1987) *Resource Allocation in the Health Service* (London, Bedford Square Press).

Mays, N. and Mulligan, J. (1998) 'Total Purchasing', in Le Grand, J., Mays, N. and Mulligan, J. (eds) *Learning from the NHS Internal Market: A Review of Evidence* (London, King's Fund), 84–99.

Mays, N., Mulligan, J-A. and Goodwin, N. (2000) The British Quasi-Market in Health Care: A Balance Sheet of the Evidence', *Journal of Health Services Research and Policy*, 5, 49–58.

Mays, N., Wyke, S., Malbon, G. and Goodwin, N. (eds) (2001) *The Purchasing of Health Care by Primary Care Organisations: An Evaluation and Guide to Future Policy* (Buckingham, Open University Press).

McColl, A. and Roland, M. (2000) 'Knowledge and Information for Clinical Governance', *British Medical Journal*, 321, 871–4.

McCormick, A., Fleming, D. and Charlton, J. (1995) *Morbidity Statistics from General Practice, 4th National Study 1991/2* (London, HMSO).

McCoy, K. (2000) *Care in the Community* (Belfast, DHSSPS).

McCulloch, S. (2001) 'Social Environments and Health: Cross-Sectional National Survey, *British Medical Journal*, 232, 208–9.

McDonald, A., Langford, F. and Boldero, N. (1997) 'The Future of Community Nursing in the UK. District Nursing, Health Visiting and School Nursing', *Journal of Advanced Nursing*, 26, 257–65.

McDonald, R. and Baughan, S. (2001) 'Rationality and Reality – Attitudes of Health Economists Working at Local Level in the UK NHS', *Critical Public Health*, 11, 319–30.

McIver, S. (1998) *Healthy Debate? An Independent Evaluation of Citizens' Juries in Health Settings* (London, King's Fund).

McKendrick, J. and McCabe, B. (1997) 'An Observers' Tale. Stonehaven Community Hospital', *Public Money and Management*, 17, 17–20.

McKeown, T. (1979) *The Role of Medicine: Dream, Mirage or Nemesis?* (Oxford, Blackwell).

McKie, L. M. (1995) 'The Art of Surveillance or Reasonable Prevention? The Case of Cervical Screening', *Sociology of Health and Illness*, 17, 441–557.

McKinlay, J. (1979) 'Epidemiological and Political Developments of Social Policies Regarding the Public Health', *Social Science and Medicine*, 13A, 541–8.

McKinlay, J. (ed.) (1988) 'The Changing Character of the Medical Profession', *Milbank Quarterly* 66, Supplement 2.

McLachlan, G. (1990) *What Price Quality? The NHS in Review* (London, Nuffield Provincial Hospitals Trust).

McLoughlin, V., Leatherman, S., Fletcher, M. and Wyn Owen, J. (2001) 'Improving performance Using Indicators. Recent Experiences in the United States, the United Kingdom, and Australia', *International Journal for Quality in Health Care*, 13, 455–62.

McMichael, A. and Haines, A. (1997) 'Global Change: The Potential Effects on Health', *British Medical Journal*, 315, 805–9.

McNulty, T. and Ferlie, E. (2002) *Reengineering Health Care* (Oxford, Oxford University Press).

Meacher, M. (1972) *Taken for a Ride* (London, Longman).

Meade, T., Dyer, S., Browne, W. and Frank, A. (1995) 'Randomised Comparison of Chiropractic and Hospital Outpatient Management for Low Back Pain: Results From

Extended Follow Up', *British Medical Journal*, 311, 349–51.

Meads, G., Killoran, A., Ashcroft, J. and Cornish, Y. (1999) *Mixing Oil and Water* (London, Health Education Authority).

Means, R., Richards, S. and Smith, R. (2003) *Community Care: Policy and Practice*, 3rd edn (Basingstoke, Palgrave).

Mechanic, D. (1961) 'The Concept of Illness Behaviour', *Journal of Chronic Diseases*, 15, 189–94.

Mechanic, D. (1991) 'Sources of Countervailing Power in Medicine', *Journal of Health Policy, Politics and Law*, 16, 485–98.

Mellor, J. and Milyo, J. (2001) 'Re-examining the Evidence of an Ecological Association between Income Inequality and Health', *Journal of Health Policy, Politics and Law*, 26 (3), 488–522.

Meltzer, H., Gill, B., Petticrew, M. and Hinds, K. (1995) *The Prevalence of Psychiatric Morbidity Among Adults Living in Private Households* (London, HMSO).

Mercer, J. and Talbot, I. C. (1985) 'Clinical Diagnosis: A Post Mortem Assessment of Accuracy in the 1980s', *Post Graduate Medical Journal*, 61, 713–16.

Micozzi, M. (1995) *Fundamentals of Complementary and Alternative Medicine* (London, Churchill Livingstone).

Miers, M. (1999) 'Nurses in the Labour Market: Exploring and Explaining Nurses' Work', in Wilkinson, G. and Miers, M. (eds) *Power and Nursing Practice* (Basingstoke, Macmillan), 83–96.

Miers, M. (2000) *Gender Issues on Nursing Practice* (Basingstoke, Macmillan).

Mihill, C. (1996) 'GPs Pay the Price for Wrong Medicine', *Guardian*, 4 June, 7.

Milburn, K. and MacAskill, S. (1994) 'Cervical Screening: Continuing Concerns in the 1990s', *Health Education Journal*, 53, 201–13.

Miles, A. (1991) *Women, Health and Medicine* (Buckingham, Open University Press).

Milewa, T. (1997) 'Community Participation and Health Care Priorities: Reflections on Policy, Theatre and Reality in Britain', *Health Promotion International*, 12, 161–8.

Milewa, T., Harrison, S., Ahmed, W. and Tovey, P. (2002) 'Citizen's Participation in Primary Healthcare Planning: Innovative Citizenship Practice in Empirical Perspective', *Critical Public Health*, 12, 39–53.

Milewa, T., Valentine, J. and Calnan, M. (1998) 'Managerialism and Active Citizenships in Britain's Reformed Health Service: Power and

Community in an Era of Decentralisation', *Social Science and Medicine*, 47, 507–17.

Milio, N. (1986) *Promoting Health through Public Policy* (Ottawa, Canadian Public Health Association).

Millar, B. (2000) 'The Directors' Cut', *Health Service Journal*, 20 April, 22–5.

Miller, E. and Gwynne, G. (1972) *A Life Apart: A Pilot Study of Residential Institutions for the Physically Handicapped and Young Chronic Sick* (London, Tavistock).

Miller, P. and Plant, M. (1996) 'Drinking, Smoking and Illicit Drug Use Among 15–16 Year Olds in the United Kingdom', *British Medical Journal*, 313, 394–7.

Ministry of Health (1954) *Report of the Committee on Economic and Financial Problems of Old Age* (The Phillips Report) (London, HMSO).

Ministry of Health (1959) *Report of the Committee on Maternity Services* (The Cranbrook Report) (London, HMSO).

Ministry of Health (1963) *The Field of Work of the Family Doctor* (The Gillie Report) (London, HMSO).

Ministry of Health (1968) *The National Health Service. The Administrative Structure of the Medical and Related Services in England and Wales* (London, HMSO).

Miu, L. (1997) *Developing Medical Directors in Clinical Directorates* (www.medg.lcs.mit.edu/people/lmui).

Mohan, J. (1995) *A National Health Service?* (Basingstoke, Macmillan).

Mohan, J. (2002) *Planning, Markets and Hospitals* (London, Routledge).

Mohan, J. and Gorsky, M. (2001) *Don't Look Back. Voluntary and Charitable Finance of Hospitals in Britain Past and Present* (London, Office of Health Economics and Association of Chartered Certified Accountants).

Monbiot, G. (2001) *Captive State – The Corporate Takeover of Britain* (London, Macmillan).

Monopolies and Mergers Commission (1993) *Private Medical Services: A Report on Agreements and Practices Relating to Charges for the Supply of Private Medical Services by NHS Consultants* (London, HMSO).

Moon, G. and Lupton, C. (1995) 'Within Acceptable Limits: Health Care Provider Perspectives on Community Health Councils in the Reformed British National Health Service', *Policy and Politics*, 23 (4), 335–46.

Moon, G. and North, N. (2000) *Policy and Place: General Medical Practice in the UK* (London, Palgrave).

Mooney, G. (1994) *Key Issues in Health Economics* (Hemel Hempstead, Harvester Wheatsheaf).

Mooney, G. H. and Healey, A. (1991) 'Strategy Full of Good Intentions', *British Medical Journal*, 303, 1119–20.

Mooney, H. (2003) 'GPs Lack a Say in PCTs', *Health Service Journal*, 22 May, 10–11.

Moore, A. (2002) 'On the Ropes', *Health Service Journal*, 21 October, 24–25.

Moore, A. (2003a) 'Partners in Time' *Health Service Journal*, 24 April, 12–13.

Moore, A. (2003b) 'A Year in Providence', *Health Service Journal*, 24 April, 10–11.

Moore, A. (2003c) 'Mixed Results for Ward Pledge', *Health Service Journal*, 20 February, 4–5.

Moore, A. (2003d) 'A Long Way to Fall', *Health Service Journal*, 23 October, 12–13.

Moore, W. (1995) 'Is Doctors' Power Shrinking?', *Health Service Journal*, 9 November, 24–7.

Moran, M. (1999) *Governing the Health Care State: A Comparative Study of the UK, the US and Germany* (Manchester, Manchester University Press).

Moran, M. and Wood, B. (1992) *States, Regulation and the Medical Profession* (Buckingham, Open University Press).

Morley, A. and Campbell, F. (2003) *A Green Paper on Democratising the NHS: People Power and Health* (London, Local Government Information Unit, Democratic Health Network).

Morris, J. K., Cook, D. and Shaper, A. (1994) 'Loss of Employment and Mortality', *British Medical Journal*, 308, 1135–9.

Morris, J. N. (1980) 'Are Health Services Important to People's Health?', *British Medical Journal*, 280, 167–8.

Morris, P. (1969) *Put Away: A Sociological Study of Institutions for the Mentally Retarded* (London, Routledge and Kegan Paul).

Moser, K., Goldblatt, P., Fox., J. and Jones, D. (1990) 'Unemployment and Mortality', in Goldblatt, P. (ed.) *Longitudinal Study: Mortality and Social Organisation* 1971–81, OPCS LS 6 (London, HMSO), 81–97.

Mossialos, E., Dixon, A., Figueras, J. and Kutzin, R. (eds) (2002) *Funding Health Care: Options for Europe* (Buckingham, Open University Press).

Mountford, L. and Rosen, R. (2001) *NHS Walk-in Centres in London* (London, King's Fund).

Muir Gray, J. (2001) *Evidence Based Health-care: How to Make Health Policy and Management decisions* (Edinburgh, Churchill Livingstone).

Muir Gray, J. and de Lusignan, S. (1999) 'National Electronic Library for Health', *British Medical Journal*, 319, 1476–9.

Muir, H. (2003) 'Preparations for Patients' Forum in Crisis', *Guardian*, 27 October, 8.

Mullan, P. (2001) *The Imaginary Time Bomb. Why an Ageing Population is not a Social Problem* (New York, IB Tauris).

Mullen, P. (1995) 'The Provision of Specialist Services Under Contracting', *Public Money and Management*, 15 (3), 23–30.

Mullen, P. (1998) 'Is it Necessary to Ration Health Care?', *Public Money and Management*, 18, 52–8.

Mullen, P. (2000) 'Public Involvement in Health Care Priority Setting: Are the Methods Appropriate and Solid?', in Coulter, A. and Ham, C. (eds) *The Global Challenge of Health Care Rationing* (Buckingham, Open University Press), 163–74.

Mulligan, J. (1998) 'Health Authority Purchasing', in Le Grand, J., Mays, N. and Mulligan, J. (eds) *Learning from the NHS Internal Market: A Review of Evidence* (London, King's Fund), 20–42.

Mulligan, J. and Appleby, J. (2001) 'The NHS and Labour's Battle for Public Opinion', in Park, A., Curtis, J., Thompson, K., Jarvis, L. and Bromley, C. (eds) *British Social Attitudes*, 18th *Report* (London, Sage).

Mulube, M. (1996) 'Myths Dispelled About Chronic Fatigue Syndrome', *British Medical Journal*, 313, 839.

Munro, J., Nicholl, J., O'Cathain, A. and Knowles, E. (2000) 'Impact of NHS Direct on Demand for Immediate Care', *British Medical Journal*, 321, 150–3.

Muntaner, C., Lynch, J. and Davey Smith, G. (2001) 'Social Capital, Disorganised Communities and the Third Way', *International Journal of Health Services*, 31 (2), 213–37.

Murray, C. and Lopez, A. (1996) *The Global Burden of Disease* (Geneva, WHO).

Nagle, D., Grail, S., Vitale, J., Woolf, E., Dussault, B. et al. (1999) 'The Mahogany Protein is a Receptor Involved in the Suppression of Obesity', *Nature*, 398, 148–52.

NAHAT (National Association of Health Authorities and Trusts) (1990) *Healthcare Economic Review* (Birmingham, NAHAT).

NAO (National Audit Office) (1987) (HC 108) *Community Care Developments 1987/88* (London, HMSO).

NAO (National Audit Office) (1989) (HC 566) *Financial Management in the NHS* (London, HMSO).

NAO (National Audit Office) (1995) (HC 261) *Contracting for Acute Health Care in England* (London, HMSO).

NAO (National Audit Office) (1996) (HC 332) *The NHS Executive: The Hospital Information Support Systems Initiative* (London, HMSO).

NAO (National Audit Office) (1999) (HC 371) *The 1992 and 1998 Information Management and Technology Strategies of the NHS Executive* (London, The Stationery Office).

NAO (National Audit Office) (2000) (HC 301) *Measuring the Performance of Government Departments* (London, HMSO).

NAO (National Audit Office) (2000a) (HC 516) *Charitable Funds Associated with NHS bodies* (London, The Stationery Office).

NAO (National Audit Office) (2000b) (HC 230) *The Management and Control of Hospital Acquired Infections in Acute NHS Trusts in England* (London, The Stationery Office).

NAO (National Audit Office) (2001a) (HC 220) *Tackling Obesity in England* (London, The Stationery Office).

NAO (National Audit Office) (2001b) (HC 375) *Managing the Relationship to Secure a Successful Partnership in PFI Projects* (London, The Stationery Office).

NAO (National Audit Office) (2001c) (HC 403) *Handling Clinical Negligence Claims in England* (London, The Stationery Office).

NAO (National Audit Office) (2002a) (HC 1288) *PFI Refinancing Update* (London, The Stationery Office).

NAO (National Audit Office) (2002b) (HC 157) *Innovation in the National Health Service: The Acquisition of the Heart Hospital* (London, The Stationery Office).

NAO (National Audit Office) (2002c) (HC 505) *NHS Direct in England 2002* (London, HMSO).

NAO (National Audit Office) (2003a) (HC 371) *PFI: Construction Performance* (London, The Stationery Office).

NAO (National Audit Office) (2003b) (HC 1055) *Achieving Improvement Through Clinical Governance: A Progress Report* (London, The Stationery Office).

NAO (National Audit Office) (2003c) (HC 255) Session 2002/03, *Safety, Quality and Efficacy: Regulating Medicines in the UK* (London, The Stationery Office).

NAO (National Audit Office) (2003d) (HC 392) *Ensuring the Effective Discharge of Older Patients from NHS Acute Hospitals* (London, The Stationery Office).

National Assembly for Wales (1998) *Strategic Framework: Better Health, Better Wales* (Cardiff, National Assembly for Wales).

National Assembly for Wales (2001a) *Improving Health in Wales: A Plan for the NHS with its Partners* (Cardiff, National Assembly for Wales).

National Assembly for Wales (2001b) *Fulfilling the Promises* (Wales, National Assembly, Learning Disability Advisory Group).

National Assembly for Wales, Office for Public Management (2001) *Signposts: A Practical Guide to Public and Patient Involvement in Wales* (Cardiff and London, NAFW, Office for Public Management).

National Association of Citizens' Advice Bureaux (2001) *Unhealthy Charges: CAB Evidence on the Impact of Health Charges* (London, National Association of Citizens' Advice Bureaux).

National Confidential Enquiry into Perioperative Deaths (1998) *1996/97 Report* (London, NCE-POD).

National Confidential Enquiry into Perioperative Deaths (2001) *The 2001 Report of the National Confidential Enquiry into Perioperative Deaths – Changing the Way We Operate* (London, NCE-POD).

National Confidential Enquiry into Perioperative Deaths (2002) *Functioning as a Team?: The 2002 Report of the National Confidential Enquiry into Perioperative Deaths (1 April 2002 to 31 March 2001)* (London, NCEPOD).

National Consumer Council (1995) *Charging Consumers for Social Services: Local Authority Policy and Practice* (London, NCC).

National Consumer Council (1997) *NHS Complaints Procedures: The First Year* (London, NCC).

National Consumer Council (1998) *Consumer Concerns 1998: A Consumer View of Health Services the Report of an RSL Survey* (London, NCC).

National Consumer Council (1999) *Self Regulation of Professionals in Healthcare – Consumer Issues* (London, NCC).

National Economic Research Associates (1994) *Financing Healthcare* (London, NERA).

National Economic Research Associates (1995) *Healthcare Report: Are Pay Beds Profitable?* (Eastleigh, Norwich Union).

National Heart Forum (1998) *Social Inequalities in Heart Disease* (London, The Stationery Office).

National Institute for Social Work (1988) *Residential Care: A Positive Choice Report of the Independent Review of Residential Care (The Wagner Report)* (London, HMSO).

Nattinger, A., Hoffman, R., Kneusel, R. and Schapira, M. (2000) 'Relation Between Appropriateness of Primary Therapy for Early

Stage Breast Carcinoma and Increased Use of Breast Conserving Surgery', *Lancet*, 356, 1148–53.

Navarro, V. (1978) *Class Struggle, the State and Medicine* (Oxford, Martin Robertson).

Nazroo, J. Y. (1997) *The Health of Britain's Ethnic Minorities: Findings from a National Survey* (London, Policy Studies Institute).

Nazroo, J. Y. (1998) 'Genetic, Cultural or Socio-economic Vulnerability? Explaining Ethnic Inequalities in Health', *Sociology of Health and Illness*, 20 (5) 710–30.

Nazroo, J. (2000) *Ethnicity, Class, and Health* (London, Policy Studies Institute).

New, B. and Le Grand, J. (1996) *Rationing in the NHS: Principles and Pragmatism* (London, King's Fund).

New Scientist (1998) 'Marijuana – A Safe High?', 21 February, 24–31.

Newhouse, J. P. and the Insurance Experiment Group (1993) *Free for All? Lessons from the RAND Health Insurance Experiment* (Cambridge, MA, Harvard University Press).

Newman, K. and Leigh, S. (1996) 'Mission Impossible: The Definition and Function of the Medical Director', *Clinicians in Management*, 5, 11–14.

NHS 24 (2002) *Annual Report and Accounts and Year Planner 2001/02* (Glasgow, NHS24).

NHS Alliance (2002) *The Vision in Practice* (Retford, NHSA).

NHS Alliance (2003) *Refocusing Commissioning for PCTs* (Retford, NHS Alliance).

NHS Confederation (2002) *Reviewing the Reviewers* (London, NHS Confederation).

NHS Confederation (2003) *Re-reviewing the Reviewers: The Second Survey of NHS Trust Experience of CHI Clinical Governance Reviews* (Birmingham, NHS Confederation).

NHS Management Executive in Scotland (1999) *Introduction of Managerial Clinical Networks in Scotland* (Edinburgh, NHSME Scotland).

NHS Trust Federation (1995) *Behind Closed Doors: Boardroom Practice in NHS Trusts* (London, NHS Trust Federation).

NHS Wales (2003) *Improving Health in Wales: Complaints in the NHS* (Cardiff, Welsh Assembly Government).

NHSE (1995) *Priorities and Planning Guidance for the NHS 1996/7* (Leeds, NHSE).

NHSE (1996) *Promoting Clinical Effectiveness* (Leeds, NHSE).

NHSE London Regional Office, SILKAP Consultants (2001) *Patient Advocacy and Liaison Services: A Review of the London PALS Pathfinder Sites* (London, NHSE London Regional Office).

NHSE/IHSM/NHS Confederation (1998) *In the Public Interest* (London, DoH).

NHSME (NHS Management Executive) (1992) *Local Voices* (London, DoH).

Nichols, L., Aronica, P. and Babe, C. (1996) 'Are Autopsies Obsolete?', *American Journal of Clinical Pathology*, 110, 210–18.

Niskanen, W. (1971) *Bureaucracy and Representative Government* (Chicago, IL, Aldine).

Nocon, A. (1993) 'Made in Heaven', *Health Service Journal*, 2 December, 24–6.

Normand, C. (1991) 'Economics, Health and the Economics of Health', *British Medical Journal*, 303, 1572–7.

North, N. (1995) 'Alford Revisited: The Professional Monopolisers, Corporate Rationalisers, Community and Markets', *Policy and Politics*, 23 (2), 115–25.

North, N. (1998) 'Implementing Strategy: The Politics of Healthcare Commissioning', *Policy and Politics*, 26, 5–14.

Nottingham, C. (2000) *The NHS in Scotland: The Legacy of the Past and Prospect of the Future* (Aldershot, Ashgate).

Nottingham, C. and O'Neill, F. (2000) 'Out of the Church and into Kwik Fit: The Nursing Profession and the Secularisation of Health Care', in Hann, A. (ed.) *Analysing Health Policy* (Aldershot, Ashgate), 183–95.

Nottingham Health Authority (1999) *Patient Partnership Strategy: The Nottingham Health Community Approach to Working with Users and Carers* (Nottingham, Nottingham Health Authority).

Nutley, S. and Smith, P. (1998) 'League Tables for Performance Improvement in Health Care', *Journal of Health Services Research and Policy*, 3, 50–8.

Oakley, A. (1980) *Women Confined* (Oxford, Martin Robertson).

Oakley, A. (1984) *The Captured Womb: A History of the Medical Care of Pregnant Women* (Oxford, Blackwell).

O'Cathain, A., Munro, J. F., Nicholl, J. P. and Knowles, E. (2000) 'How Helpful is NHS Direct? Postal Survey of Callers', *British Medical Journal*, 135, 320.

O'Connor, J. (1973) *The Fiscal Crisis of the State* (New York, St Martin's Press).

O'Donnell, O., Propper, C. and Upward, R. (1991) *An Empirical Study of Equity in the Finance and Delivery of Health Care in Britain*, Discussion Paper No. 85 (Centre for Health Economics, University of York).

OECD (2001) OECD Health Data (Paris, OECD).

OECD (2003) *OECD Health Data 2003: A Comparative Analysis of 30 Countries* (Paris, OECD).

Offe, C. (1984) *The Contradictions of the Welfare State* (London, Hutchinson).

Office for National Statistics (1998) *Social Trends 1997* (London, The Stationery Office).

Office for National Statistics (2000) *Social Trends 2000* (London, The Stationery Office).

Office for National Statistics (2003) *Social Trends 2003* (London, The Stationery Office).

Office of Fair Trading (2003) *The Private Dentistry Market in the UK* (London, Office of Fair Trading).

Office of Government Commerce and Commission for Architecture and the Built Environment (2000) *Improving Standards of Design in the Procurement of Public Buildings* (London, CABE/OGC).

Office of Health Economics (1997) *Hospital Acquired Infection* (London, OHE).

Office of Health Economics (2003) *15th Compendium of Health Statistics* (London, OHE).

Office of the Commissioner for Public Appointments (2000) *Public Appointments to NHS Trusts and Health Authorities* (London, Cabinet Office).

Oliver, A. (2002) 'Reforming Public Sector Dentistry in the UK', *British Journal of Health Care Management*, 8, 212–6.

Oliver, M. (1990) *The Politics of Disablement* (Basingstoke, Macmillan).

O'Neill, O. (2002) *Reith Lectures*, April–May.

Ong, B., Boaden, M. and Cropper, S. (1997) 'Analysing the Medicine-Management Interface in Acute Trusts', *Sociology of Management in Medicine*, 11 (2), 88–95.

ONS/CRC/London School of Hygiene and Tropical Medicine (1999) *Cancer Survival Trends in England and Wales 1971–95* (London, The Stationery Office).

Orbach, S. (1978) *Fat is a Feminist Issue* (London, Hamlyn).

Orchard, C. (1993) 'Strained Legacy', *Health Service Journal*, 2 December, 27.

O'Reilly, D., Steele, K., Merriman, B., Gilliland, A. and Brown, S. (1998) 'Effect of Fundholding on Removing Patients from General Practitioners Lists: Retrospective study', *British Medical Journal*, 317, 785–68.

Orme, J., Powell, J., Taylor, P., Harrison, T. and Greg, M. (2003) *Public Health for the 21st Century: New Perspectives on Policy, Participation and Practice* (Buckingham, Open University Press).

Osborne, D. and Gaebler, T. (1992) *Reinventing Government* (Reading, MA, Addison-Wesley).

Osler, M., Prescott, E., Gronbaek, M., Christensen, U., Due, P. and Engholm, G. (2002) 'Income Inequality, Individual Income, and Mortality in Danish Adults: Analysis of Pooled Data from Two Cohort Studies', *British Medical Journal*, 324, 13–16.

Ottewill, R. and Wall, A. (1990) *The Growth and Development of the Community Health Services* (Sunderland, Business Education Publishers).

Ovretveit, J. (1992) *Health Service Quality – An Introduction to Quality Measures for Health Services* (Oxford, Blackwell Scientific).

Ovretveit, J. (1998) *Evaluating Health Interventions* (Buckingham, Open University Press).

Ovretveit, J., Thompson, T. and Mathias, P. (eds) (1997) *Interprofessional Working for Health and Social Care* (Basingstoke, Macmillan).

Owen, D. (1988) *Our NHS* (London, Pan).

Packwood, T., Keen, J. and Buxton, M. (1991) *Hospitals in Transition. The Resource Management Experiment* (Buckingham, Open University Press).

Packwood, T., Kerrison, S. and Buxton, M. (1994) 'The Implementation of Medical Audit', *Social Policy and Administration*, 28 (4), 299–315.

Packwood, T., Pollitt, C. and Roberts, S. (1998) 'Good Medicine? A Case Study of Business Process Reengineering in a Hospital', *Policy and Politics*, 26, 401–15.

Palfrey, C. (2000) *Key Concepts in Health Care Policy and Planning – An Introductory Text* (Basingstoke, Macmillan).

Pamuk, E. R. (1985) 'Social Class Inequality in Mortality from 1971–72 in England and Wales', *Population Studies*, 39, 17–31.

Parry, G. J., Gould, C., McCabe, C. J. and Tarnow-Mordi, W. O. (1998) 'Annual League Tables of Mortality in Neonatal Intensive Care Units: Longitudinal Study', *British Medical Journal*, 316, 1931–5.

Parsons, T. (1951) *The Social System* (New York, Free Press of Glencoe).

Paton, C. (1993) 'Devolution and Centralism in the National Health Service', *Social Policy and Administration*, 27 (2), 83–108.

Paton, C. (1995) 'Present Dangers and Future Threats: Some Perverse Incentives in the NHS Reforms', *British Medical Journal*, 310, 1245–8.

Paton, C. (1998) *Competition and Planning in the NHS* (Cheltenham, Thornes).

Patten, T. and Brandreth, M. (2001) 'Fast Forward', *Health Service Journal*, 21 June, 28–9.

Patterson, L. (2001) 'Let's Get on with It', *Health Matters*, 44, 8–9.

Patterson-Brown, S. (1998) 'Should Doctors Perform an Elective Caesarean Section on request? Yes, as Long, as the Woman, is Fully Informed', *British Medical Journal*, 317, 462–3.

Payer, L. (1989) *Medicine and Culture* (London, Gollancz).

Payne, M. (2000) *Teamwork in Multiprofessional Care* (Basingstoke, Macmillan).

Payne, N. and Saul, C. (1997) 'Variations in the Use of Cardiology Sources in a Health Authority: Comparison of Coronary Artery Revascularisation Rates with Prevalence of Angina and Coronary Mortality', *British Medical Journal*, 257, 314.

Payne, S. (1996) 'Masculinity and the Redundant Male: Explaining the Increasing Incarceration of Young Men', *Social and Legal Studies*, 5, 159–78.

Payne, S. (1998) 'Hit and Miss, the Success and Failure of Psychiatric Services for Women', in Doyal, L. (ed.) *Women and Health Services* (Buckingham, Open University Press), 83–99.

Pearson, A., Punton, S. and Durant, I. (1992) *Nursing Beds – An Evaluation of the Effects of Therapeutic Nursing* (London, Scutari Press).

Peck, E. (1995) 'The Performance of an NHS Trust Board: Actors Accounts, Minutes and Observation', *British Journal of Management*, 6, 135–56.

Peck, E. and Parker, E. (1998) 'Mental Health – the NHS: Policy and Practice 1979–98', *Journal of Mental Health*, 7, 241–59.

Peck, E., Towell, D. and Gulliver, P. (2001) 'The Meanings of Culture in Health and Social Care: A Study of the Combined Trust in Somerset', *Journal of Interprofessional Care*, 15, 319–27.

Peckham, S. and Exworthy, M. (2003) *Primary Care in the UK: Policy, Organisation and Management* (Basingstoke, Palgrave).

Pell, J. P., Pell, A. C. H., Norrie, J., Ford, I. and Cobbe, S. (2000) 'Effect of Socioeconomic Deprivation on Waiting Time for Cardiac Surgery: Retrospective Cohort Study', *British Medical Journal*, 320, 15–19.

Pereira, J. (1993) 'What Does Equity in Health Mean?', *Journal of Social Policy*, 22 (1), 19–48.

Perkin, H. (1989) *The Rise of Professional Society* (London, Routledge).

Petchey, R. (1987) 'Health Maintenance Organisations: Just What the Doctor Ordered?', *Journal of Social Policy*, 16 (4), 489–507.

Peters, T. and Waterman, R. (1982) *In Search of Excellence* (New York, Harper and Row).

Pettigrew, A., Ferlie, E., Fitzgerald, L. and Wensley, R. (1991) *Research in Action:*

Authorities in the NHS (University of Warwick, Centre for Corporate Strategy and Change).

Phillips, A. and Rakusen, J. (1989) *The New 'Our Bodies Ourselves'* (Harmondsworth, Penguin).

Pickard, S. (1997) 'The Future Organisation of Community Health Councils', *Social Policy and Administration*, 31, 274–89.

Pickard, S. (1998) 'Citizenship and Consumerism in Health Care: A Critique of Citizens' Juries', *Social Policy and Administration*, 32, 226–44.

Pickin, M., Sampson, F., Munro, J. and Nicholl, J. (2001) 'General Practitioners' Reasons for Removing Patients from their Lists: Postal Survey in England and Wales', *British Medical Journal*, 322, 1158–9.

Pietroni, P. (1991) *The Greening of Medicine* (London, Gollancz).

Platt, S. D., Martin, C. J. and Hunt, S. M. (1989) 'Damp Housing, Mould Growth and Symptomatic Health State', *British Medical Journal*, 298, 1673–8.

Player, S. and Pollock, A. (2001) 'Long-Term Care: From Public Responsibility to Private Good', *Critical Social Policy*, 21, 231–55.

PMS National Evaluation Team (2002) *National Evaluation of First Wave NHS Personal Medical Pilots. Summaries of Findings from Four Research Projects* (University of Birmingham, University of Manchester, Queen Mary College, University of London, University of Nottingham, University of Southampton).

Political and Economic Planning (1937) *Report on the British Health Services* (London, Political and Economic Planning).

Pollitt, C. (1993a) *Managerialism and the Public Services: The Anglo American Experience*, 2nd edn (Oxford, Blackwell).

Pollitt, C. (1993b) 'The Struggle for Quality: The Case of the NHS', *Policy and Politics*, 21 (3), 161–70.

Pollock, A. (2000) 'Will Intermediate Care be the Undoing of the NHS?', *British Medical Journal*, 321, 393–4.

Pollock, A., Player, S. and Godden, S. (2001) 'How Private Finance is Moving Primary Care into Corporate Ownership', *British Medical Journal*, 322, 960–3.

Pollock, A., Shaoul, J. and Vickers, N. (2002) 'Private Finance and Value for Money in NHS Hospitals: A Policy in Search of a Rationale?' *British Medical Journal*, 324, 1205–9.

Pollock, A. M. (1999) 'Devolution and Health: Challenges for Scotland and Wales', *British Medical Journal*, 318, 1195–8.

Pollock, A. M., Dunnigan, M., Gaffrey, D., Macfarlan, A. and Majeed, F. (1997) 'What Happens When the Private Sector Plans Hospitals Services for the NHS – Three Case Studies under the Private Finance Initiative, *British Medical Journal*, 314, 1266–71.

Popay, J. and Williams, G. (1994) 'Local Voices in the Health Service: Needs, Effectiveness and Sufficiency', in Oakley, A. and Williams, A. (eds) *The Politics of the Welfare State* (London, UCL Press).

Porter, S. (1999) 'Working with Doctors', in Wilkinson, G. and Miers, M. (eds) *Power and Nursing Practice* (Basingstoke, Macmillan), 97–110.

Powell, M. (1990) 'Need and Provision in the NHS: An Inverse Care Law?', *Policy and Politics*, 18, 31–8.

Powell, M. (1992) 'A Tale of Two Cities: A Critical Evaluation of the Geographical Provision of Health Care Before the NHS', *Public Administration*, 70 (1), 67–80.

Powell, M. (1997) *Evaluating the National Health Service* (Buckingham, Open University Press).

Powell, M. (1998) 'In What Sense a National Health Service?', *Public Policy and Administration*, 13, 56–9.

Powell, M. and Moon, G. (2001) 'Health Action Zones: The Third Way of a New Area-Based Policy', *Health and Social Care in the Community*, 9, 43–50.

Power, C. (1994) 'Health and Social Inequality in Europe', *British Medical Journal* 308, 1153–6.

Power, C., Matthews, S. and Manor, O. (1996) 'Inequalities in Self-Related Health in the 1958 Birth Cohort: Lifetime Social Circumstance or Social Mobility?', *British Medical Journal*, 313, 449–53.

Power, M. (1994) *The Audit Explosion* (London, Demos).

Powles, J. (1973) 'On the Limitations of Modern Medicine', *Science, Medicine and Man*, 1, 1–30.

Poxton, R. (1994) *Joint Commissioning: The Story So Far*, Briefings nos 1 and 2 (London, King's Fund).

Prentice, A. and Jebb, S. (1995) 'Obesity in Britain: Gluttony or Sloth?', *British Medical Journal*, 311, 437–9.

Price, D. (1996) 'Lessons for Health Care Rationing from the Case of Child B', *British Medical Journal*, 312, 167–9.

Price, D. and Pollock, A. (2002) 'Extending Choice in the NHS', *British Medical Journal*, 325, 293–4.

Pritchard, C. (1992) 'What Can We Afford for the NHS?', *Social Policy and Administration*, 26 (1), 40–54.

Pritchard, P. (1978) *Manual of Primary Care: Its Nature and Organisation* (Oxford, Oxford University Press).

Pritchard, P. (ed.) (1981) *Patient Participation in General Practice* (London, Royal College of General Practitioners).

Propper, C. (1998) *Who Pays For and Who Gets Health Care? Delivery of Health Care in the UK*, Health Economics Series Paper 5 (London, Nuffield Trust).

Propper, C., Burgess, S. and Abraham, D. (2002) *Competition and Quality: Evidence from the Internal Market 1991–1999*, Paper presented at a conference of the National Institute of Economic and Social Research, London, 19 November.

Propper, C. and Green, K. (2001) 'A Larger Role for the Private Sector in Financing UK Health Care: The Arguments and the Evidence', *Journal of Social Policy*, 30, 685–704.

Propper, C. and Söderlund, N. (1998) 'Competition in the NHS Internal Market: An Overview of its Effects on Hospital Prices and Costs', *Health Economics*, 7, 187–97.

Propper, C. and Upward, R. (1992) 'Need, Equity and the NHS: The Distribution of Health Care Expenditure', *Fiscal Studies*, 13, 1–21.

Propper, C., Wilson, D. and Söderlund, N. (1998) 'The Effects of Regulation and Competition in the NHS Internal Market: The Case of GP Fundholding Prices' *Journal of Health Economics*, 17, 645–73.

Public Accounts Committee (1993) (HC 485) *63rd Report 1992/3. Wessex Regional Health Authority: Regionally Managed Services Organisation* (London, HMSO).

Public Accounts Committee (1996a) (HC 146) *6th Report 1995/6: The Private Finance Initiative* (London, HMSO).

Public Accounts Committee (1996b) (HC 97) *7th Report 1996/97. Hospital Information Supports Systems Initiative* (London, The Stationery Office).

Public Accounts Committee (1996c) (HC 304) *31st Report 1995/6: Clinical Audit in England* (London, HMSO).

Public Accounts Committee (1998) (HC 657) *62nd Report 1997/98. The Purchase of Read Codes* (London, The Stationery Office).

Public Accounts Committee (2002) (HC 517) *46th Report 2001/2. Inappropriate Adjustments to NHS Waiting Lists* (London, HMSO).

Public Administration Select Committee (2000) (HC 410) *2nd report 1999/2000. Appointments to NHS Boards: Report of the Commission for Public Appointments* (London, The Stationery Office).

Public Administration Select Committee (2003) (HC 62) *5th Report 2002/03. On Target? Government by Measurement* (London, The Stationery Office).

Putnam, R. (2000) *Bowling Alone: The Collapse and Revival of American Commonality* (London and New York, Simon and Schuster).

Quennell, P. (2001) 'Getting their Say or Getting their Way?', *Journal of Management in Medicine*, 15, 201–19.

Radical Statistics Health Group (1977) *RAWP Deals: A Critique of 'Sharing Resources for Health in England'* (London, Radical Statistics Health Group).

Raine, R. (2000) 'Does Gender Bias Exist in the Use of Specialist Health Care?', *Journal of Health Services Research and Policy*, 5, 237–9.

Raine, R., Hutchings, A. and Black, N. (2003) 'Is Publicly Funded Health Care Really Distributed According to Need? The Example of Cardiac Rehabilitation in the UK', *Health Policy*, 63, 63–72.

Ramsey, M., Baker, P., Goulden, C., Sharp, C. and Sondhi, A. (2001) *Drug Misuse Declared in 2000: Results from the British Crime Survey* (London, Home Office).

Rea, D. (1995) 'Unhealthy Competition: The Making of a Market for Mental Health', *Policy and Politics*, 23 (2), 141–55.

Read, S. and Graves, K. (1994) *Reduction of Junior Doctors' Hours in Trent Region: The Nursing Contribution* (Sheffield, Sheffield Centre for Health and Related Research, Trent Regional Health Authority).

Redmayne, S. (1996) *Small Steps: Big Goals* (Birmingham, NAHAT).

Redwood, H. (2000) *Why Ration Health Care?: An International Study of the United Kingdom, France, Germany and Public Sector Health Care in the USA* (London, Institute for Civil Society).

Redwood, J. (1988) *In Sickness and in Health: Management Change in the NHS* (London, Centre for Policy Studies).

Regen, E., Smith, J., Goodwin, N., McLeod, H. and Shapiro, J. (2001) *Passing on the Baton: Final Report of a National Evaluation of Primary Care Groups and Trusts* (Birmingham, HSMC).

Reid, F., Cook, D. and Whincup, P. (2002) 'Use of Statins in the Secondary Prevention of Coronary Heart Disease: Is Treatment Equitable?', *Heart*, 88, 15–19.

Reilly, J. and Dorosty, A. (1999) 'Epidemic of Obesity in UK Children', *The Lancet*, 354, 1874.

Reinhardt, U. (1996) 'A Social Contract for 21st Century Health Care: Three Tier Health Care With Bounty Hunting', *Health Economics*, 5, 479–99.

Relman, A. (1980) 'The New Medical-Industrial Complex', *New England Journal of Medicine*, 303 (17), 963–70.

Rhodes, P. and Small, N. (2001) *Too Ill to Talk? User Involvement and Palliative Care* (London, Routledge).

Richards, S. and Brown, C. (2001) 'Tony Blair: Yes I Agree with Gordon Brown. Raising Taxation is the Way to Fund a Better NHS', *Independent on Sunday*, 2 December, 5.

Riddell, P. (1991) *The Thatcher Era and its Legacy* (Oxford, Blackwell).

Rimm, E., Klatsky, A., Grobee, D. and Stampfer, M. (1996) 'Review of Moderate Alcohol Consumption and Reduced Risk of Coronary Heart Disease: Is the Effect Due to Beer, Wine or Spirits?', *British Medical Journal*, 312, 731–6.

Ritchie, J. (2000) *The Report of the Inquiry into Quality and Practice Within the National Health Service Arising from the Actions of Rodney Ledward* (London, NHS Executive South East Regional Office).

Rivett, G. (1998) *From Cradle to Grave: Fifty Years of the NHS* (London, King's Fund).

Robb, B. (1967) *Sans Everything* (London, Nelson).

Roberts, E., Robinson, J. and Seymour, L. (2002) *Old Habits Die Hard: Tackling Age Discrimination in Health and Social Care* (London, King's Fund).

Roberts, H. (ed.) (1992) *Women's Health Matters* (London, Routledge).

Roberts, H. (1997) 'Children, Inequalities and Health', *British Medical Journal*, 314, 1122–3.

Roberts, I. and Power, C. (1996) 'Does the Decline in Child Injury Mortality Vary By Social Class? A Comparison of Class Specific Mortality in 1981 and 1991', *British Medical Journal*, 313, 784–6.

Robinson, D. (1971) *The Process of Becoming Ill* (London, Routledge).

Robinson, D., Bell, C., Moller, H. and Basnett, I. (2003) 'Effect of the UK Government's Two Week Target on Waiting Times in Women with Breast Cancer in South East England', *British Journal of Cancer*, 89, 492–6.

Robinson, J. (1992) 'Introduction: Beginning the Study of Nursing Policy', in Robinson, J., Gray, A. and Elkan, R. (eds) *Policy Issues in Nursing* (Milton Keynes, Open University Press), 1–8.

Robinson, R. (2002a) *The Finance and Provision of Long Term Care for Elderly People in the UK: Recent Trends, Current Policy and Future Prospects*, http://www.ipss.go.jp/English/WebJournal.files/SocialSecurity/2002/02Dec/robinsonpdf.

Robinson, R. (2002b) 'User Charges for Health Care', in Mossialos, E., Dixon, A., Figueras, J. and Kutzin, R. (eds) (2002) Funding Health care: Options for Europe (Buckingham, Open University Press), 161–83.

Robinson, R. (2002c) 'NHS Foundation Trusts', *British Medical Journal*, 325, 506–7.

Robinson, R. and Chalkley, M. (1998) *Theory and Evidence on Cost-Sharing in Health Care* (London, OHE).

Robinson, R. and Exworthy, M. (2001) *Three at the Top: Working Relationships between Chairs and Chief Executives at First Wave Primary Care Trusts. Preliminary Report for the NHS Executive Leadership Programme* (London, LSE).

Robinson, R. and Steiner, A. (1998) *Managed Health Care: US Evidence and Lessons for the NHS* (Buckingham, Open University Press).

Roderick, P., Clements, S., Shona, N., Martin, D. and Diamond, I. (1999) 'What Determines Geographic Variation in Rates of Acceptance on to Renal Replacement Therapy in England?', *Journal of Health Services Research and Policy*, 4, 139–46.

Roe, B., Walsh, N. and Huntington, J. (2000) *Breaking the Mould: Nurses Working in PMS Pilots* (Birmingham, HSMC).

Rogers, A. and Pilgrim, D. (2001) *Mental Health Policy in Britain: A Critical Introduction* (London, Palgrave).

Roland, M. and Shapiro, J. (1998) *Specialist Outreach Clinics in General Practice* (Oxford, Radcliffe Medical Press).

Rose, R. (2000) 'How Much Does Social Capital Add to Individual Health: A Survey Study of Russia', *Social Science and Medicine*, 51, 1421–35.

Rosen, G. (1993) *A History of Public Health*, expanded edn (New York, Johns Hopkins).

Rosen, R., Florin, D. and Dixon, J. (2001) *Access to Health Care – Taking Forward the Findings from the Scoping Exercise* (London, National Coordinating Centre for NHS Service Delivery and Organisation).

Rosen, R. and Jenkins, C. (2003) *Mental Health Services in Primary Care: A Review of Recent Development in London* (London, King's Fund).

Rosenthal, M., Mulcahy, L. and Lloyd-Bostock, S. (1999) *Medical Mishaps: Pieces of the Puzzle* (Buckingham, Open University Press).

Rosser, R. and Kind, P. (1978) 'A Scale of Valuations of States of Illness: Is There A Social Consensus?', *International Journal of Epidemiology*, 7, 347–58.

Rosser, R. and Watts, V. (1972) 'The Measurement of Hospital Output', *International Journal of Epidemiology*, 1, 361–8.

Rose, R. and Davies, P. (1995) Inheritance in Public Policy: Change Without Choice in Britain (New Haven, CT, Yale University Press).

Rowe, R. and Bond, M. (2003) 'Hitting the Big Time', *Health Service Journal*, 20 March, 30–1.

Rowe, R. and Shepherd, M. (2002) 'Public Participation in the New NHS', *Social Policy and Administration*, 36, 275–90.

Royal College of Obstetricians and Gynaecologists, Royal College of Midwives, Royal College of Anaesthetists, National Childbirth Trust (2002) *National Sentinel Caesarean Section Audit* (London, RCOG, RCM and NCT).

Royal College of Physicians (1981) *Medical Aspects of Dietary Fibre* (London, Pitman).

Royal College of Physicians (1994) *Ensuring Equality and Quality of Care for Elderly People* (London, Royal College of Physicians of London).

Royal College of Physicians (1995) *Setting Priorities for the NHS: A Framework for Decision-Making* (London, Royal College of Physicians).

Royal College of Physicians (2000) *Nicotine Addiction in Britain* (London, Royal College of Physicians).

Royal College of Psychiatrists (1995) *Report of the Confidential Inquiry into Homicides and Suicides by Mentally Ill People* (London, Royal College of Psychiatrists).

Royal Liverpool Children's Inquiry, The (2001) *The Report of the Royal Liverpool Children's Inquiry Chair: M Redfern (QC)* (London, The Stationery Office).

Royal Pharmaceutical Society of Great Britain (1997) *Building for the Future: A Strategy for 21st Century Pharmaceutical Service* (London, Royal Pharmaceutical Soceity).

Ruane, S. (2000) 'Acquiescence and Opposition the Private Finance Initiative in the NHS' *Policy and Politics*, 28, 411–24.

Ruggie, M. (1996) *Realignments in the Welfare State: Health Policy in the United States, Canada and Britain* (New York, Columbia University Press).

Rummery, K. and Glendinning, C. (2000) *Primary Care and Social Services. Developing New Partnerships for Older People* (London, Radcliffe Medical).

Sabo, D. and Gordon, G. (1993) *Men's Health and Illness: Gender, Power and the Body* (London, Sage).

Sagan, L. A. (1987) *The Health of Nations* (New York, Basic Books).

Sainsbury Centre for Mental Health (2003) *Money for Mental Health* (London, SCMH Publications).

Saks, M. (2003) *Orthodox and Alternative Medicine: Politics, Professionalisation and Health Care* (London, Continuum).

Saks, M. (1995) *Professions and the Public Interest: Medical Power, Altruism and Alternative Medicine* (London, Routledge).

Salisbury, C. (1989) 'How Do People Choose Their Doctor?', *British Medical Association*, 299, 608–10.

Salmon, J. W. (1995) 'A Perspective on the Corporate Transformation of Health Care', *International Journal of Health Studies*, 25 (1), 11–42.

Salter, B. (1994) 'The Politics of Community Care: Social Rights and Welfare Limits', *Policy and Politics*, 22 (2), 119–31.

Salter, B. (1995) 'The Private Sector and the NHS: Redefining the Welfare State', *Policy and Politics*, 23 (1), 17–30.

Salter, B. (1996) 'Medicine and the State: Redefining the Concordat', *Public Policy and Administration* 10 (3), 60–87.

Salter, B. (1998) *The Politics of Change in the Health Service* (Basingstoke, Macmillan).

Salter, B. (1999) 'Change in the Governance of Medicine – The Politics of Self Regulation', *Policy and Politics*, 27, 143–58.

Salter, B. (2000) *Medical Regulation and Public Trust: An International Review* (London, King's Fund).

Salter, B. (2003) 'Patients and Doctors: Reformulating the UK Health Policy Community', *Social Science and Medicine*, 57, 927–36.

Saltman, R., Figueras, J. and Sakellarides, C. (eds) (1998) *Critical Challenges for Health Care Reform in Europe* (London, WHO and Open University Press).

Salvage, J. (1985) *The Politics of Nursing* (Oxford, Heinemann).

Salvage, J. and Wright, S. (1995) *Nursing Development Units: A Force for Change* (London, Scutari).

Sashidaran, S. and Francis, E. (1993) 'Epidemiology, Ethnicity and Schizophrenia', in Ahmad, W. (ed.) *Race and Health in Contemporary Britain* (Buckingham, Open University Press), 96–113.

Sassi, F. and Le Grand, J. (2001) 'Equity versus Efficiency: A Dilemma for the NHS', *British Medical Journal*, 323, 762–3.

Saxena, S., Majeed, A. and Jones, M. (1999) 'Socio-economic Differences in Childhood Consultation Rates in General Practice in England and Wales: Prospective cohort study', *British Medical Journal*, 318, 642–6.

Scally, G. and Donaldson, L. (1998) 'Clinical Governance and the Drive for Quality Improvement in the New NHS in England', *British Medical Journal*, 317, 61–5.

Scambler, A., Scambler, G. and Craig, D. (1981) 'Kinship and Friendship Networks and Women's Demand for Primary Care', *Journal of Royal College of General Practitioners*, 26, 746–50.

Schieber, G. and Poullier, J. (1992) 'International Health Spending', *Health Affairs*, 10 (1), 106–16.

Schneider, E. and Epstein, A. (1996) 'Influence of Cardiac Surgery Performance Reports on Referral Practices and Access to Care', *New England Journal of Medicine*, 335(4), 251–6.

Scitovsky, A. (1988) 'Medical Care in the Last 12 Months of Life: The Relation Between Age, Functional Status, and Medical Care Expenditure', *The Milbank Quarterly*, 66 (4), 640–60.

Scope (1995) *Disabled in Britain: Behind Closed Doors – The Carer's Experience* (London, Scope).

Scott, C. (2001) *Public and Private Roles in Health Care Systems. Reform Expenses in Seven OECD Countries* (Buckingham, Open University Press).

Scott-Samuel, A. (1996) 'Health Impact Assessment', *British Medical Journal*, 313, 183–4.

Scottish Association of Health Councils (1998) *Report of Health Councils' Complaints Project* (Edinburgh, Scottish Association of Health Councils).

Scottish Executive (2000a) *Our National Health: A Plan for Action, A Plan for Change* (Edinburgh, Scottish Executive).

Scottish Executive (2000b) *The Same As You* (Edinburgh, Scottish Executive).

Scottish Executive (2000c) *For Scotland's Children. Better Integrated Services for Children* (Edinburgh, Scottish Executive).

Scottish Executive (2001) *Patient Focus and Public Involvement* (Edinburgh, Scottish Executive).

Scottish Executive (2003a) *Partnership for Care: Scotland's Health White Paper* (Edinburgh, Scottish Executive).

Scottish Executive (2003b) *Reforming the NHS Complaints Procedures Patient Focus and Public Involvement. A Draft for Consultation* (Edinburgh, Scottish Executive).

Scottish Executive (2003c) *A New Public Involvement Structure for NHS Scotland: Proposals* (Edinburgh, Scottish Executive).

Scottish Executive (2003d) *Improving Health in Scotland: The Challenge* (Edinburgh, The Scottish Executive).

Seale, C., Pattison, S. and Davey, B. (2001) *Medical Knowledge, Doubt and Certainty* (Buckingham, Open University Press).

Secretary of State for Scotland (1997) *Designed to Care* (Edinburgh, The Stationery Office).

Seddon, D. and Robinson, C. (2001) 'Carers of Older People with Dementia: Assessment and the Carers Act' *Health and Social Care in the Community*, 9, 151–8.

Select Committee on Public Adminsitration (2000) (HC 410) *2nd Report 1999/2000: Appointment to NHS Bodies* (London, The Stationery Office).

Shackley, P. and Ryan, M. (1994) 'What is the Role of the Consumer in Health Care?', *Journal of Social Policy*, 23 (4), 517–41.

Shapiro, J. (1994) *Shared Purchasing and Collaborative Commissioning within the NHS* (Birmingham, NAHAT).

Sharma, U. (1995) *Complementary Medicine Today: Practitioners and Patients*, revised edn (London, Routledge).

Shaw, M., Dorling, D. and Brimblecombe, N. (1998) 'Changing the Map: Health in Britain 1951–91', *Sociology of Health and Illness*, 20 (5), 694–709.

Shaw, M., Dorling, D., Gordon, D. and Davey-Smith, G. (1999) *The Widening Gap: Health Inequalities and Policy in Britain* (Bristol, Policy Press).

Shaw, R. and Smith, P. (2001) 'Allocating Health Care Resources to Reduce Health Inequalities', in Appleby, J. and Harrison, A. (eds) *Health Care UK*, Spring (London, King's Fund), 7–14.

Shaw, S. and Abbott S. (2002) 'Too Much to handle', *Health Service Journal*, 27 June, 28–30.

Sheaff, R. and Lloyd-Kendall, A. (2000) 'Principal–Agent Relationships in General Practice: The First Wave of English Personal Medical Services Pilot Contracts', *Journal of Health Services Research and Policy*, 5, 156–63.

Sheaff, R., Smith, K. and Dickson, M. (2002) 'Is GP Restratification Begging in England?', *Social Policy and Administration*, 36 (7), 765–79.

Shekelle, P., Eccles, M., Grimshaw, J. and Woolf, S. H. (2001) 'When Should Clinical Guidelines be Updated?', *British Medical Journal*, 323, 155.

Shepperd, S., Harwood, D., Jenkinson, C., Gray, A., Vessey, M. and Morgan, P. (1998a) 'Randomised Controlled Trial Comparing Hospitals at Home Care with Inpatient Hospital Care I: 3 Month Follow up of Health Outcomes', *British Medical Journal*, 316, 1786–91.

Shepperd, S., Harwood, D., Jenkinson, C., Gray, A., Vessey, M. and Morgan, P. (1998b) 'Randomised Controlled Trial Comparing Hospitals at Home Care with Inpatient Hospital Care II: Cost Minimisation Analysis', *British Medical Journal*, 316, 1791–6.

Shibuya, K., Hashimoto, H. and Yano, E. (2002) 'Individual Income, Income Distribution and Self-rated Health in Japan', *British Medical Journal*, 324, 16–19.

Shipman Inquiry, The (2001) *First Report* (London, The Stationery Office).

SHM (2002) *NHS Beacon Programme Evaluation – Synopsis of Key Findings, Recommendations and Next Steps* (London, Modernisation Agency).

Shum, C., Humphreys, A., Wheeler, D., Cochrane, M., Skoda, S. and Clement, S. (2000) 'Nurse Management of Patients with Minor Illnesses in General Practice: Multicentre, Randomised Controlled Trial', *British Medical Journal*, 320, 1038–43.

Sibbald, B. (2000) 'Primary Care: Background and Policy Issues', in Williams, A. (ed.) *Nursing, Medicine and Primary Care* (Buckingham, Open University Press), 14–27.

Siddall, R. (2002) 'Cardiac Arrested?', *Health Service Journal*, 112, 28 March, 36–7.

Simpson, J. and Scott, T. (1997) 'Beyond the Call of Duty', *Health Service Journal*, 8 May, 22–4.

Singleton, C. and Aird, B. (2002) 'As Good As New', *Health Service Journal*, 27 June, 28–30.

Singleton, N., Bumpstead, R., O'Brien, M., Lee, A. and Meltzer, H. (2001) *Psychiatric Morbidity among Adults Living in Private Households* (London, The Stationery Office).

Sloan, F. (2001) 'Arrow's Concept of the Health Care Consumer: A 40 Year Retrospective', *Journal of Health Politics, Policy and Law*, 26 (5), 899–911.

Smaje, C. (1995) *Health, Race and Ethnicity: Making Sense of the Evidence* (London, King's Fund).

Smaje, C. and Le Grand, J. (1997) 'Ethnicity, Equity and the Use of Health Services in the British NHS', *Social Science and Medicine*, 45, 485–96.

Smith, A. (1987) 'Qualms about QALYs', *The Lancet*, 1, 1134–6.

Smith, A. and Jacobson, B. (1988) *The Nation's Health: A Strategy for the 1990s* (London, King Edward's Hospital Fund).

Smith, C. (1999) *Making Sense of the Private Finance Initiative* (Oxford, Radcliffe Medical Press).

Smith, F. B. (1979) *The People's Health* (London, Croom Helm).

Smith G. and Wales, C. (1999) 'The Theory and Practice of Citizens' Juries', *Policy and Politics*, 27, 295–308.

Smith, J., Walshe, K. and Hunter, D. (2001) 'The Redisorganisation of the NHS', *British Medical Journal*, 323, 1263–4.

Smith, P. (1995) 'On the Unintended Consequences of Publishing Performance Data in the Public Sector', *International Journal of Public Administration*, 18, 277–310.

Smith, P. (2003) 'Master Mind', *Health Service Journal*, 2 October, 22–7.

Smith, R. (2001) 'Why are Doctors so Unhappy?', *British Medical Journal*, 322, 1073–4.

Smith, R. (2002) 'In Search of "Non-disease" ', *British Medical Journal*, 324, 883–5.

Snashall, D. (1996) 'Hazards of Work', *British Medical Journal*, 313, 161–3.

Snelgrove, S. and Hughes, D. (2000) 'Interprofessional Relations between Doctors and Nurses: Perspectives from South Wales', *Journal of Advanced Nursing*, 31, 661–7.

Social Exclusion Unit (1999) *Teenage Pregnancy* (London, Cabinet Office).

Social Services Committee (1985) (HC13) *2nd Report 1958/6. Community Care with Special Reference to Adult Mentally Ill and Mentally Handicapped People* (London, HMSO).

Social Services Committee (1986) (HC 387) *4th Report 1985/6. Public Expenditure in the Social Services* (London, HMSO).

Social Services Inspectorate (1996) *Caring for People at Home: Part II. Report of a Second Inspection of Arrangements for Assessment and Delivery of Home Care Services* (London, DoH).

Social Services Inspectorate (2001) *Improving Older People's Services: Inspection of Social Care Services for Older People* (London, DoH).

Social Services Inspectorate (2002) *Improving Older People's Services: Policy into Practice. The Second Phase of Inspections into Older People's Services* (London, DoH).

Soderlund, N. (1999) 'Do Managers Pay their Way? The Impact of Management Input on Hospital Productivity in the NHS Internal Market', *Journal of Health Services Research and Policy*, 4, 6–15.

Soderlund, N., Csaba, I., Gray, A., Milne, R. and Raftery, J. (1997) 'Impact of the NHS Reforms on English Hospital Productivity: An Analysis of the First Three Years', *British Medical Journal*, 315, 1126–9.

Soni Raleigh, V. and Kiri, V. (1997) 'Life Expectancy in England: Variations and Trends by Gender, Health Authority and Level of Deprivation', *Journal of Epidemiology and Community Health*, 51 (6), 649–58.

Soothill, K., Mackay, L. and Webb, C. (eds) (1995) *Interprofessional Relations in Health Care* (London, Edward Arnold).

Sorell, T. (1997) 'Morality, Consumerism and the Internal Market in Healthcare', *Journal of Medical Ethics*, 23, 71–6.

South, J. (1999) 'Eligibility Criteria and Entitlements: Defining Need for NHS Continuing Care', *Social Policy and Administration*, 33, 132–49.

Spencer, N. (1996) *Poverty and Child Health* (London, Radcliffe Medical Press).

Stacey, M. (1992) *Regulating British Medicine: The General Medical Council* (Chichester, John Wiley).

Stanistreet, D., Scott-Samuel, A. and Bellis, M. A. (1999) 'Income Inequality and Mortality in England', *Journal of Public Health Medicine*, 21 (2), 205–7.

Starfield, B. (1998) *Primary Care: Balancing Health Needs, Services and Technology* (New York, Oxford University Press).

Starr, P. and Immergut, E. (1987) 'Health Care and the Boundaries of Politics', in Maier, C. S. (ed.) *Changing Boundaries of the Political* (Cambridge, Cambridge University Press), 221–54.

Stein, L. (1978) 'The Doctor-Nurse Game', in Dingwall, R. and McIntosh, J. (eds) *Readings in the Sociology of Nursing* (Edinburgh, Churchill Livingstone), 107–17.

Steiner, A., Walsh, B., Pickering, R., Wiles, R., Ward, J. and Broking, J. (2001) 'Therapeutic Nursing or Unblocking Beds: A Randomised Controlled Trial of a Post-Acute Intermediate Care Unit', *British Medical Journal*, 322, 453–60.

Stephenson, P. (2003) 'Only 62 Targets Now', *Health Service Journal*, 8 February, 8.

Stern, J. (1983) 'Social Mobility and the Interpretation of Social Class Mortality Differentials', *Journal of Social Policy*, 12 (1), 27–49.

Stern, R., Martin, V. and Cray, S. (1995) *Developing the Role and Purpose of NHS Boards Part One: Where Are We Now?* (Southborough, Salomons Centre).

Stevens, A. and Gillam, S. (1998) 'Needs Assessment: From Theory to Practice', *British Medical Journal*, 316, 1448–52.

Stewart, A. (1999) 'Cost Containment and Privatisation', in Drache, D. and Sullivan, T. (eds) *Market Limits in Health Reform: Public Success, Private Failure* (London, Routledge), 64–84.

Stewart, J., Kendall, E. and Coote, A. (1996) *Citizens' Juries* (London, Institute for Public Policy Research).

Stewart, M. and Brown, J. (2001) 'Patient Centredness in Medicine', in Edwards, A. and Elwyn, G. (eds) *Evidence Based Patient Care* (Oxford, Oxford University Press), 98–117.

Stewart-Brown, S., Surender, R., Bradlow, J., Coulter, A. and Doll, H. (1995) 'The Effects of Fundholding in General Practice on Prescribing Habits Three Years After Introduction of the Scheme', *British Medical Journal*, 311, 1543–7.

Stowe, K. (1989) *On Caring for the National Health* (London, Nuffield Provincial Hospitals Trust).

Straw, P., Bruster, P., Richards, N. and Lilley, S. (2000) 'Sit Up and Take Notice', *Health Service Journal*, 19 May, 24–6.

Strong, P. and Robinson, J. (1990) *The NHS: Under New Management* (Buckingham, Open University Press).

Sturm, R. and Gresenz, C. (2002) 'Relations of Income Inequality and Family Income to Chronic Medical Conditions and Mental Health Disorders: National Survey in USA', *British Medical Journal*, 324, 20–3.

Sullivan, H. and Skelcher, C. (2002) *Working Across Boundaries – Collaboration in Public Services* (Basingstoke, Palgrave Macmillan).

Sunkin, M. (2001) 'Trends in Judicial Review and the Human Rights Act', *Policy Money and Management*, 21 (3), 9–12.

Sussex, J. (2001) *The Economics of the Private Finance Initiative* (London, Office of Health Economics).

Sussex, J. and Goddard, M. (2002) 'Flexible Friends', *Health Service Journal*, 23 May, 28–9.

Sutherland, H. and Piachaud, D. (2001) 'Reducing Child Poverty in Britain: An Assessment of Government Policy 1997–2001', *The Economic Journal*, 111, 85–101.

Svensson, R. (1996) 'The Interplay between Doctors and Nurses – A Negotiated Order Perspective', *Sociology of Health and Illness*, 18, 379–8.

Swage, T. (2000) *Clinical Governance in Health Care Practice* (Oxford, Butterworth-Heinemann).

System Three Social Research/York Health Economics Consortium (2001) *NHS Complaints Procedure National Circulation* (London, DoH).

Szasz, T. S. and Hollender, M. H. (1956) 'A Contribution to the Philosophy of Medicine: The Basic Models of the Doctor–Patient Relationship', *American Medical Association, Archives of Internal Medicine*, 97, 585–92.

Szreter, S. (1988) 'The Importance of Social Intervention in Britain's Mortality Decline c.1850–1914', *Social History of Medicine*, 1 (1), 1–38.

Tallis, R. (ed.) (1997) *Increasing Longevity: Medical, Social and Political Implications* (London, Royal College of Physicians).

Tam, H. (1998) *Communitarianism: A New Agenda for Politics and Citizenship* (Basingstoke, Macmillan).

Taxis, K. and Barber, N. (2003) 'Ethnographic Study of Incidence and Severity of Intravenous Drug Error', *British Medical Journal*, 326, 684–7.

Taylor, D. (1988) 'Primary Care Services', in Maxwell, R. (ed.) *Reshaping the National Health Service* (Oxford, Policy Journals), 2–47.

Taylor, D. (1998) *Improving Health Care: The Political and Professional Challenges of Raising Health Care Quality* (London, King's Fund).

Taylor, F. W. (1911) *Scientific Management* (New York, Harper and Row).

Thane, P. (1987) 'The Growing Burden of an Ageing Population', *Journal of Public Policy*, 7 (4), 373–87.

Thatcher, M. (1982) *Speech to Conservative Party Conference*, Brighton, 8 October.

Thatcher, M. (1993) *The Downing Street Years* (London, Harper Collins).

Thomas, K., Fall., M., Parry., G. and Nicholl, J. (1995) *National Survey of Access to Complementary Health Care via General Practice* (Sheffield, Sheffield Centre for Health and Related Research, University of Sheffield).

Thomas, K., Nicholl, J. and Coleman, P. (1995) 'Assessing the Outcome of Making it Easier for Patients to Change General Practitioner: Practice Characteristics Associated with Patient Movements', *British Journal of General Practice*, 45, 581–6.

Thompson, J. (1984) 'Compliance', in Fitzpatrick, R., Hinton, J., Newman, S., Scambler, G. and Thompson, J. (eds) (1984), *The Experience of Illness* (London, Tavistock).

Thomson, H., Petticrew, M., and Morrison, D. (2001) 'Health Effects of Housing Improvement: Systematic Review of International Studies', *British Medical Journal*, 323, 187–90.

Thorne, S., Ternulf Nyhlin, K. and Paterson, B. (2000) 'Attitudes towards Patient Expertise in Chronic Illness', *International Journal of Nursing Studies*, 37, 303–11.

Timmins, N. (1988) *Cash, Crisis and Cure: The Independent Guide to the NHS Debate* (Oxford, Alden Press).

Timmins, N. (1995) *The Five Giants: A Biography of the Welfare State* (London, Harper Collins).

Tinsley, R. and Luck, M. (1998) 'Fundholding and the Community Nurse', *Journal of Social Policy*, 27, 471–87.

Toke, D. (2001) 'GM Crops: Science, Policy and Environmentalists', *Environmental Politics*, 10 (4), 115–20.

Tomlinson, B. (1992) *Report of the Inquiry into London's Health Service* (London, HMSO).

Townsend, P. (1962) *The Last Refuge* (London, Routledge and Kegan Paul).

Townsend, P., Davidson, N. and Whitehead, M. (1992) *Inequalities in Health*, revised edn (Harmondsworth, Penguin).

Towse, A. and Sussex, J. (2000) 'Getting the UK Health Expenditure up to the European Union Mean – What Does that Mean?', *British Medical Journal*, 320, 640–2.

Toynbee, P. and Walker, D. (2001) *Did Things Get Better?* (Harmondsworth, Penguin).

Traynor, M. (1999) *Managerialism and Nursing: Beyond Oppression and Profession* (London, Routledge).

Treasury/DoH (Department of Health) (2002) *Tackling Health Inequalities: Summary of the 2002 Cross Cutting Review* (London, DoH).

Trevett, N. (1997) 'Injecting New Life into the Wirral', *Healthlines*, 39, 20–1

Tritter, J., Barley, V., Daykin, N., Evans, S., McNeill, J., Rimmer, J., Sanidas, M. and Turton, P. (2003) 'Divided Care and the Third Way: User Involvement in Statutory and Voluntary Sector Cancer Services', *Sociology of Health and Illness*, 25, 429–56.

Tsouros, A. and Draper, R. (1992) 'The Healthy Cities Project: New Development and Research Needs', in Davies, M. P. and Kelly, J. K. (eds) *Healthy Cities* (London, Routledge), 25–33.

Tuckett, D., Bolton, M., Olson, C. and Williams, A. (1985) *Meetings Between Experts: An Approach to Sharing Ideas in Medical Consultation* (London, Tavistock).

Tudor Edwards, R. (1997) *NHS Waiting Lists: Towards the Elusive Solution* (London, Office of Health Economics).

Tudor-Hart, J. (1971) 'The Inverse Care Law', *Lancet*, 27 February, 405–12.

Tudor-Hart, J. (1981) 'A New Kind of Doctor', *Journal of the Royal Society of Medicine*, 74, 871–83.

Tudor-Hart, J. (1994) *Feasible Socialism. The National Health Service: Past Present and Future* (London, Socialist Health Association).

Tuohy, C. (1999) *Accidental Logics: The Dynamics of Change in the Health Care Arena in the United States, Britain and Canada* (Oxford, Oxford University Press).

Turner, B. (1987) *Medical Power and Social Knowledge* (London, Sage).

Turrell, A. R., Castleden, C. M. and Freestone, B. (1998) 'Long Stay Care and the NHS: Discontinuities between Policy and Practice', *British Medical Journal*, 317, 942–4.

Twaddle, A. C. (1974) 'The Concept of Health Status', *Social Science and Medicine*, 8 (1), 29–38.

Twigg, J. (2000) 'The Changing Role of Users and Carers', in Hudson, B. (ed.) *The Changing Role of Social Care* (London, Jessica Kingsley).

Tymms, P. and Wiggins, A. (2000) 'School Experience of League Tables Should Make Doctors Think Again', *British Medical Journal*, 321, 1467.

UK Climate Change Impacts Review Group (1996) *Review of the Potential Effects of Climate Change in the UK* (London, HMSO).

UKCC (UK Central Council for Nursing, Midwifery and Health Visiting) (1992a) *The Code of Professional Conduct for Nurses, Midwives and Health Visitors* (London, UKCC).

UKCC (UK Central Council for Nursing, Midwifery and Health Visiting) (1992b) *The Scope of Professional Practice* (London, UKCC).

UKCC (UK Central Council for Nursing, Midwifery and Health Visiting) (1996) *Guidelines for Professional Practice* (London, UKCC).

UKCC (UK Central Council for Nursing, Midwifery and Health Visiting) (1999) *Fitness for Practice* (London, The UKCC Commission for Nursing and Midwifery Education).

UNICEF (2002) *We the Children: Meeting the Promises of the World Summit for Children* (Geneva, Unicef).

United Nations (2002) *Report of the Second World Assembly on Ageing* (New York, UN).

Utting, W. (1997) *People Like Us: The Report of the Review of Safeguards for Children Living Away from Home* (London, The Stationery Office).

van de Mheen, H., Stronks, K. and Mackenbach, J. (1998) 'A Lifecourse Perspective on Socio-Economic Inequalities in Health', *Sociology of Health and Illness*, 20, 754–77.

van Herk, R., Klazinger, N., Schepers, R. and Casparie, A. (2001) 'Medical Audit: Threat or Opportunity for the Medical Profession. A Comparative Study of Medical Audit among Medical Specialists in General Hospitals in the Netherlands and England 1970–1999', *Social Science and Medicine*, 53, 1721–2.

Vaughan, B. and Lathlean, J. (1999) *Intermediate Care Models in Practice* (London, King's Fund).

Verschuren, W., Jacobs, D., Bloemberg, B., Kromhout, D., Menotti, A., Aravanis, C., Blackburn, H., Buzina, R., Dontas, A. S. and Fidanza, F. (1995) 'Serum Total Cholesterol and Long Term Coronary Heart Disease Mortality in Different Cultures. Twenty-Five Year Follow Up of the 7 Countries Study', *Journal of the American Medical Association*, 274 (2), 131–6.

Vincent, C., Neale, G. and Woloshynowych, M. (2001) 'Adverse Events in British Hospitals: Preliminary Retrospective Record Review', *British Medical Journal*, 322, 517–9.

Vrijheid, M., Dolk, H., Armstrong, B., Ambransky, L., Bianchi, F., Fazarine, I., Garne, E., Ide, R., Nelen, V., Rober, E., Scott, J., Stone, D. and Tencani, R. (2002) 'Chromosomal Congenital Anomalies and Residence Near Hazardous Waste Landfill Sites', *The Lancet*, 359, 320–2.

Wagstaff, A., van Doorslaer, A., van der Burg, H., Calonge, S., Christiansen, T. et al. (1999)

'Equity in the Finance of Health Care: Some Further Comparisons', *Journal of Health Economics*, 18, 263–90.

Walby, S. and Greenwell, J. (1994) *Medicine and Nursing: Professions in a Changing Health Service* (London, Sage).

Walker, A., Maher, J., Coulthard, M., Goddard, E. and Thomas, M. (2001) *Living in Britain. Results from the 2000/01 General Household Survey* (London, The Stationery Office).

Wall, A. and Baddeley, S. (1998) 'Chair–Chief Executive Relationships in the National Health Service', in Coulson, A. (ed.) *Trust and Contracts: Relationships in Local Government, Health and Public Services* (Bristol, Policy Press), 79–93.

Wall, A. and Owen, B. (1999) *Health Policy: Health Care and the NHS* (Eastbourne, The Gildredge Press).

Wallace, H. and Mulcahy, L. (1999) *Cause for Complaint: An Evaluation of the Effectiveness of the NHS Complaints Procedure* (London, The Public Law Project).

Wallace, L. and Stoten, B. (2002) 'The Late Show', in Health Service Journal (ed.), *Clinical Governance and Risk Management* (London, HSJ Management Collections – EMAP Public Sector Management), 12–13.

Walshe, K. (2002a) 'Power with Responsibility', *Health Service Journal*, 7 June, 25.

Walshe, K. (2002b) 'The Rise of Regulation in the NHS', *British Medical Journal*, 324, 967–70.

Walshe, K. (2003a) *Regulating Healthcare: A Prescription for Improvement?* (Buckingham, Open University Press).

Walshe, K. (2003b) 'Foundation Hospitals – A New Direction for NHS Reform?', *Journal of the Royal Society of Medicine*, 96, 106–10.

Walshe, K. (2003c) 'Lead in their Pencils', *Health Service Journal*, 30 October, 18–19.

Walshe, K., Freeman, T., Latham, L., Wallace, L. and Spurgeon, P. (2000) *Clinical Governance: From Policy to Practice* (Manchester, HSMC).

Walshe, K. and Higgins, J. (2002) 'The Use and Impact of Inquiries in the NHS', *British Medical Journal*, 325, 895–950.

Walston, S., Burns, L. and Kimberly, J. (2000) 'Does Re-engineering Really Work. An Examination of the Context and Outcome of Hospital Reengineering Initiation', *Health Services Research*, 34, 1363–88.

Walt, G. (1994) *Health Policy: An Introduction to Process and Power* (London, Zed Books).

Wanless, D. (2001) *Securing Our Future Health: Taking a Long Term View – Interim Report* (London, HM Treasury).

Wanless, D. (2002) *Securing Our Future Health: Taking a Long Term View – Final Report* (London, HM Treasury).

Wanless, D. (2003) *Securing Good Health for the Whole Population: Population Health Trends* (London, HM Treasury).

Wanless, D. (2004) *Securing Health for the Whole Population* (London, HM Treasury).

Ward, S. (2001) 'On the Wrong Foot?', *Health Service Journal*, 9 August, 24–7.

Watkins, S. (1987) *Medicine and Labour. The Politics of a Profession* (London, Lawrence and Wishart).

Watterson, A. (1994) 'Threats to Health and Safety in the Workplace in Britain', *British Medical Journal*, 308, 1115–16.

Webster, C. (1988) *Health Services Since the War, Volume I: Problems of Health Care. The National Health Service before 1957* (London, HMSO).

Webster, C. (1996) *The Health Services Since the War*. Vol. II: *Government and Health Care. The British National Health Service 1958–79* (London, HMSO).

Webster, C. (1998) *The National Health Service: A Political History* (Oxford, Oxford University Press).

Webster, C. (2002) *The National Health Service: A Political History*, 2nd edn (Oxford, Oxford University Press).

Weingart, S. N., Wilson, McL. R., Gibberd, R. W. and Harrison, B. (2000) 'Epidemiology of Medical Error', *British Medical Journal*, 320, 774–7.

Wells, J. (1999) 'The Growth of Managerialism and its Impact on Nursing and the NHS', in Norman, I. and Cowley, S. (eds) *The Changing Nature of Nursing in a Managerial Age* (Oxford, Blackwell Science), 57–81.

Welsh Assembly Government (2002a) *Health and Social Care Guide for Wales* (Cardiff, Welsh Assembly Government).

Welsh Assembly Government (2002b) *Wellbeing in Wales* (Cardiff, National Assembly for Wales).

Welsh Assembly Government (2003a) *Signposts Two: Putting Public and Patient Involvement into Practice* (Cardiff, Welsh Assembly Government).

Welsh Assembly Government (2003b) *Health, Social Care and Wellbeing Strategies* (Cardiff, Welsh Assembly Government).

Welsh Assembly Government (2003c) *Healthy and Active Lifestyles in Wales: A Framework for Action* (Cardiff, Welsh Assembly Government).

Welsh Office (1997) *Health Gain Targets for Wales, DGM (97) 50* (Cardiff, Welsh Office).

Welsh Office (1998) *Involving the Public: Putting Patients First* (Cardiff, Welsh Office).

Welsh Office, NHS Directorate (1989) *Welsh Health Planning Forum: Strategic Intent and Direction for the NHS in Wales* (Cardiff, Welsh Office).

West, P. (1998) *Managed Care: A Model for the UK?* (Office of Health Economics, London).

White, D., Leach, K. and Christensen, L. (1996) 'Self-fulfilling Prophecies', *Health Service Journal*, 23 May, 31.

White, T. (1993) *Management for Clinicians* (London, Edward Arnold).

Whitehead, M. (1987) *The Health Divide* (London, Health Education Council).

Whitehead, M. (1994) 'Who Cares About Equity in the NHS?', *British Medical Journal*, 308, 1284–7.

Whitney, R. (1988) *National Health Crisis: A Modern Solution* (London, Shepherd-Walwyn).

WHO (World Health Organisation) (1946) *Constitution: Basic Documents* (Geneva, WHO).

WHO (World Health Organisation) (1978) *Alma Ata 1977: Primary Health Care* (Geneva, WHO/Unicef).

WHO (World Health Organisation) (1981) *Global Strategy for Health for All by the Year 2000* (Geneva, WHO).

WHO (World Health Organisation) (1986) *Ottawa Charter for Health Promotion* (Ottawa, WHO).

WHO (World Health Organisation) (1995) *The World Health Report: Bridging the Gaps* (Geneva, WHO).

WHO (World Health Organisation) (1998a) *The World Health Report: Life in the 21st Century: A Vision for All* (Geneva, WHO).

WHO (World Health Organisation) (1998b) *Obesity and Diet-Related Non-Communicable Diseases* (Geneva, WHO).

WHO (World Health Organisation) (1998c) *Health for All for the 21st Century* (Geneva, WHO).

WHO (World Health Organisation) (1999) *The World Health Report: Making a Difference* (Geneva, WHO).

WHO (World Health Organisation) (2000) *The World Health Report 2000: Health Systems* (Geneva, WHO).

WHO (World Health Organisation) Regional Office for Europe (1985) *Targets for Health for All: Targets in Support of the European Regional Strategy for Health for All* (Copenhagen, WHO Regional Office for Europe).

WHO (World Health Organisation) Regional Office for Europe (1993) *Health For All Targets: The Health Policy For Europe*, updated edn 1991 (Copenhagen, WHO Regional Office for Europe).

WHO Regional Office for Europe (1994) *Declaration on the Promotion of Patients' Rights in Europe* (Amsterdam, WHO).

WHO Regional Office for Europe (1998) *Health 21: The Health Policy Framework for the WHO European Region* (Copenhagen, WHO).

Whynes, D. (1997) *Can the NHS Reforms Make GPs into Entrepreneurs?* ESRC Briefing Paper No. 3 (Nottingham, ESRC Programme on Economic Beliefs and Behaviour).

Wicks, D. (1998) *Nurses and Doctors at Work: Rethinking Professional Boundaries* (Buckingham, Open University Press).

Widgery, D. (1988) *The National Health: A Radical Perspective* (London, Hogarth).

Wild, S. and McKeigue, P. (1997) 'Cross-Sectional Analysis of Mortality by Country of Birth in England and Wales 1970–92', *British Medical Journal*, 314, 305–10.

Wilding, J. (1997) 'Obesity Treatment', *British Medical Journal*, 315, 997–1000.

Wilding, P. (1982) *Professional Power and Social Welfare* (London, Routledge).

Wilkin, D., Coleman, A., Dowling, B. and Smith, K. (2002) *The National Tracker Survey of Primary Care Groups and Trusts 2001/02: Taking Responsibility?* (University of Manchester, National Primary Care Research and Development Centre).

Wilkin, D., Gillam, S. and Smith, K. (2001) 'Tackling Organisational Change in the New NHS', *British Medical Journal*, 322, 1464–7.

Wilkin, D., Gillam, S. and Toleman, A. (2001) *The National Tracker Survey of Primary Care Groups: Progress and Challenges 1999/2000* (University of Manchester, National Primary Care Research and Development Centre).

Wilkinson, D. (1999) *Poor Housing and Health: A Summary of Research Evidence* (Edinburgh, Scottish Office).

Wilkinson, R. (1996) *Unhealthy Societies – The Affliction of Inequality* (London, Routledge).

Wilkinson, R. G. (1997) 'Health Inequalities: Relative or Absolute Material Standards?', *British Medical Journal*, 314, 591–5.

Wilkinson, S. and Kitzinger, C. (eds) (1994) *Women and Health* (London, Taylor and Francis).

Wilkinson, S. and Kitzinger, C. (1999) 'Towards a Feminist Approach to Breast Cancer', in Wilkinson, S. and Kitzinger, C. (eds) *Women and Health* (London, Taylor and Francis), 124–40.

Williams, A. (1985) 'The Cost of Coronary Artery Bypass Grafting', *British Medical Journal*, 291, 326–9.

Williams, A. (1988) 'Health Economics: The End of Clinical Freedom?', *British Medical Journal*, 297, 183–8.

Williams, A. (2000) *Nursing, Medicine and Primary Care* (Buckingham, Open University Press).

Williams, B. (1997) 'Utilisation of NHS Hospitals in England by Private Patients 1989–95', *Health Trends*, 29, 21–5.

Williams, B. and Pearson, J. (1999) 'Private Patients in NHS Hospitals: Comparison of Two Sources of Information', *Journal of Public Health Medicine*, 21, 70–3.

Williams, B., Whatmough, P., McGill, J. and Rushton, L. (2000) 'Private Funding of Elective Hospitals Treatment in England and Wales 1997–98: National Survey', *British Medical Journal*, 320, 904–5.

Williams, D., Lavizzo-Mourey, R. and Warren, R. (1994) 'The Concept of Race and Health Status in America', *Public Health Reports*, 109 (1), 26–41.

Williams, S. (2000) 'NHS Direct Investigated', *Health Which?*, August, 12–16.

Williams, S. and Calnan, M. (eds) (1996) *Modern Medicine: Lay Perspectives and Experiences* (London, UCL Press).

Williamson, C. (1992) *Whose Standards? Consumer and Professional Standards in Health Care* (Buckingham, Open University Press).

Williamson, C. (2000) 'Consumer and Professional Standards Working Towards Consensus', *Quality in Health Care*, 9, 190–4.

Wilsford, D. (1991) *Doctors and the State: The Politics of Health Care in France and the United States* (London, Duke University Press).

Wilsford, D. (1994) 'Path Dependency – Why History Makes it Difficult but not Impossible to Reform Health Care Systems In a Big Way', *Journal of Public Policy*, 14, 251–83.

Wilson, A. and Parker, H. (2003) 'Guest Editorial: Intermediate Care and General Practitioners An Uncertain Relationship', *Health and Social Care in the Community*, 11, 81–4.

Wilson, A., Parker, H., Wynn, A., Jagger, C., Spiers, N., Jones, J. and Parker, G. (1999) 'Randomised Controlled Trial of Effectiveness of Leicester Hospital at Home Scheme Compared with Hospital Care', *British Medical Journal*, 319, 1542–6.

Wilson, P. (2001) 'A Policy Analysis of the Expert Patient in the UK. Self Care as an Expression of Pastoral Power?', *Health and Social Care in the Community*, 9, 134–42.

Wilson, R., Buchan, I. and Whalley, T. (1995) 'Alterations in Prescribing by General

Practitioner Fundholders: An Observational Study', *British Medical Journal*, 311, 1347–50.

Wilson, R. M., Runciman, W. B., Gibberd, R. W., Harrison, B. T., Newby, L. and Hamilton, J. D. (1995) 'The Quality in Australian Health Care Study', *Medical Journal of Australia*, 163, 458–71.

Winkler, F. (1987) 'Consumerism in Health Care: Beyond the Supermarket Model', *Policy and Politics*, 15 (1), 1–8.

Winslow, C., Kosekoff, J., Chassin, M., Kanouse, D. and Brook, R. (1988) 'The Appropriateness of Performing Coronary Artery Bypass Graft Surgery', *Journal of the American Medical Association*, 260, 505–9.

Wistow, G. and Hardy, B. (1999) 'The Development of Domiciliary Care: Mission Accomplished', *Policy and Politics*, 27.

Wistow, G. and Harrison, S. (1998) 'Rationality and Rhetoric: The Contribution to Social Care Policy: Making of Sir Roy Griffiths 1986–1991', *Public Administration*, 76, 649–68.

Wistow, G., Knapp, M., Hardy, B. and Allen, C. (1994) *Social Care in a Mixed Economy* (Buckingham, Open University Press).

Wittenberg, R., Sandhu, B. and Knapp, M. (2002) 'Funding Long Term Care: The Public and Private Options' in Mossialos, E., Dixon, A., Figueras, J. and Kutzin, J. (eds) *Funding Health Care: Options for Europe* (Buckingham, Open University Press), 226–49.

Witz, A. (1992) *Professions and Patriarchy* (London, Routledge).

Witz, A. (1994) 'The Challenge of Nursing', in Gabe, J., Kelleher, D. and Williams, G. (eds) *Challenging Medicine* (London, Routledge), 23–45.

Wohl, A. S. (1984) *Endangered Lives: Public Health in Victorian Britain* (London, Unwin Methuen).

Wolfson, M., Kaplan, G., Lynch, J., Ross, N. and Backlund, E. (1999) 'Relation Between Income Inequality and Mortality: Empirical Demonstration', *British Medical Journal*, 319, 953–7.

Wolk, A., Manson, J. E., Stampfer, M. J., Colditz, G. A., Hu, F. B., Speizer, F. E., Hennekens, C. H. and Willett, W. C. (1999) 'Long-Term Intake of Dietary Fibre and Decreased Risk of Coronary Heart Disease Among Women', *Journal of the American Medical Association*, 281 (21) 1990–2004.

Wood, B. (1989) 'The Information Revolution, Health Reform and Doctor – Manager Relations', *Public Policy and Administration*, 14, 1–13.

Wood, B. (2000) *Patient Power?: The Politics of Patients' Associations in Britain and America* (Buckingham, Open University Press).

Woods, K. (2001) 'The Development of Integrated Health Care Models in Scotland', *International Journal of Integrated Care*, 1 (3), http://www.ijic.org

Woolhandler, S., Himmelstein, D. and Lewontin, J. (1993) 'Administrative Costs in US Hospitals', *New England Journal of Medicine*, 329, 400–3.

Wordsworth, S., Donaldson, C. and Scott, A. (1996) *Can We Afford the NHS?* (London, Institute of Public Policy Research).

Wright, J., Williams, R. and Wilkinson, J. (1998) 'Development and Importance of Health Needs Assessment', *British Medical Journal*, 316, 1310–13.

Wyke, A. (1996) *21st Century Miracle Medicine* (New York, Plenum Publishing).

Yates, J. (1995) *Private Eye, Heart and Hip* (London, Churchill Livingstone).

Yates, J. (2002a) 'Blank Checks', *Health Service Journal*, 10 January, 30–1.

Yates, J. (2002b) 'Mixed Message', *Health Service Journal*, 19 September, 21.

Yates, J. (2003) 'Take Heart', *Health Service Journal*, 6 March, 27.

Yates, J. R. W. (1996) 'Medical Genetics', *British Medical Journal*, 312, 1021–5.

York Health Economics Consortium and MSA Health and Social Research Consultancy (1999) *NHS Trust and Speciality Unit Cost Benchmarking in the NHS* (London, DoH (Department of Health)).

Young, H. (1991) *One of Us*, final edn (London, Macmillan).

Zola, I. K. (1975) 'Medicine as an Institution of Social Control', in Cox, G. and Mead, A. (eds) *A Sociology of Medical Practice* (London, Collier Macmillan).

Index